Thyroperoxidase and Thyroid Autoimmunity

Thyroperoxydase et auto-immunité thyroïdienne

Colloques INSERM
ISSN 0768-3154

Other *Colloques* published as co-editions by John Libbey Eurotext and INSERM

133 Cardiovascular and Respiratory Physiology in the Fetus and Neonate. *Physiologie Cardiovasculaire et Respiratoire du Fœtus et du Nouveau-né.*
Scientific Committee : P. Karlberg,
A. Minkowski, W. Oh and L. Stern;
Managing Editor : M. Monset-Couchard.
ISBN : John Libbey Eurotext 0 86196 125 0
INSERM 2 85598 340 1

134 Porphyrins and Porphyrias. *Porphyrines et Porphyries.*
Edited by Y. Nordmann.
ISBN : John Libbey Eurotext 0 86196 087 4
INSERM 2 85598 281 2

137 Neo-Adjuvant Chemotherapy. *Chimiothérapie Néo-Adjuvante.*
Edited by C. Jacquillat, M. Weil and D. Khayat.
ISBN : John Libbey Eurotext 0 86196 125 0
INSERM 2 85598 340 1

139 Hormones and Cell Regulation (10th European Symposium). *Hormones et Régulation Cellulaire (10ᵉ Symposium Européen).*
Edited by J. Nunez, J.E. Dumont and R.J.B. King.
ISBN : John Libbey Eurotext 0 86196 125 0X
INSERM 2 85598 340 1

147 Modern Trends in Aging Research. *Nouvelles Perspectives de la Recherche sur le Vieillissement.*
Edited by Y. Courtois, B. Faucheux, B. Forette, D.L. Knook and J.A. Tréton.
ISBN : John Libbey Eurotext 0 86196 126 0X
INSERM 2 85598 340 1

149 Binding Proteins of Steroid Hormones. *Protéines de liaison des Hormones Stéroïdes.*
Edited by M.G. Forest and M. Pugeat.
ISBN : John Libbey Eurotext 0 86196 125 0
INSERM 2 85598 340 1X

151 Control and Management of Parturition. *La Maîtrise de la Parturition.*
Edited by C. Sureau, P. Blot, D. Cabrol, F. Cavaillé and G. Germain.
ISBN : John Libbey Eurotext 0 86196 125 0
INSERM 2 85598 340 1

Thyroperoxidase and Thyroid Autoimmunity

Thyroperoxydase et auto-immunité thyroïdienne

Proceedings of the International Symposium on Thyroperoxidase and Thyroid Autoimmunity, held in Marseille (France), June 28-30, 1990

Sponsored by the Institut National de la Santé et de la Recherche Médicale (INSERM)

Edited by

Pierre Carayon
Jean Ruf

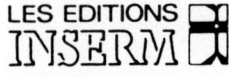

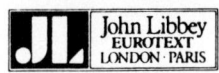

British Library Cataloguing in Publication Data
International Symposium on Thyroperoxidase and
Thyroid Autoimmunity, (1990; Marseille, France)
Thyroperoxidase and thyroid autoimmunity.
  1. Man. Thyroid. Diseases. Immunological aspects
  I. Title II. Carayon, Pierre III. Ruf, Jean
  606.44079

ISBN 0 86196 277-X
ISBN 0768-3154

First published in 1990 by

Editions John Libbey Eurotext
6 rue Blanche, 92120 Montrouge, France. (1) 47 35 85 52
ISBN 0 86196 277-X

John Libbey & Company Ltd
13 Smiths Yard, Summerley Street, London SW18 4HR,
England.
(1) 947 27 77

Institut National de la Santé et de la Recherche Médicale
101 rue de Tolbiac, 75654 Paris Cedex 13, France.
(1) 45 84 14 41
ISBN 2 85 598 440-8

ISSN 0768-3154

© 1990 Colloques INSERM/John Libbey Eurotext Ltd,
All rights reserved
Unauthorized publication contravenes applicable laws

Preface

Autoantibodies to the thyroid microsomal antigen have been recognized for more than thirty years. Evidence has accumulated on the important role of these autoantibodies in the autoimmune process directed to the thyroid gland. However, the exact nature of the microsomal antigen remained, for years, a matter of controversy. In 1985, a major finding was achieved which considerably aroused the interest of the scientific community in this antigen. In our laboratory, in Marseille, we identified the thyroid microsomal antigen to thyroperoxidase (TPO) a key enzyme of thyroid hormone biosynthesis. Our finding was soon confirmed by several other laboratories and followed by a rapid growth of work on TPO. This research area has undoubtedly exploded in the last five years leading to an accumulation of data on the TPO structure and regulation and role in the autoimmune process. Development of molecular probes by biochemistry, immunology and molecular biology opened the way to new approaches in the study of the mechanisms involved in autoimmunity. Furthermore, the identification of TPO as the thyroid microsomal antigen raised the hypothesis that microsomal antigens from other target organs might be membrane enzymes as has been already confirmed for gastric parietal cells.

The large quantity of results collected within a few years, demanded systematization : an international symposium on TPO was imperative, and the idea was received graciously by scientific investigators, biologists and physicians. This book, containing the communications held during the symposium, sets out the main progress achieved in the knowledge of biochemical and immunological properties of TPO, and tries to bring to light the potentialities of TPO in human pathology.

Pierre Carayon
Jean Ruf

Préface

L'existence de l'antigène microsomal thyroïdien est connue depuis plus de trente ans. Au cours des années, s'est précisé le rôle important des auto-anticorps microsomaux dans le processus auto-immun dirigé contre la thyroïde. La nature précise de l'antigène microsomal, cependant, n'avait pu être élucidée. En 1985, une découverte importante va considérablement accroître l'intérêt porté à cet antigène. Notre équipe identifie l'antigène microsomal thyroïdien à la thyroperoxydase (TPO), enzyme clé de la biosynthèse des hormones thyroïdiennes. Cette découverte a suscité de par le monde un très grand nombre de travaux. En cinq ans les connaissances sur la TPO se sont prodigieusement développées. Le gène de la TPO a été cloné, sa structure et sa régulation mieux précisées. L'obtention de sondes nucléotidiques, immunologiques et peptidiques a ouvert la voie à une nouvelle approche du rôle de la TPO dans les affections auto-immunes de la thyroïde. De plus, l'identification de la TPO à l'antigène microsomal a suscité l'hypothèse que les antigènes microsomaux d'autres organes cibles de l'auto-immunité puissent être des enzymes membranaires.

L'ensemble considérable de résultats amassés en quelques années, nécessitait de les confronter et de les mettre en ordre. L'idée d'un symposium international sur la TPO, s'imposait. Chercheurs, biologistes et cliniciens l'ont accueillie avec intérêt.

Ce livre, qui contient les communications présentées lors du symposium, rassemble l'essentiel des progrès accomplis dans la connaissance des propriétés biochimiques et immunologiques de la TPO et tente de mettre à jour l'intérêt potentiel de la TPO en pathologie humaine.

Pierre Carayon
Jean Ruf

Acknowledgments/*Remerciements*

The International Symposium on Thyroperoxidase and Thyroid Autoimmunity was organized by an international committee formed by/ *Le Symposium International sur la Thyroperoxydase et l'Auto-Immunité Thyroïdienne a été organisé par un comité international composé de :*

    Chairman/*Président*
        René Mornex (Lyon)

    Members/*Membres*
        Gian-Franco Bottazzo (London),
        Lewis Braverman (Worcester),
        Pierre Carayon (Marseille),
        Jeannine Charreire (Paris),
        Jean-Louis Codaccioni (Marseille),
        Barbara Czarnocka (Warsaw),
        Paul Czernichow (Paris),
        Jan De Vijlder (Amsterdam),
        Aldo Pinchera (Pisa),
        Bernard Rousset (Lyon),
        Jean Ruf (Marseille),
        Peter Scriba (Lübeck),
        Gilbert Vassart (Bruxelles).

The meeting was held with the scientific sponsorship of/*La réunion était placée sous le patronage scientifique de :*

- Institut National de la Santé et de la Recherche Médicale (INSERM);
- Centre National de la Recherche Scientifique (CNRS);
- Université Aix-Marseille II;
- Faculté de Médecine de Marseille;
- Assistance Publique de Marseille;
- Institut de Médecine tropicale du Service de Santé des Armées;
- Société Française de Biochimie et Biologie Moléculaire;
- Société Française de Biologie Clinique;
- Société Française d'Endocrinologie;

— Société Française d'Immunologie;
— Commission de Radio-Analyse et Techniques Associées.

Valuable financial help was obtained from/*Une aide financière a été obtenue de* :

— Institut National de la Santé et de la Recherche Médicale (INSERM);
— Université Aix-Marseille II;
— Association pour la Recherche en Biologie Cellulaire;
— Conseil Régional Provence-Alpes-Côte-d'Azur;
— Conseil Général des Bouches-du-Rhône;
— Ville de Marseille;
— Henning-Berlin;
— Behring-Diagnostic.

The publication of this volume would have not been possible without the generous financial support/*La publication du présent ouvrage n'aurait pas été possible sans le support financier de* :

— Institut National de la Santé et de la Recherche Médicale (INSERM);

We are much grateful to these institutions for their commitment. We are also thankful to the chairman and the members of the program organizing committee, the registrants and invited faculty and all of whom contributed in diverse ways in the Symposium / *Nous remercions vivement toutes ces institutions pour leur participation. Nous remercions également le président et les membres du comité scientifique, les participants, les conférenciers invités, et tous ceux qui, d'une façon ou d'une autre, ont contribué à l'élaboration et à la tenue de ce symposium ainsi qu'à la réalisation de cet ouvrage.*

The diffusion of this volume was supported by / *La diffusion de cet ouvrage a été facilitée par* :

— Henning-Berlin;

— Behring-Diagnostic.

Contents
Sommaire

V   Preface
VI   *Préface*
VII Acknowledgments
VIII *Remerciements*

MOLECULAR BIOLOGY AND REGULATION
BIOLOGIE MOLÉCULAIRE ET RÉGULATION

3 **S. Kimura**
Structure and regulation of the human thyroid peroxidase gene
Structure et régulation du gène de la thyroperoxydase humaine

11 **M.J. Abramowicz, D. Christophe and G. Vassart**
Regulation of the TPO gene transcription
Régulation de la transcription du gène de la TPO

17 **K.D. Kaufman, S. Filetti, P. Seto and B. Rapoport**
Expression of recombinant, enzymatically-active, human thyroid peroxidase in eukaryotic cells
Expression d'une thyroperoxydase humaine recombinante active dans les cellules eucaryotes

25 **H. Francis-Lang, M. Price, U. Martin and R. Di Lauro**
The thyroid specific nuclear factor, TTF-1, binds to the rat thyroperoxidase promoter
Le facteur nucléaire thyroïdien TTF-1 se fixe sur le promoteur de la thyroperoxydase de rat

33 **B. Corvilain, C. Gerard, E. Raspe, A. Lefort, J. Mockel, J. Van Sande and J.E. Dumont**
Hormonal regulation of iodination
Régulation hormonale de l'iodation

43 **L. Chiovato, P. Vitti, C. Mammoli, F. Santini, M. Tonacchera, P. Lapi, P. Cucchi, P. Carayon and A. Pinchera**
Regulation by TSH and thyroid stimulating antibodies of TPO expression
Régulation de l'expression de la TPO par la TSH et les anticorps stimulant de la thyroïde

53 **R. Zarrilli, S. Formisano and B. Di Jeso**
Thyroglobulin, thyroid peroxidase and iodide carrier display different sensitivities to hormonal induction and to neoplastic transformation
La thyroglobuline, la thyroperoxydase et le transporteur d'iode montrent des sensibilités différentes à l'induction hormonale et à la transformation maligne

55 **P.S. Barnett, B. Bhatt, A. Pagliuca, G. Mufti, A.M. Mc Gregor and J.P. Banga**
The thyroid peroxidase gene : accurate localisation by non-isotopic *in situ* hybridisation to chromosome 2p13
Le gène de la thyroperoxydase : sa localisation précise sur le chromosome 2p13 par hybridation in situ *non isotopique*

STRUCTURE AND FUNCTION
STRUCTURE ET FONCTION

59 **B. Czarnocka, J. Ruf, M. Ferrand and P. Carayon**
Immunochemical properties of hTPO
Propriétés immuno-chimiques de la TPO humaine

69 **A.B. Rawitch, G. Pollock, S.X. Yang and A. Taurog**
The location and nature of the N-linked oligosaccharide units in porcine thyroid peroxidase : studies on the tryptic glycopeptides
Nature et localisation des unités N-oligosaccharidiques dans la thyroperoxydase porcine : études sur les glycopeptides trypsiques

77 **M. Nakamura, I. Yamazaki and S. Ohtaki**
Thyroperoxidase selects either one-or two- electron oxidations of iodotyrosine and thyroglobulin, depending on their iodine contents
La thyroperoxydase selectionne des oxydations de tyrosine iodée et de thyroglobuline à un ou deux électrons suivant leur contenu en iode

85 **A. Taurog**
Thyroid peroxidase as the target for the mechanism of action of the thioureylene antithyroid drugs

La thyroperoxydase comme cible du mécanisme d'action des drogues anti-thyroïdiennes dérivées du thiouracile

95 **C. Dupuy, A. Virion, J. Kaniewski, D. Dème and J. Pommier**
Thyroid NADPH-dependent H_2O_2 generating system : mechanism of H_2O_2 formation and regulation by Ca^{2+}
Le système producteur d'H_2O_2 thyroïdien NADPH-dépendant : mécanisme de la formation d'H_2O_2 régulé par Ca^{2+}

103 **Y. Long, J.L. Franc and A. Giraud**
Effect of deglycosylation on human and porcine thyroperoxidase activity
Effet de la deglycosylation sur l'activité des thyroperoxydases humaine et porcine

LOCALIZATION AND TRAFFIC
LOCALISATION ET TRANSPORT

107 **L.E. Ericson, V. Johanson, J. Mölne, M. Nilsson and T. Ofverholm**
Intracellular transport and cell surface expression of thyroperoxidase
Transport intracellulaire et expression sur la surface cellulaire de la thyroperoxydase

117 **B. Rousset, Z. Kostrouch, J. Pommier and Y. Munari-Silem**
Immunolocalization of functionnal thyroperoxidase and expression of thyroid cell differentiation
Immunolocalisation de la thyroperoxydase fonctionnelle et expression de la différenciation des cellules thyroïdiennes

127 **P. Fragu, S. Halpern, J.C. Olivo and E. Kahn**
Microscopic imaging of human thyroid hormonosynthesis : digital correlation of ion and optical microscopic images
Imagerie microscopique de l'hormonosynthèse thyroïdienne humaine : corrélation digitale d'images obtenues par microscopie optique et ionique

133 **C. de Micco, J. Ruf, M.A. Chrestian, N. Gros, J.F. Henry and P. Carayon**
TPO as marker of malignancy in thyroid tumors : immunohistochemical study
Etude immuno-histochimique de la TPO dans les tumeurs thyroïdiennes : intérêt comme marqueur de malignité

137 **D. Gruffat, S. Gonzalvez and O. Chabaud**
Long term iodination of thyroglobulin by porcine thyroid cells cultured in porous bottom culture chambers. Regulation by thyrotropin

Suivi de l'iodation de la thyroglobuline par des cellules thyroïdiennes porcines cultivées en chambre poreuse. Régulation par la thyrotropine

INHERITED DEFECTS
ANOMALIES CONGÉNITALES

141 **J. Léger, N. Hoog and P. Czernichow**
Iodine organification defect. Permanent and transient cases diagnosed early in infancy
Défaut de l'organification de l'iode. Cas permanents et transitoires diagnostiqués précocement dans l'enfance

149 **J.J.M. De Vijlder, H. Bikker and T. Vulsma**
DNA polymorphisms in the TPO gene and hereditary defects in iodide organification
Polymorphisme du DNA dans le gène de la TPO et défauts héréditaires dans l'organification de l'iode

157 **G. Medeiros-Neto, A. Mangklabruks, N.J. Cox, D. Rosenthal, D.P. Carvalho-Guimarães and L.J. DeGroot**
Defective expression of the thyroid peroxidase gene
Expression défectueuse du gène de la thyroperoxydase

165 **M.T. den Hartog, B.E. Sjollema, A. Rijnberk, J.E. van Dijk and J.J.M. de Vijlder**
Loosely anchored peroxidase. A possible explanation for an iodide organification defect in a hypothyroid cat
Ancrage faible de la peroxydase. Une explication possible du défaut d'organification de l'iode chez un chat hypothyroïdien

CIRCULATING TPO
LA TPO CIRCULANTE

169 **T.J. Wilkin and J.L. Diaz**
Approaches to the measurement of TPO in serum
Tentatives de dosage de la TPO circulante

173 **U. Feldt-Rasmussen, M. Hoier-Madsen, J. Date and M. Blichert-Toft**
Acute release of thyroid peroxidase during subtotal thyroidectomy
Relargage aigu de thyroperoxydase lors de la thyroïdectomie subtotale

CHARACTERIZATION OF TPO AUTOANTIBODIES
CARACTÉRISATION DES AUTO-ANTICORPS ANTI-TPO

177 **L.J. DeGroot**
Heterogeneity of human autoantibodies to TPO
Hétérogénéité des auto-anticorps anti-TPO humains

183 **J. Ruf, M. Ferrand and P. Carayon**
Cross-reactivity between antibodies to thyroglobulin and thyroperoxydase
Réactivité croisée entre anticorps anti-thyroglobuline et anti-thyroperoxydase

195 **N. Fukuma, D. Sarsero, J. Furmaniak, C.A.S. Pegg, S.M. McLachlan and B. Rees Smith**
B and T cell epitopes on thyroid peroxidase
Epitopes de cellules B et T sur la thyroperoxydase

203 **R. Elisei, S. Swillens, G. Vassart and M. Ludgate**
Molecular characterization of thyroid peroxidase epitopes
Caractérisation des épitopes de la thyroperoxydase au niveau moléculaire

209 **R. Finke, P. Seto, M. Derwahl and B. Rapoport**
Identification of nine amino acids as the epitope for two monoclonal anti-peroxidase antibodies
Identification de neuf acides aminés correspondant à un épitope reconnu par deux anticorps monoclonaux anti-thyroperoxydase

211 **D.L. Ewins, J.P. Banga, R.W.S. Tomlinson, P.S. Barnett and A.M. McGregor**
Determination of epitope specificities of monoclonal antibodies to thyroid peroxidase using recombinant antigen preparations
Détermination des spécificités épitopiques d'anticorps monoclonaux anti-thyroperoxydase au moyen de préparations d'antigène recombinant

EFFECTS OF TPO AUTOANTIBODY ON THE THYROID CELL
EFFETS DES AUTO-ANTICORPS ANTI-TPO SUR LA CELLULE THYROIDIENNE

215 **Y. Kohno, N. Naito, F. Yamaguchi, K. Saito, H. Niimi and T. Hosoya**
Autoantibodies inhibiting thyroid peroxidase enzyme activity : specificities of anti-thyroid peroxidase antibodies in healthy subjects and patients with systemic lupus erythematosus

Les auto-anticorps inhibiteurs de l'activité enzymatique de la thyroperoxydase : spécificités des anticorps anti-thyroperoxydase chez les sujets normaux et les patients atteints de lupus érythémateux

225 **R. Winand and P. Wadeleux**
Is TPO the only thyroid antigen involved in the complement dependent cytotoxicity ?
La TPO est-elle le seul antigène thyroïdien impliqué dans la cytotoxicité dépendante du complément

233 **U. Bogner, H. Peters and H. Schleusener**
Thyroid cytotoxic antibodies are not identical with thyroid microsomal/peroxidase antibodies
Les anticorps thyroïdiens cytotoxiques ne sont pas les anticorps anti-microsome thyroïdien/anti-peroxydase

CELLULAR IMMUNOLOGY AND EXPERIMENTAL MODELS
IMMUNOLOGIE CELLULAIRE ET MODELES EXPÉRIMENTAUX

243 **F. Akasu, Y. Kasuga, S. Matsubayashi, P. Carayon and R. Volpé**
Induction of CD^{4+} T cells from autoimmune thyroid disease by thyroperoxidase (TPO) *in vitro*
Induction in vitro, *par la thyroperoxydase (TPO), de cellules T CD^{4+} dans les cas de maladies thyroïdiennes auto-immunes*

251 **H. Tang, E. Baudin and J. Charreire**
Localization in tryptic fragments from thyroglobulin of epitope(s) related to Hashimoto's thyroiditis or experimental autoimmune thyroiditis
Localisation, dans des fragments trypsiques de thyroglobuline, d'épitope(s) impliqué(s) dans la thyroïdite d'Hashimoto ou dans la thyroïdite expérimentale auto-immune

257 **N. Yokoyama, A. Taurog, S. Alex, R. Rajatanavin and L.E. Braverman**
Do TPO antibodies play a role in lymphocytic thyroiditis in the BB/Wor rat ?
Les anticorps anti-TPO jouent-ils un rôle dans la thyroïdite lymphocytaire du rat BB/Wor ?

267 **C.M. Dayan, M. Londei, A.E. Corcoran, B. Rapoport and M. Feldmann**
Specific recognition of thyroid peroxidase by thyroid infiltrating T cell clones in human autoimmune thyroiditis

Reconnaissance spécifique de la peroxydase thyroïdienne par des clones de cellules T infiltrant la thyroïde dans la thyroïdite auto-immune humaine

TPO AUTOANTIBODIES IN HUMAN
AUTO-ANTICORPS ANTI-TPO CHEZ L'HOMME

271 **D.I.W. Phillips, L. Prentice, D. Sarsero, S.M. McLachlan, M. Upadhyaya, P.W. Lunt and B. Rees Smith**
Autoantibodies to thyroid peroxidase and thyroglobulin are inherited as an autosomal dominant characteristic in families not selected for autoimmune thyroid disease
Les auto-anticorps anti-thyroperoxydase et anti-thyroglobuline sont transmis comme un trait caractéristique autosomique dominant dans des familles non sélectionnées pour une maladie auto-immune thyroïdienne

275 **S. Mariotti, P. Caturegli, G. Barbesino and A. Pinchera**
Serum anti-thyroid peroxidase autoantibody in autoimmune thyroid disease
Les auto-anticorps anti-thyroperoxydase sériques dans la maladie thyroïdienne auto-immune

285 **F. Doullay, J. Ruf, P. Carayon and J.L. Codaccioni**
Autoantibodies to thyroperoxidase in various thyroid and autoimmune diseases
Les auto-anticorps anti-thyroperoxydase dans diverses maladies thyroïdiennes et auto-immunes

297 **U. Feldt-Rasmussen, M. Hoier-Madsen, K. Bech, L. Hegedüs, H. Perrild, H. Bliddal, B. Danneskiod-Samso, B. Rasmusson, N.J. Kriegbaum, K. Müller, A. Schouboe and E. Hippe**
Anti-TPO antibodies in non-thyroid autoimmune diseases
Les anticorps anti-TPO dans les maladies auto-immunes non thyroïdiennes

303 **D. Glinoer, P. de Nayer, B. Lejeune, J. Kinthaert, J. Ruf, G. Servais and P. Carayon**
Antithyroid peroxidase antibodies in normal pregnancy
Les anticorps anti-thyroperoxydase lors de grossesse normale

INVESTIGATION OF THYROID AUTOIMMUNITY
EXPLORATION DE L'AUTO-IMMUNITÉ THYROÏDIENNE

315 H. Bornet, A.M. Madec, P. Rodien, R. Latter, P. Haond, H. Allannic and J. Orgiazzi
Evaluation of anti-TPO antibody determination in various clinical situations
Evaluation du dosage des anticorps anti-TPO dans différents cas cliniques

321 R. Gutekunst, W. Hafermann, U. Löhrs and P.C. Scriba
The value of ultrasonography in the detection of lymphocytic thyroiditis
Valeur de l'échographie dans le dépistage des thyroïdites lymphocytaires

329 K. Weber and H. Schatz
Autoantibodies to thyroid peroxidase and microsomal antigen in autoimmune thyroid diseases
Les auto-anticorps anti-thyroperoxydase et anti-antigène microsomal dans les maladies thyroïdiennes auto immunes

331 L. Baldet, J. Faure and C. Jaffiol
Auto-anticorps anti-thyroperoxydase (anti-TPO) en pathologie thyroïdienne
Anti-thyroperoxidase autoantibodies (anti-TPO) in thyroid diseases

333 P. Caron, T. Babin and M. Hoff
Etude comparative des méthodes de dosage des auto-anticorps anti-thyroïdiens en pathologie thyroïdienne
Anti-thyroid autoantibodies : comparative study in thyroid diseases

335 C. Massart, I. Guilhem, J. Gibassier, M. Nicol and H. Allannic
Anticorps anti-thyroperoxydase et maladie de Basedow : intérêt dans la surveillance du traitement par anti-thyroïdiens de synthèse
Anti-thyroperoxidase antibodies and Graves' disease : interest in the follow-up of patients treated with anti-thyroid drugs

337 C. Poustis-Delpont, S. Altare, S. Hieronimus, A.M. Guedj, M. Harter and P. Sudaka
Evaluation d'une technique de dosage des anticorps anti-thyroperoxydase par radiocompétition

Evaluation of a radiocompetition assay for anti-thyroperoxidase antibodies

339 **C. Schvartz, H. Larbre, B. Maes, M.J. Delisle and G. Deltour**
Dosage des anticorps anti-TPO et anti-microsomes dans différentes pathologies thyroïdiennes
Anti-TPO and anti-microsomal antibody assays in several thyroid diseases

341 **M. Izembart and G. Vallée**
Intérêt clinique de la détermination des anticorps anti-thyroperoxydase : résultats préliminaires
Clinical interest of anti-thyroperoxidase antibody : preliminary results

343 **Y. Fulla, L. Nonnenmacher and B. Weill**
Comparaison entre le dosage des anticorps anti-TPO en radioimmunologie et le dosage des anticorps anti-microsomes en immunofluorescence
Comparison between radioimmunoassay or anti-TPO auto-antibodies and indirect immunofluorescence assay for anti-microsomal antibodies

345 **S. Dimackie, P. Courrière, A. Boneu and G. Soula**
Intérêt du dosage des anticorps anti-récepteurs de la TSH (TBII) dans la maladie de Basedow
Usefulness of anti-TSH receptor antibody assay (TBII) in Graves' disease

347 **V.J.M. Pop, H.A.M. de Rooy, H.L. Vader and D. Van der Heide**
Prevalence of postpartum thyroid dysfunction in The Netherlands
Prévalence du dysfonctionnement thyroïdien au cours post-partum aux Pays-Bas

MISCELLANEOUS
DIVERS

351 **J.P. Banga, D.L. Ewins, P.S. Barnett, R.W.S. Tomlinson, D. Mahadevan, G.J. Barton, B.J. Sutton, J.W. Saldanha, E. Odell and A.M. McGregor**
Thyroid peroxidase autoantigen : localization of autoantigenic epitopes on recombinant protein and prediction of secondary structure
L'auto-antigène thyroperoxydase : localisation des épitopes auto-antigéniques sur la protéine recombinante et prédiction de la structure secondaire

Molecular biology and regulation

Biologie moléculaire et régulation

Structure and regulation of the human thyroid peroxidase gene

S. Kimura

Laboratory of Molecular Carcinogenesis, National Cancer Institute, National Institutes of Health, Bethesda, MD 20892, USA

INTRODUCTION

Strategy for isolating human TPO cDNAs and gene

The molecular biology of the thyroid peroxidase (TPO) gene is a new frontier in thyroid research related to thyroid endocrinology and autoimmune thyroid disorders. Especially, analysis of human TPO by direct cloning, sequencing, and expression of its cDNA can circumvent problems associated with enzyme purification from human thyroid samples, mainly due to a lack of availability of the tissues. Purified human TPO protein, however, has been obtained (Czarnocka et al., 1985; Ohtaki et al., 1986).

Our approach to the study of human TPO was to use oligonucleotides whose sequences were derived from partial amine acid sequences of tryptic fragments of the purified enzyme, to screen a human thyroid cDNA library prepared from thyroid mRNA of a patient with Graves' disease. Full-length cDNAs were isolated, completely sequenced, and subjected to cDNA expression. They were then used to isolate the TPO gene from human genomic libraries, and the gene was characterized. In these ways, human TPO can be compared structurally, at both the protein and gene levels, with other peroxidases, leading to the understanding of common structure-function relationships of peroxidases. Sequences present upstream of the TPO gene can also be examined for promoter and enhancer activities responsible for regulating human TPO gene expression. A rat TPO cDNA was also isolated using the human cDNA as probe, in order to study the regulation of TPO gene expression using FRTL-5 rat thyroid cells as a model system of thyroid function.

RESULTS AND DISCUSSION

Structure and evolution of human TPO

Two different size TPO cDNAs, designated hTPO-1 (3048bp) and hTPO-2 (2877bp), were isolated from a human thyroid cDNA library (Kimura et al., 1987). The hTPO-1 and hTPO-2 cDNAs are almost identical except that the hTPO-2 has 171 bp deletion in the middle of the hTPO-1 coding sequence without any reading frame disruption, resulting in a 57 amino acid shorter open reading frame. This 171 bp sequence starts with GT and ends with AG, which are in good agreement with the donor and acceptor splice site consensus sequences, respectively (Fig. 1). These results suggest that hTPO-

1 and hTPO-2 are alternatively spliced products of the primary TPO gene transcript.

Computer analysis revealed that the hTPO-1 has 46% nucleotide and 44% deduced amino acid sequence similarities with human myeloperoxidase (MPO) cDNA (3213 bp) (Kimura and Ikeda-Saito, 1988). This latter enzyme is found in granulocytes and monocytes and plays a major role in H_2O_2-dependent microbicidal system of neutrophils. The 171 bp segment that is not present in the hTPO-2 sequence (Fig. 1) is also aligned very well with MPO sequence. These results clearly indicated that TPO and MPO are members of the same gene family and diverged from a common ancestral gene. This is rather surprising since both enzymes were thought to be quite different in terms of biochemical and physicochemical properties and physiological functions.

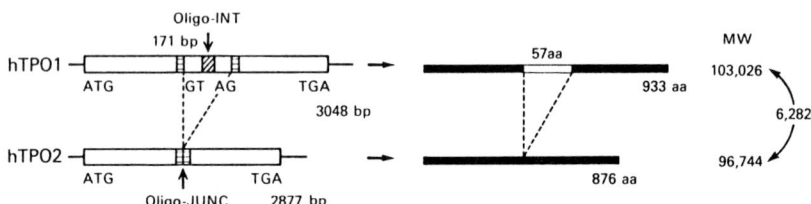

Fig. 1. Schematic relationships of hTPO-1 and hTPO-2 cDNAs, and their protein products. Two cDNAs are shown by solid line and open reading frames by open boxes. Their protein products are indicated by closed boxes and the calculated molecular weights are shown at the right. The value of 6,282 is the molecular weight difference between hTPO-1 and hTPO-2 proteins. The 171 bp sequence coding for 57 amino acids, which is missing in hTPO 2, is also shown. Oligonucleotides specific to only hTPO-1 or hTPO-2 mRNAs, designated Oligo-INT or Oligo-JUNC, respectively, have complementary sequences to the indicated regions.

Based on the amino acid sequence comparisons with other known peroxidases, we predicted in TPO and MPO, the location of a proximal histidine residue which is linked to the iron center of the enzyme and those of two possible distal histidine residues, one of which is actually important in serving as an acid-base catalyst during the reaction (Fig. 2; Kimura and Ikeda-Saito, 1988). Of interest is that one of the possible distal histidine-containing regions is located within the 171 bp coded protein sequence which is absent in the hTPO-2 sequence (Fig. 1). This suggests that the hTPO-2 protein would not have any peroxidase activity if the deleted portion contains a critical sequence for the activity. In the predicted proximal histidine-containing region, 74% amino acid sequence similarity is found between TPO and MPO. Furthermore, some common features are observed between animal peroxidases and other plant, yeast, and fungi peroxidases in spite of the fact that there are no significant global sequence similarities among them. These data may even suggest the existence of a peroxidase gene superfamily.

The evolutionary relationship between TPO and MPO becomes more evident when both gene structures are compared. The TPO gene spans at least 150 kbp on human chromosome 2p (short arm) (Kimura et al., 1987; de Vijlder et al., 1988) and contains 17 exons (Kimura et al., 1989a) whereas human MPO gene spans about 10 kbp on chromosome 17 and consists of 12 exons (Fig. 2; Morishita et al, 1987). The 171 bp segment which is absent in hTPO-2 (Fig. 1), is entirely contained within exon 10. In both genes, the position of the exon-intron junctions and the amino acid codon separation patters at the junctions are very well conserved. These results confirmed that these genes diverged from a common ancestor.

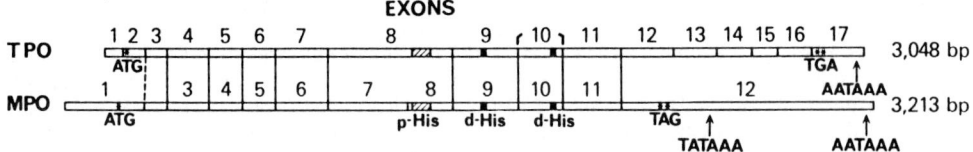

Fig. 2. Schematic comparison of the cDNA structures between human TPO and MPO. TPO and MPO cDNAs are divided into 17 and 12 exons, respectively. The positions of homologous exon-intron junctions between TPO and MPO are shown by a **solid line** extending between the genes. The exon-intron junctions that are not precisely aligned are denoted by a **dotted line**. Initiation codon, termination codon, and poly(A) addition signals are indicated. The alternatively spliced sequence in TPO, which is absent in hTPO-2 sequence, is marked by a **bracket**. The conserved putative proximal histidine-containing region (p-His) and two of the possible distal histidine-containing regions (d-His) are shown (modified from Kimura et al., 1989a).

Intron insertion and/or deletion, and exon shuffling seem to have played a very important role in the evolution of the peroxidase gene family. The former events can be clearly seen at the 1st exon-intron junction in TPO and the 7th junction in MPO which do not have any counterparts in the other gene (Fig. 2). The latter phenomena are observed in only TPO gene and can explain the origin of exons 13, 14, 15, and 16, each encoding a different protein module. Whether intron deletion or the insertion events played important roles in evolution of the TPO and MPO genes should become more evident once other peroxidase genes, that share the same ancestral gene as TPO and MPO, are isolated and sequenced, if there are any.

Expression and regulation of human TPO

Expression of two mRNAs corresponding to hTPO-1 and hTPO-2 was examined by Northern blot analyses using oligonucleotides specific to each mRNA (Oligo-INT and Oligo-JUNC in Fig. 1); Oligo-INT and Oligo-JUNC are specific to only mRNAs corresponding to hTPO-1 and hTPO-2, respectively. Two mRNA bands corresponding to the two cDNAs were detected in all human thyroid tissues examined, not only diseased but also normal thyroid tissues (Kimura et al. 1987). The relative expression level of the two mRNAs, however, varied in each sample. Other tissues such as liver did not show any mRNA band, suggesting tissue specific expression.

Human TPO has been shown to have two distinct protein bands of about 100 and 107 kDa on SDS-polyacrylamide gels and by Western blotting (Czarnocka et al., 1985; Kotani et al., 1986; Ohtaki et al. 1986; Hamada et al., 1987). These two protein bands might be explained by the presence of two alternately spliced mRNAs since the relative molecular weight difference between the two proteins are close to that of the expressed hTPO-1 and hTPO-2 proteins (Fig.1). Hamada et al. (1987) has reported, however, that the 100 kDa protein could be a degradative product of 107 kDa protein, suggesting the existence of only one TPO species. We do not know at this moment whether indeed the two mRNAs expressed in thyroid tissues are translated into proteins in vivo, and whether they appear as two protein bands as detected on SDS-polyacrylamide gels and Western immunoblots, or only one protein exists. The relationship between the expression of two mRNAs and the corresponding protein(s), and their biological and functional significances, remain to be understood.

In order to explore the mechanism of regulating TPO gene expression, we have taken two approaches. One is to use a rat FRTL-5 thyroid cell line as a model system since no normal human thyroid cell lines are presently available that retain most of thyroid functions. To this end, we isolated a partial cDNA clone to FRTL-5 TPO and used this cDNA to study the effect of various hormones and growth factors on TPO gene expression in FRTL-5 cells. Expression of the thyroglobulin gene was also examined in parallel with that of the TPO gene. The results are summarized in Table 1. Among the differences, two most interesting ones observed between TPO and thyroglobulin gene expressions are followings: 1) A nuclear "run-on" assay detected transcriptional activation of the thyroglobulin gene by TSH, insulin, or IGF-I whereas this does not appear to be the case in TPO gene expression; 2) Cycloheximide pre-treatment of cells inhibited TSH-induced increases in thyroglobulin but not TPO mRNA levels (Isozaki et al., 1989).

Table 1. Effect of noted ligands on TPO and thyroglobulin mRNA levels in FRTL-5 thyroid cells.

		TPO	Thyroglobulin
1.	TSH (in the presence of insulin or IGF-I)	Increase within 3 hr, at 10^{-11}M through 10^{-9}M TSH	Increase at 10 hr, reach maximum at 10^{-10}M TSH
	Mimicked by cAMP?	Yes	Yes
	Transcriptional activation?	No	Yes
2.	TSH (in the absence of insulin or IGF-I)	Readily increased by 10^{-10}M TSH	No increase Require insulin, or IGF-I
	Mimicked by cAMP?	Yes	No
3.	Insulin or IGF-I	Small increase	Similar or greater increase than TSH
	Transcriptional Activation?	No	Yes
4.	Cycloheximide	No inhibition of TSH-induced increase	Inhibition of TSH-induced increase
5.	Methimazole	No change of TSH-induced increase	Further increase of TSH-induced increase
6.	Phorbol 12-myristate 13-acetate	Decrease of TSH-induced increase Greater than thyroglobulin	Decrease of TSH-induced increase Smaller than TPO

FRTL-5 cells were maintained without TSH (1, 4, 5, and 6), or without TSH, insulin, and IGF-I (2 and 3) for 3 days, and the TPO and thyroglobulin mRNA levels were assayed by Northern blotting or slot blot analyses 24 hr after addition of the noted ligands alone (1, 2, and 3) or together with TSH (4, 5, and 6), except experiments 1 and 4. In experiment 1, the time course of TSH-induced mRNA level increase was monitored whereas in the experiment 4, cycloheximide was added to the medium 30 min before TSH addition (Isozaki et al., 1989).

The latter results suggest that thyroglobulin gene expression may require the mediation of newly synthesized proteins. This possibility agrees very well with the time course of TSH-induced thyroglobulin mRNA level where an increase of the mRNA level appears only after 10 hr of TSH treatment. Thus, genes of two most important proteins in thyroid hormone synthesis, TPO and thyroglobulin, are regulated quite differently under multi-hormonal and multi-factoral controls.

A second approach to study the regulation of TPO gene expression is to directly examine the human TPO gene upstream sequence for promoter and/or enhancer activities. CAT (chloramphenicol acetyl transferase) constructs driven by various length of human TPO gene upstream sequences can be transfected into rat FRTL-5 cells and the promoter and/or enhancer activities determined by analyses of CAT activities. We believe that the characteristics of DNA sequences and protein factors involved in TPO gene regulation are conserved between human and rat since TPO is one of the essential proteins for the thyroid functions. In these ways, DNA sequences responsible for tissue specificity may also be determined.

cDNA expression of human TPO

The cDNA expression of human TPO was carried out by using vaccinia-virus expression system. Recombinant virus carrying hTPO-1 cDNA (Fig. 1), designated vhTPO-1, was constructed and was used to infect Hep G2 cells. The human hepatoma Hep G2 cell line was chosen to express hTPO-1 because this liver-derived cell line is known to possess ample intracellular membrane and to express a variety of heme proteins, and therefore to contain an adequate amount of heme. Expressed protein appeared as early as 6 hrs after infection and the expression level reached maximum approximately 24 hrs after infection. The expressed protein level remained elevated at 24 hr through 72 hr post-infection, suggesting that the expressed hTPO-1 protein is not particularly labile. This hTPO-1 cDNA expressed protein had the same molecular weight as the purified TPO corresponding to a higher molecular weight species (about 107 kDa), as determined by immunoblotting (Kimura et al., 1989b).

Table 2. Guaiacol oxidation activity of vaccinia virus expressed hTPO-1 protein.

	Post infection time hr	Guaiacol oxidation activity (Specific activity)	(fold increase)
vWT	48	ND	
vhTPO-1	11	ND	
	24	0.032	1
	48	0.181	5.7
	72	0.256	8.0
hTPO-1 after immunoaffinity column		80.8	316 (relative to 72 hr activity)

Guaiacol oxidation activity was determined in 0.1M Tris, pH 7.4 at 20°C, by following absorbance changes at 470 nm in the presence of 30 mM guaiacol and 0.5 mM H_2O_2 using an Aminco DW-2000 spectrophotometer. A mean value of specific activities from three determinations is expressed in ΔO.D.470/min/mg protein. "ND" indicates no detectable activity (modified from Kimura et al., 1989b).

Peroxidase activity was determined by guaiacol oxidation using vhTPO-1 expressed protein (Table 2). Cells infected with wild type viruses or recombinant viruses carrying vector only, did not have any peroxidase activity. These data suggest that measurable peroxidase activity was indeed derived from the cDNA-expressed hTPO-1. A lag time of about 24 hr was apparent between expressed protein level (reaching maximum at about 24 hr) and activity expression (Table 2), suggesting that post-translational modification of the protein such as glycosylation or signal peptide cleavage might be a necessary requirement for enzymatic activity. Alternatively, heme incorporation may not occur during, or soon after, protein synthesis.

Monoclonal antibody-assisted immunoaffinity column chromatography was used to partially purify vaccinia-expressed hTPO-1 (Ohtaki et al., 1986). The immunoenriched hTPO-1 exhibited the characteristic difference spectrum of a hemeprotein, when complexed with cyanide, with a maximum absorbance at 433 nm and a more than 300-fold higher specific activity in guaiacol oxidation (Table 2).

CONCLUSION

Two human TPO cDNAs that are produced by alternative splicing, and the genomic clones were isolated and characterized. Similarities in amino acid sequences and gene structures found between human TPO and MPO uncovered an evolutionary relationship between these two peroxidases. Based on the amino acid sequence comparisons among known peroxidases, the locations of proximal and distal histidine residues which compose a putative common enzyme active site of peroxidases, were predicted in TPO and MPO. The cDNA expression of TPO, in conjunction with site-directed mutagenesis, can be used to further understand the common active site structure and the structure-function relationships of peroxidases. Related to this, it is very interesting to know whether hTPO-2 expressed protein has peroxidase activity since hTPO-2 sequence lacks one of the possible distal histidine-containing regions. This is also relevant to understanding the meanings of hTPO-2 mRNA and/or protein expression(s) relative to hTPO-1 in thyroid tissues. The regulation of TPO gene expression can be studied by using rat FRTL-5 thyroid cells as a model system and transfection of human TPO promoter driven-CAT constructs into FRTL-5 cells. A variety of approaches such as described herein, hopefully lead us to understand the role of TPO in thyroid function and autoimmunity as well as the mechanism of thyroid hormone synthesis.

ACKNOWLEDGEMENTS

I wish to thank my collaborators, Drs. Sachiya Ohtaki, Tomio Kotani, Masao Ikeda-Saito, Osamu Isozaki and Leonard Kohn.

REFERENCES

Czarnocka, B., Ruf, J., Ferrand, M., Carayon, P., and Lissitzky, S. (1985): Purification of the human thyroid peroxidase and its identification as the microsomal antigen involved in autoimmune thyroid diseases. *FEBS Lett.* 190, 147-152.

de Vijlder, J.J.M., Dinsart, C., Libert, F., Geurts van Kessel, A., Bikker, H., Bolhuis, P.A., and Vassart, G. (1988): Regional localization of the gene for thyroid peroxidase to human chromosome 2pter → p12. *Cytogenet. Cell Genet.* 47, 170-172.

Hamada, N., Portmann, L., and DeGroot, L.J. (1987): Characterization and isolation of thyroid microsomal antigen. *J. Clin. Invest.* 79, 819-825.

Isozaki, O., Kohn, L.D., Kozak, C.A., and Kimura, S. (1989): Thyroid peroxidase: rat cDNA sequence, chromosomal localization in mouse, and regulation of gene expression by comparison to thyroglobulin in rat FRTL-5 cells. *Mol. Endocrinol.* 3, 1681-1692.

Kimura, S., Kotani, T., McBride, O.W., Umeki, K., Hirai, K., Nakayama, T., and Ohtaki, S. (1987): Human thyroid peroxidase: complete cDNA and protein sequence, chromosome mapping, and identification of two alternately spliced mRNAs. *Proc. Natl. Acad. Sci. USA* 84, 555-5559.

Kimura, S. and Ikeda-Saito, M. (1988): Human myeloperoxidase and thyroid peroxidase, two enzymes with separate and distinct physiological functions, are evolutionarily related members of the same gene family. *Proteins: Struct., Funct., Genet.* 3, 113-120.

Kimura, S., Hong, Y.-S., Kotani, T., Ohtaki, S., and Kikkawa, F. (1989a): Structure of the human thyroid peroxidase gene: comparison and relationship to the human myeloperoxidase gene. *Biochemistry* 28, 4481-4489.

Kimura, S., Kotani, T., Ohtaki, S., and Aoyama, T. (1989b): cDNA-directed expression of human thyroid peroxidase. *FEBS Lett.* 250, 377-380.

Kotani, T., Umeki, K., Matsunaga, S., Kato, E., and Ohtaki, S. (1986): Detection of autoantibodies to thyroid peroxidase in autoimmune thyroid diseases by micro-ELISA and immunoblotting. *J. Clin. Endocrinol. Metab.* 62, 928-933.

Morishita, K., Tsuchiya, M., Asano, S., Kaziro, Y. and Nagata, S. (1987): Chromosomal gene structure of human myeloperoxidase and regulation of its expression by granulocyte colony-stimulating factor. *J. Biol. Chem.* 262, 15208-15213.

Ohtaki, S., Kotani, T., and Nakamura, Y. (1986): Characterization of human thyroid peroxidase purified by monoclonal antibody-assisted chromatography. *J. Clin. Endocrinol. Metab.* 63, 570-576.

ABSTRACT

Two different size thyroid peroxidase (TPO) cDNAs, that are generated through alternative splicing of the same gene primary transcript, were isolated from a human thyroid library. Using specific oligonucleotides, two mRNAs corresponding to the two cDNAs were found to be expressed in all thyroid tissues examined. Comparison of cDNA nucleotide and deduced amino acid sequences of human TPO with those of human myeloperoxidase (MPO) revealed that the two enzymes belong to the same gene family and diverged from a common ancestral gene. By further comparison of the amino acid sequences of TPO and MPO with other known peroxidases, the location of proximal and distal histidine-containing regions, those composing a putative common active site of peroxidases, were predicted. The human TPO gene was also isolated and characterized. The gene spans at least 150 kbp on human chromosome 2p and contains 17 exons. A comparison of the gene structure between TPO and MPO further confirmed that they evolved from a common ancestral gene. Furthermore, these data suggested that exon shuffling and intron insertion and/or deletion played important roles in the evolution of the TPO gene. A rat TPO cDNA clone was used to study and compare the regulation of the TPO and thyroglobulin gene expressions in FRTL-5 cells. Results suggest that thyroid hormone synthesis is a complex process under multi-hormonal and multi-factoral controls. Finally, a human TPO was successfully expressed as an enzymatically active protein in human Hep G2 cells using a vaccinia-virus cDNA expression system.

Résumé

Deux ADN complémentaires de la thyropéroxydase, de taille différente, générés par épissage alternatif d'un même gène primaire transcrit, ont été isolés d'une banque de thyroïdes humaines. En utilisant des oligonucléotides spécifiques, on a pu montrer que deux ARN messagers correspondant aux deux ADN complémentaires s'exprimaient dans tous les tissus thyroïdiens examinés. La comparaison des séquences nucléotidiques de cADN et des séquences de TPO humaine avec celles de la myélopéroxydase humaine (MPO), a révélé que les deux enzymes appartiennent à la même famille de gènes et dérivent d'un gène ancestral commun. Une comparaison plus approfondie entre les séquences amino-acides de TPO et de MPO avec les autres péroxydases connues, a permis de localiser le domaine responsable de l'activité enzymatique. Par ailleurs, le gène de la TPO humaine a été isolé et caractérisé. Le gène mesure au moins 150 kb sur le chromosome humain 2p et contient 17 exons. La comparaison de la structure des gènes de la TPO et de la MPO a confirmé qu'ils s'étaient différenciés à partir d'un gène ancestral commun. De plus, ces résultats suggèrent qu'un réarrangement des exons ainsi que l'insertion et/ou la délétion des introns, jouent un rôle important dans l'évolution du gène de la TPO. Nous avons étudié et comparé la régulation de la TPO et les expressions du gène de la thyroglobuline dans les cellules FRTL-5, à partir de clones de cADN de thyropéroxydase du rat. Les résultats montrent que la synthèse des hormones thyroïdiennes est un processus complexe qui s'opère sous contrôle multi-hormonal et multi-factoriel. Nous avons finalement réussi à exprimer la TPO humaine par recombinaison génétique, dans les cellules Hep G2.

Regulation of the TPO gene transcription

M.J. Abramowicz, D. Christophe and G. Vassart*

*Institut de Recherche Interdisciplinaire, Université Libre de Bruxelles, Campus Erasme, and * Service de Génétique, Hôpital Erasme, Route de Lennik 808, B1070 Brussels, Belgium*

ABSTRACT

In contrast with thyroglobulin, transcription of the thyroperoxidase gene after TSH or cyclic AMP agonist activation, is rapid and occurs whether or not protein synthesis has been blocked. The promoter of the TPO gene has been analyzed. In transfection experiments of dog thyroid cells in primary culture, this promoter confers strong TSH and cyclic AMP responsiveness to fused reporter genes. Unexpectedly, it does not contain a canonical cAMP Responsive Element.
When compared to the evolutionary related myeloperoxidase gene, the TPO gene contains an additional first intron. This genetic fragment doesn't seem to enhance transcription of the gene.
No length polymorphism was detected among European Caucasians using a probe corresponding to the first intron of the gene.
Molecular mechanisms of TPO and thyroglobulin genes transcriptional activation by cyclic AMP agonists are currently being investigated.

INTRODUCTION

The availability of thyroperoxidase (TPO) complementary DNA (cDNA) (Libert, et al., 1987; Kimura et al., 1987) led to the demonstration that its messenger RNA (mRNA) accumulates in the cytoplasm of thyrocytes after thyrotropin (TSH) stimulation (Chazenbalk et al., 1987).
It was shown by in vitro run-on transcription assays that this control occurs at least in part at the level of the transcription of the gene, and that it is most likely mediated by cyclic AMP (cAMP), as it is mimicked by forskolin, a universal activator of adenyl-cyclase (Gerard et al., 1988).

Cyclic AMP-responsive genes are currently divided in two groups (Roesler et al., 1988). Interestingly, the thyroid follicular cell in primary culture specifically expresses two genes which behave as typical examples of each of those two types:
the stimulation by cAMP of the transcription of the TPO gene is rapid and insensitive to the protein synthesis-blocking agent

cycloheximide ("type I"), while that of thyroglobulin (TG) is delayed in time and requires on-going protein synthesis ("type II") (Gerard et al., 1989).

The aim of our work is to analyse the molecular mechanisms involved in the regulation of the TPO gene transcription by TSH and cAMP. As a first step, the promoter of this gene was isolated.

Cloning of the 5'region of the TPO gene

A human genomic library in (λ phage) was screened using a 30-mer oligonucleotide complementary to the 5' end of human TPO cDNA as a probe, and one clone, λhpTPOD51, was isolated. It contains three exons of the human TPO gene, including the first one, as was demonstrated by S_1 nuclease analysis (Abramowicz et al.,1990).

The lengths of the two first intervening sequences that the recombinant λ phage encompasses, as determined by restriction mapping analysis and Southern blotting, differ from those recently reported by another group of authors who extensively studied the human TPO gene organisation (Kimura et al., 1989): 0.9 versus 1.6 Kb and 7.5 versus 22 Kb, for introns 1 and 2 respectively.

A possible explanation to that discrepancy is length polymorphism (in which case a variable number of tandem repeats [VNTR] would likely be responsible). However,we couldn't objectivate any such polymorphism amongst 22 unrelated subjects, using a probe complementary to the 0.9 Kb first intron. It must be emphasized that this preliminary result does not rule out the length polymorphism hypothesis, as the subjects we studied, although unrelated, were all European Caucasians.

Sequence at the 5'end of the TPO gene

A (3.2 Kb) EcoRI fragment from the λhpTPOD51 recombinant phage DNA, containing the first exon of TPO and 2.7 Kb of 5'-flanking region, was subcloned in M13 phage vector end partially sequenced on both strands by the dideoxy method (Sanger et al., 1977).
In contrast with the length discrepancy discussed above, the sequence data are strictly identical to those of Kimura et al.

Interestingly, by comparison with the myeloperoxidase (MPO) gene, the sequence identifies an additional intron (9 bp downstream from the 30-mer probe), and the first (84 bp long) exon of TPO is thus entirely non-coding.

A TATA motif was found at -21 to -27 bp upstream from the cap-site.

As the stimulation of the TPO gene transcription by cAMP is rapid (one hour) and doesn't require on-going protein synthesis, it may be classified as a "Type I" cAMP-responsive gene (Roesler et al., 1988) and its proximal promoter region is therefore expected to harbor a CRE or an AP-2 site (Imagawa et al., 1987).
Sequencing of 0.9 Kb of the proximal promoter does not reveal a canonical cAMP Responsive Element (CRE) consensus TGACGTCA (Montminy et al., 1986) nor any of its functional variants described to date (Roesler et al., 1988).

However, a decameric GC-rich motif GGCCCGGCGC found at -132 to -123 relative to the cap-site might correspond to an AP-2 site.

Of potential significance is another decameric motif found immediately upstream from the GC-rich one (at -154 to -145), **TGAC**CA**GTCA**, corresponding to a perfect CRE split in the middle by an intervening dinucleotide. As CRE-Binding proteins (CREBs) are thought to recognize one half of the CRE consensus and to activate DNA transcription as dimers (Yamamoto et al., 1988), it will be of interest to test this CRE-like decamer for involvement in cAMP-dependent transcriptional control. Furthermore, considering its similarity with a nonamer TGACCAGCA found in the TG gene promoter in a region (-112 to -104 relative to transcriptional start site in the human) that is highly conserved between species, the CRE-like decamer might play a role in tissue-specificity of thyroid genes expression.

Before testing such working hypothesis, it is mandatory to demonstrate that the TPO gene 5' flanking region we isolated actually functions as a cAMP-activated gene promoter in the thyrocyte. This was done by transient expression analysis, using two independent reporter genes.

TPO promoter functional analysis by transfection experiments

Recombinant plasmids containing the same (PCR-generated) 0.9 Kb fragment of the TPO gene 5' flanking DNA fused to promoterless reporter genes coding for bacterial Chloramphenicol Acetyl Transferase (CAT) and human Growth Hormone (GH) were constructed and named pTPOCAT and pTPOGH, respectively.
Dog thyroid cells were primocultured as described (Roger and Dumont, 1984): after overnight seeding in control medium supplemented with 1 % foetal calf serum (FCS), follicles were allowed to multiply for three days in control medium containing EGF (25 ng/ml) and FCS (10 %) and to redifferentiate for three days in control medium containing forskolin 10^{-5} M [control medium is DMEM/MCDB 104/Ham's F12 (2:1:1) supplemented with Penicillin (100 IU/ml), Streptomycin (100 µg/ml), Amphotericin B (2.5 µg/ml), Glutamine (2 mM), Ascorbic acid (40 µg/ml) and Insulin (5 µg/ml)].
Cells were then transfected with pTPOCAT, pTPOGH or pbTGCAT3 plasmid DNA in DEAE-Dextran (Christophe et al., 1989)(pbTGCAT3 contains 470 bp of the TG gene promoter and displays full promoter activity (Christophe et al., 1989)).
p0GH and pSV0CAT, containing promoterless GH and CAT reporter genes respectively, and PXGH5 and pRSVCAT, where those reporter genes are fused to strong constitutive promiscuous promoters (of mouse metallothionein gene, and Rous Sarcoma Virus long terminal repeat, respectively) were used as negative and positive controls of promoter activity.
Cells were then maintained for three more days in control medium alone, or supplemented with TSH (1mU/ml) or forskolin (10^{-5} M), and CAT or GH assays were performed.

As expected from in-vitro run-on transcription experiments, basal expression (i.e., expression in control medium) was low (in both reporter gene systems); around background value in CAT assays and below the detection limit in GH immunoradiometric assays. Both TSH and forskolin induced a strong stimulation of TPO promoter activity in transfected thyrocytes, with CAT as well as GH constructions. Much lower transcriptional activation was observed from control plasmids, indicating that the effect on TPO constructs was indeed essentially promoter-specific (Abramowicz et al., 1990).

The low trancriptional activation by TSH or forskolin we observed from control plasmids transfections may result from non specific activation of the transcription machinery by cAMP.

In our primary cultures, basal transcription from the TG gene promoter was measurable, and TSH-and forskolin-stimulated expression of CAT reporter gene was superior to that from the TPO gene promoter. The proximal promoter region of the TG gene thus appears more powerful than that of TPO.

No enhancer in the first intron of the TPO gene

As the latter gene displays an extra-intron when compared to homologous MPO gene, it was of interest to test this region for the presence of a tissue-specific enhancer of transcriptional activation.

IpTPOCAT and IpTPOGH plasmids were constructed, which contain the first intron (0.9 Kb) fused upstream from the proximal promoter (0.6 Kb), in front of the reporter gene, and functional promoter activity was tested in transient expression experiments.
Addition of the first intron to proximal promoter did not seem to enhance promoter activity in TSH-or-forskolin stimulated cells.

CONCLUSION

Our data demonstrate that the 0.9 Kb segment flanking the human thyroperoxidase gene contains (a) cis element(s) implicated in the transcriptional regulation of the gene by cAMP-dependent mechanisms. Further studies will aim at the identification of the trans-acting factors involved and of their precise targets.

Acknowledgements

We are grateful to Pr.J.E.Dumont for continuous support and pertinent advice. This work was supported by grants from the F.R.S.M., the Belgian Ministère de la Politique Scientifique, Solvay S.A. and ARBD asbl.
M.J.A. is a Research Assistant and D.C. a Research Associate at the National Fund for Scientific Research, Belgium.

REFERENCES

Abramowicz,M.J. et al.(1990): Thyroid peroxidase gene promoter confers TSH responsiveness to heterologuous reporter genes in transfection experiments. Biochem.Biophys.Res.Com. 166,1257-1264.

Chazenbalk,G. et al.(1987): Thyrotropin Stimulation of Cultured Thyroid Cells Increases Steady State Levels of the Messenger Ribonucleic Acid for Thyroid Peroxidase. Mol.Endo. 1,913-917.

Gerard,C.M. et al.(1988): Transcriptional regulation of the thyroperoxidase gene by thyrotropin and forskolin. Mol.Cell.Endocr.

60,239-242.

Gerard,C.M. et al.(1989): Control of Thyroperoxidase and Thyroglobulin by cAMP: Evidence for Distinct Regulatory Mechanisms. Mol.Endo. 3(12),2110-2118.

Imagawa,M. et al.(1987): Transcription Factor AP-2 Induction by Two Different Signal-Transduction Pathways: Protein Kinase C and cAMP. Cell 51,251-260.

Kimura,S. et al.(1987): Human thyroid peroxidase: Complete cDNA and protein sequence, chromosome mapping, and identification of two alternately spliced mRNAs. Proc.Natl.Acad.Sci.USA. 84,5555-5559.

Kimura,S. et al.(1989): Structure of the Human Thyroid Peroxidase Gene: Comparison and Relationship to the Human Myeloperoxidase Gene. Biochemistry 28,4481-4489.

Libert,F. et al.(1987): Complete nucleotide sequence of the human thyroproxidase-microsomal antigen cDNA. Nucleic Ac.Res. 15,6735.

Montminy,M.R. et al.(1986): Identification of a cyclic-AMP-responsive element within the rat somatostatin gene. Proc.Natl.Acad.Sci.USA. 83,6682-6686.

Roesler,W.J.et al.(1988): Cyclic AMP and the Induction of Eukaryotic Gene Transcription. J.Biol.Chem. 263,9063-9066.

Roger,P.P. and Dumont,J.E.(1984): Factors controlling proliferation and differentiation of canine thyroid cells cultured in reduced serum conditions: effect of thyrotropin, cyclic AMP and growth factors. Mol.Cel.Biol. 36,79-93.

Sanger,F. et al.(1977): DNA sequencing with chain-terminating inhibitors. Proc.Natl.Acad.Sci USA. 74,5463-5467.

Yamamoto,K.K. et al.(1988): Phosphorylation-induced binding and transcriptional efficacy of nuclear factor CREB. Nature 334,494-498.

Résumé

Contrairement à celle de la thyroglobuline, l'activation transcriptionnelle du gène de la thyroperoxydase par la TSH ou les agonistes de l'AMP cyclique est rapide et insensible aux agents bloquant la synthèse protéique.
Dans des expériences de transfections de cellules thyroïdiennes de chien en culture primaire, le promoteur du gène de la TPO confère à des gènes rapporteurs qui lui ont été fusionnés, une forte inductibilité par la TSH et l'AMP cyclique. De façon inattendue, sa séquence ne contient pas le classique Elément de Réponse au cAMP. Comparé au gène de la myéloperoxydase qui lui est homologue, celui de la TPO possède un intron supplémentaire à son début. Celui-ci ne paraît pas impliqué dans l'activation transcriptionnelle. Sa longueur n'est pas polymorphe dans la population européenne que nous avons étudiée.
Les mécanismes moléculaires des activations transcriptionnelles des gènes de la TPO et de la thyroglobuline sont actuellement à l'étude.

Expression of recombinant, enzymatically-active, human thyroid peroxidase in eukaryotic cells

K.D. Kaufman, S. Filetti, P. Seto and B. Rapoport

The University of California, San Francisco, Thyroid Molecular Biology Laboratory (111T), Veteran' Administration Medical Center, 4150 Clement Street, San Francisco, California, 94121, USA

INTRODUCTION

A major recent discovery regarding Hashimoto's thyroiditis is that the microsomal antigen (MSA) is, at least in part, thyroid peroxidase (TPO). This conclusion was based on immunologic evidence (Czarnocka et al., 1985; Portmann et al., 1985; Kotani et al., 1986; Mariotti et al., 1987), and subsequently confirmed by the molecular cloning of the cDNA for TPO (Magnusson et al., 1987a; Magnusson et al., 1987b; Kimura et al., 1987; Libert et al., 1987) and the MSA (Libert et al., 1987; Seto et al., 1987) that showed that their derived amino acid sequences are the same. A suitable preparation of recombinant TPO is not yet available for studies on the immunological abnormalities in Hashimoto's thyroiditis. Fragments of hTPO have been generated as recombinant bacterial fusion proteins (Libert et al., 1987; Ludgate et al., 1989). However no combination of fragments has been found that react with all Hashimoto's sera. As an alternative approach, we expressed recombinant hTPO in Chinese hamster ovary cells (Kaufman et al., 1989). Like native hTPO, this recombinant TPO is enzymatically-active, is expressed on the cell surface, and is not a fusion protein.

METHODS

Expression of hTPO: A full-length hTPO cDNA clone was isolated from a Graves' thyroid cDNA library in lambda-Zap. The Bluescript plasmid generated from this clone contained bases 5-3060 of hTPO cDNA, including the start of translation and the poly-A tail. The hTPO cDNA, sub-cloned into the eukaryotic expression vector pECE (Fig. 1), was stably expressed in Chinese hamster ovary cells (Kaufman et al., 1989).

Preparation of microsomes containing recombinant hTPO: Confluent dishes of CHO cells expressing hTPO were homogenized in 10 mM Tris, pH 7.4, containing 0.25 M sucrose, 2 mM phenylmethyl sulfonyl fluoride, 10 ug/ml leupeptin, 0.5 mg/ml bacitracin (Buffer A). The 10,000 - 100,000 x g microsomal pellet (100-200 ug protein per 100 mm dish of cells) was stored at -80°C until use.

ELISA of anti-MSA and anti-TPO antibodies: Sera from 51 individuals were kindly provided by Dr. S. M. McLachlan (University of Wales College of Medicine, Cardiff,

U.K.). Forty seven of these sera were from patients with autoimmune thyroid disease, selected to represent a balanced spectrum of anti-MSA titers from low to very high. Four sera were from normal individuals. Anti-MSA and anti-TGA antibodies were measured in Dr. McLachlan's laboratory (Schardt et al., 1982; Endo et al., 1980; McLachlan et al., 1982). In order to avoid cross-reactivity of patients' sera with any Tg remaining in the microsomal preparation, sera were pre-adsorbed with Tg. Antibodies against recombinant TPO were measured according to Schardt et al. (Schardt et al., 1982), with minor modifications. Serum samples were diluted 1/100, 1/1000 or 1/10,000 in PBS, 5 g/L BSA.

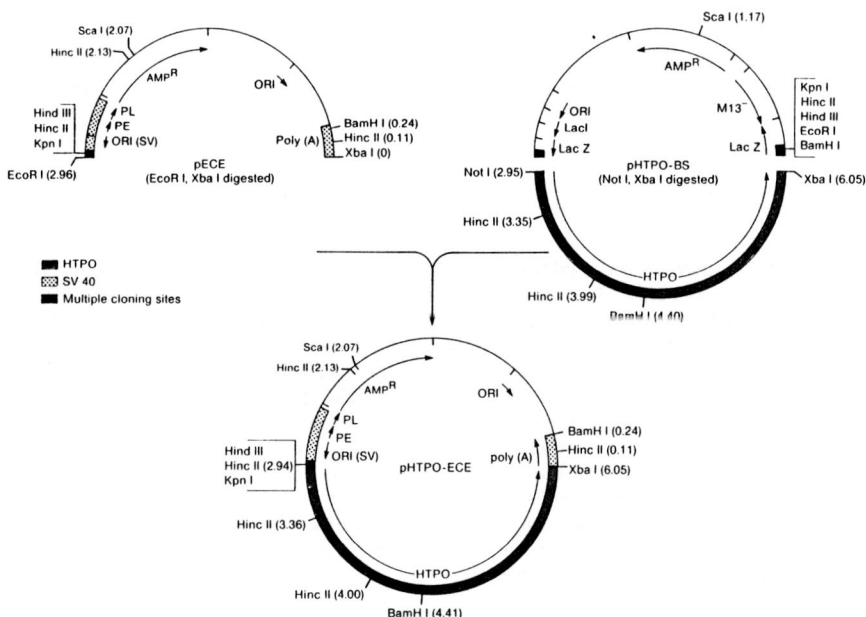

Fig. 1. Construction of the expression plasmid pHTPO-ECE. pHTPO-BS (upper right) was digested with Not I, the ends blunted with the Klenow fragment of DNA polymerase I, and the DNA subsequently digested with Xba I. The recovered hTPO cDNA was ligated into the Eco RI (blunted) Xba I site of pECE (upper left).

RESULTS

Recombinant hTPO expressed in eukaryotic cells was compared with Graves' thyroid microsomes as a source of antigen in an ELISA procedure. In comparing 51 sera at a standard (1/100) dilution in both the recombinant hTPO and the thyroid microsomal assay, a moderately good correlation was observed ($r=0.668$; $p<0.001$) (Fig. 2A). Clearly, however, there were some widely discrepant values. In particular, two sera (sera #11 and 27, Fig. 2A, large circle and square, respectively) that were very potent in the anti-MSA assay gave values in the anti-hTPO antibody assay similar to the four normal sera (Fig. 2A, four data points within rectangle near the origin). A number of other sera, primarily in the high range of activity, also gave significantly higher values with the thyroid microsomal preparation than with recombinant hTPO (Fig. 2A). At the same serum dilution, there was a poor correlation between the values obtained with Tg and recombinant hTPO as antigen (r=0.315; p<0.05; data not shown).

In an autoimmune serum containing antibodies against multiple antigens, the different antibodies are likely to have varying affinities for their respective antigens. If hTPO is the primary autoantigen in the thyroid microsomal preparation, the same serum dilution curve should be observed in assays using thyroid microsomes and recombinant hTPO. In support of this hypothesis, at serum dilutions of 1/1000 or 1/10,000, the correlation in ELISA values between thyroid microsomes and hTPO was much greater (r=0.906 and 0.902, respectively; p<0.001) (Figs. 2B and 2C). Dramatically, the two sera that were strongly positive with the thyroid microsomal but not with the recombinant hTPO antigen (Fig. 2A) were no longer significantly discrepant between the two assays (Fig. 2B and 2C). The dilution curves for these two sera were quite different in the anti-MSA and anti-hTPO antibody assays (Fig. 3A and 3B), confirming that these sera were reacting with low affinity to an antigen other than hTPO. Of interest, these two sera were also distinguished by their extremely high levels of anti-Tg antibody. In contrast, other sera with similar anti-MSA levels (at 1/100 serum dilution) yield normal dilution curves in both assays (sera #12 and 28, Fig. 3A and 3B).

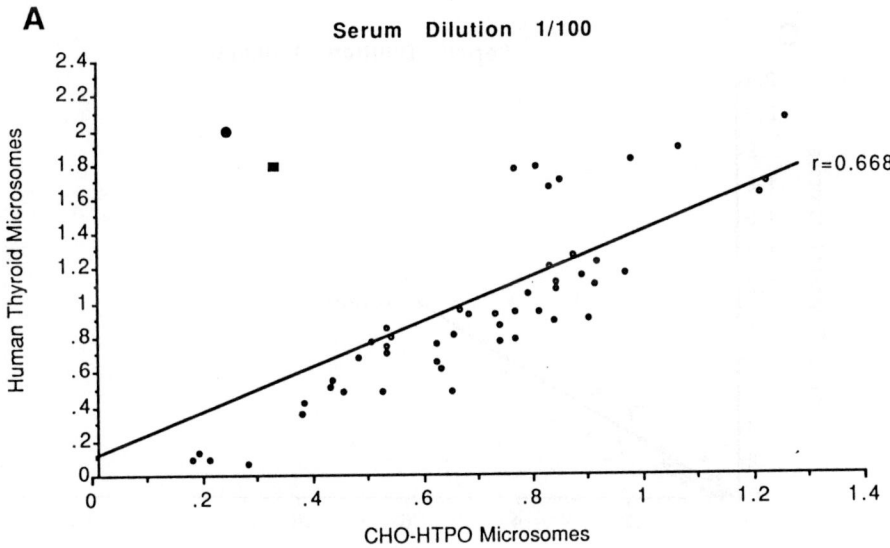

Fig. 2: Comparison of 51 sera, selected to provide a spectrum of anti-MSA levels, in terms of their reactivity with Graves' thyroid microsomes and recombinant hTPO generated in non-thyroidal eukaryotic cells. The anti-MSA assay data are expressed as an ELISA index, relative to a standard serum. Data for the anti-hTPO antibody assay are expressed as absolute O.D. units, normalized to a blank well value of 0.000. (A) serum dilution 1/100 (sera from four normal patients are enclosed within the rectangle);

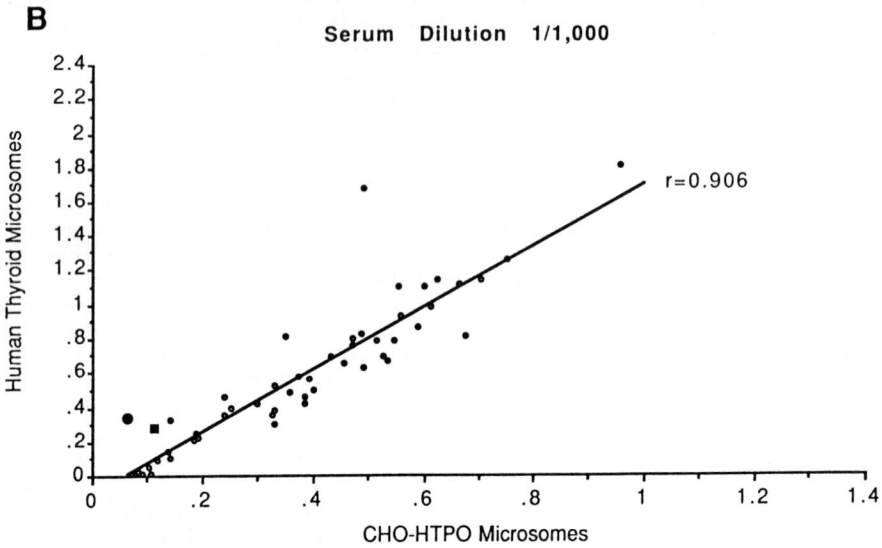
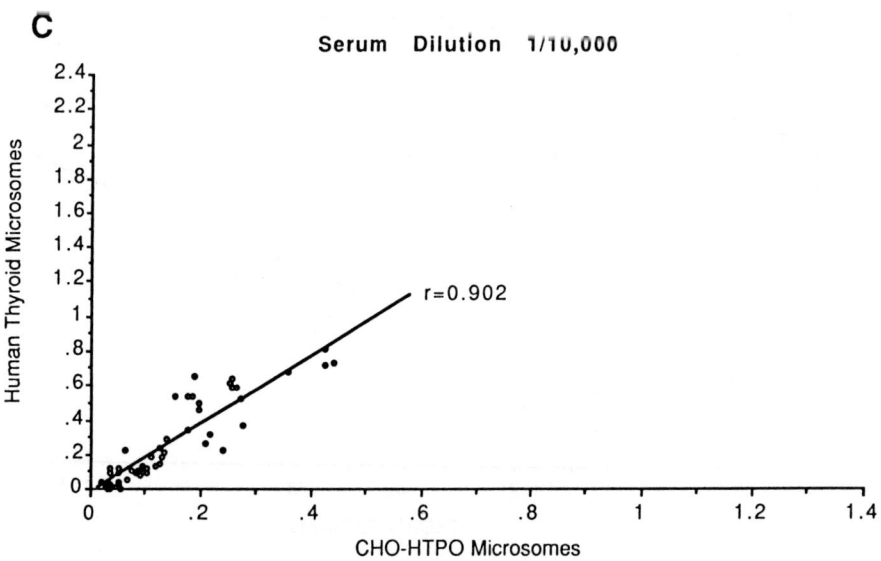

Fig. 2. (continued) (B) serum dilution 1/1,000; (C) serum dilution 1/10,000.

We also expressed our anti-hTPO antibody ELISA data as the difference between values obtained using the CHO-HTPO microsomes and the CHO-K1 microsomes as antigen to correct for possible interference by anti-CHO cell antibodies (Kaufman et al., 1989) (data not shown). We found no significant change in the correlation between the thyroid microsomal and the recombinant hTPO assays using these revised data at each of the three serum dilutions. Anti-CHO-K1 antibody ELISA values for the 47 sera of patients with autoimmune thyroid disease tested, at standard (1/100) dilution,

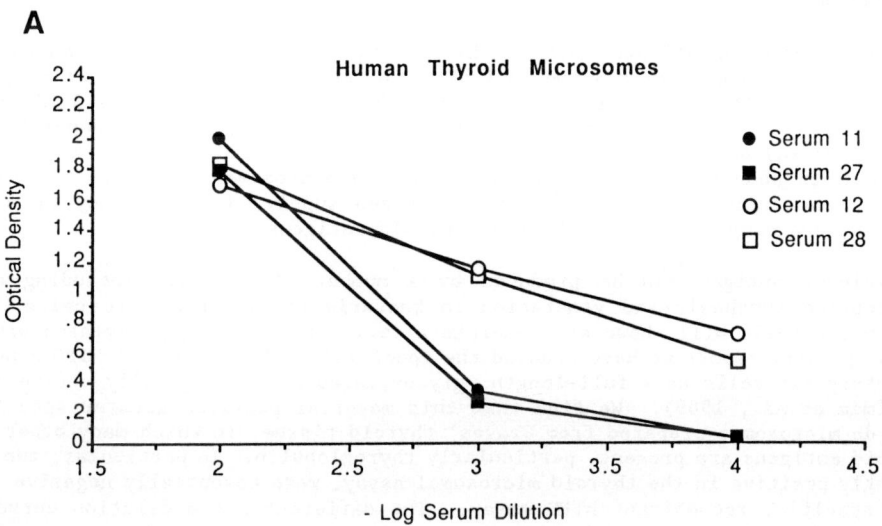

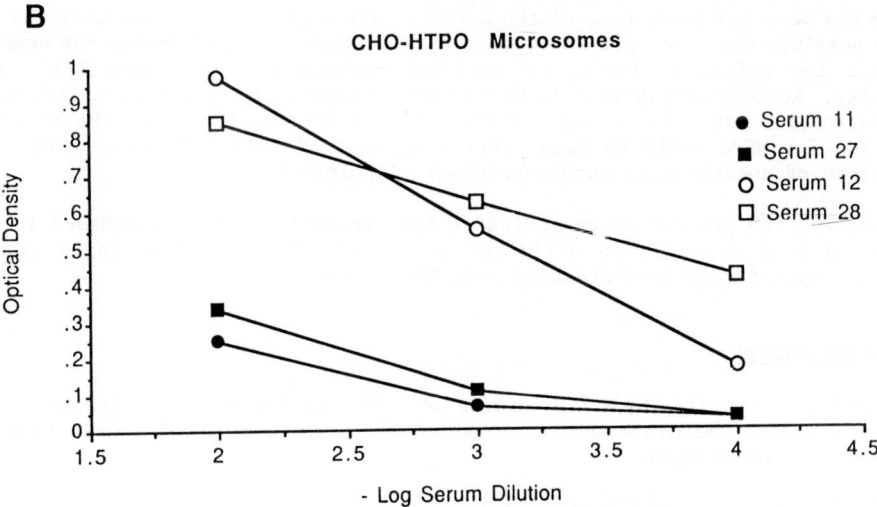

Fig. 3: Two sera (#11 and 27) reacting discrepantly with human thyroid microsomes (A) and recombinant hTPO (B) are reacting with an antigen other than hTPO in panel A at standard (1/100) serum dilution. Dilution curves are also shown for two other sera (#12 and 28) with similar anti-MSA activity at standard serum dilution.

were 0.164 ± 0.066 SD (mean ± SD). Intra-assay variability (10 iterations for each serum) at standard (1/100) serum dilution, expressed as mean ± SD (Fig. 3), was 0.346 ± 0.018 (low-potency serum), 0.599 ± 0.044 (medium-potency serum), and 0.923 ± 0.094 (high-potency serum). The intra-assay coefficients of variation (CV) for these sera were 5.12%, 7.39%, and 10.2%, respectively. The inter-assay CV's (7 iterations for each serum) were 5.36%, 7.63%, and 7.29%, respectively.

DISCUSSION

Studies using immunoaffinity-purified hTPO have previously demonstrated an excellent correlation between anti-MSA and anti-hTPO antibody values (Mariotti et al., 1987; Ruf et al., 1988). However, the supply of human thyroid glands is limited, the antigen is of variable quality (Schardt et al., 1982), and immunopurification procedures may not always yield hTPO free of other thyroid antigens, particularly Tg which is abundantly present even in thyroid microsomes. Recombinant hTPO is clearly a solution to the problems of antigen supply, inconsistency of antigen quality, and contamination with other thyroid antigens.

Recombinant antigen can be produced by a number of methods, including direct polypeptide synthesis and generation in bacteria or in eukaryotic cells. Only eukaryotic cells will, however, generate a fully-processed, glycosylated protein. In the present report we have studied the specificity of recombinant hTPO generated in eukaryotic cells as a full-length, glycosylated and biologically-active enzyme (Kaufman et al., 1989). We find that this material provides greater specificity than do microsomes prepared from Graves' thyroid tissue, in which many other human thyroid antigens are present, particularly thyroglobulin. In particular, two sera, strongly positive in the thyroid microsomal assay, were essentially negative in the more specific, recombinant hTPO assay. The different serum dilution curves for these two sera between the thyroid microsomal and recombinant hTPO assays clearly indicate that these sera are reacting with lesser affinity to an antigen other than hTPO. The identity of this other antigen(s) is unknown, but it should be noted that these two sera contained some of the highest levels of anti-TGA levels in the group. It is possible that even pre-adsorption with a large excess of Tg may not completely inhibit low affinity binding of anti-TGA binding to an antigen (Tg) of high capacity. Another possibility is that of cross-reactivity between anti-TGA and hTPO (Kohno et al., 1988; Ruf et al., 1989). But if that is the case, the affinity of anti-TGA for hTPO would be much lower than that of anti-hTPO antibodies, and is therefore of questionable pathophysiologic importance.

In summary, the present study indicates that recombinant hTPO expressed in a non-thyroidal cell provides an unlimited source of hTPO for immunologic assays of improved specificity over standard anti-MSA assays.

ACKNOWLEDGEMENTS

This work was supported by N.I.H. grants DK-36182, DK-19289 and the Research service of the Veterans' Administration. The expert assistance of Gil dela Calzada is gratefully acknowledged.

REFERENCES

Czarnocka, B., Ruf, J., Ferrand, M., Carayon, P. & Lissitzky, S. (1985): Purification of the human thyroid peroxidase and identification as the microsomal antigen in thyroid diseases. FEBS Letters 109, 147-152.
Endo, Y., Nakano, J., Horinouchi, K., Ohtaki, S., Izumi, M. & Ishikawa, E.

(1980): An enzyme immunoassay for the measurement of anti-thyroglobulin autoantibody in human serum. Clin. Chim. Acta 103, 67-77.

Kaufman, K.D., Rapoport, B., Seto, P., Chazenbalk, G.D. & Magnusson, R.P. (1989): Generation of recombinant, enzymatically-active, human thyroid peroxidase and its recognition by antibodies in the sera of patients with Hashimoto's thyroiditis. J. Clin. Invest. 84, 394-403.

Kimura, S., Kotani, T., McBride, O.W., Umeki, K., Hirai, K., Nakayama, T. & Ohtaki, S. (1987): Human thyroid peroxidase: Complete cDNA and protein sequence, chromosome mapping, and identification of two alternately spliced mRNAs. Proc. Natl. Acad. Sci. USA 84, 5555-5559.

Kohno, Y., Naito, N., Hiyama, Y., Shimojo, N., Suzuki, N., Tarutani, O., Niimi, H., Nakajima, H. & Hosoya, T. (1988): Thyroglobulin and thyroid peroxidase share common epitopes recognized by autoantibodies in patients with chronic autoimmune thyroiditis. J. Clin. Endocrinol. Metab. 67, 899-907.

Kotani, T., Umeki, K., Matsunga, S., Kato, E. & Ohtaki, S. (1986): Detection of autoantibodies to thyroid peroxidase in autoimmune thyroid diseases by micro-ELISA and immunoblotting. J. Clin. Endocrinol. Metab. 62, 928-933.

Libert, F., Ruel, J., Ludgate, M., Swillens, S., Alexander, N., Vassart, G. & Dinsart, C. (1987): Thyroperoxidase, an auto-antigen with a mosaic structure made of nuclear and mitochondrial gene modules. EMBO J. 6, 4193-4196.

Ludgate, M., Mariotti, S., Libert, F., Dinsart, C., Piccolo, P., Santini, F., Ruf, J., Pinchera, A. & Vassart, G. (1989): Antibodies to human thyroid peroxidase in autoimmune thyroid disease: Studies with a cloned recombinant complementary deoxyribonucleic acid epitope. J. Clin. Endocrinol. Metab. 68, 1091-1096.

Magnusson, R.P., Gestautas, J., Taurog, A. & Rapoport, B. (1987a): Molecular cloning of the structural gene for porcine thyroid peroxidase. J. Biol. Chem. 262, 13885-13888.

Magnusson, R.P., Chazenbalk, G.D., Gestautas, J., Seto, P., Filetti, S., DeGroot, L.J. & Rapoport, B. (1987b): Molecular cloning of the complementary deoxyribonucleic acid for human thyroid peroxidase. Mol. Endocrinol. 1, 856-861.

Mariotti, S., Anelli, S., Ruf, J., Bechi, R., Czarnocka, B., Lombardi, A., Carayon, P. & Pinchera, A. (1987): Comparison of serum thyroid microsomal and thyroid peroxidase autoantibodies in thyroid disease. J. Clin. Endocrinol. Metab. 65, 987-993.

McLachlan, S.M., Clark, S., Stimson, W.H., Clark, F. & Rees Smith, B. (1982): Studies of thyroglobulin autoantibody synthesis using a micro-ELISA assay. Immunol. Letters 4, 27-33.

Portmann, L., Hamada, N., Heinrich, G. & DeGroot, L.J. (1985): Anti-thyroid peroxidase antibody in patients with autoimmune thyroid disease: Possible identity with antimicrosomal antibody. J. Clin. Endocrinol. Metab. 61, 1001-1003.

Ruf, J., Czarnocka, B., Ferrand, M., Doullais, F. & Carayon, P. (1988): Novel routine assay of thyroperoxidase autoantibodies. Clin. Chem. 34, 2231-2234.

Ruf, J., Ferrand, M. & Carayon, P. (1989): Cross-reactivity of antibodies to thyroglobulin and thyroperoxidase. Program, 18th Annual Meeting of the European Thyroid Association, 127 (Abstract)

Schardt, C.W., McLachlan, S.M., Matheson, J. & Rees Smith, B. (1982): An enzyme-linked immunoassay for thyroid microsomal antibodies. J. Immunol. Methods 55, 155-168.

Seto, P., Hirayu, H., Magnusson, R.P., Gestautas, J., Portmann, L., DeGroot, L.J. & Rapoport, B. (1987): Isolation of a cDNA clone for the thyroid microsomal antigen: Homology with the gene for thyroid peroxidase. J. Clin. Invest. 80, 1205-1208.

ABSTRACT

Recombinant, enzymatically-active human thyroid peroxidase (hTPO) generated in non-thyroidal eukaryotic cells was compared with Graves' thyroid microsomes as a source of antigen for the immunologic detection of anti-microsomal/anti-hTPO antibodies. Enzyme-linked immunosorbent assay (ELISA) of 51 sera, selected to produce a balanced distribution of anti-microsomal antibody (anti-MSA) levels, revealed (at 1/100 serum dilution) a moderately good correlation between anti-MSA and anti-hTPO antibody levels ($r=0.668$; $p<0.001$). However, a number of sera, with high anti-MSA levels, yielded markedly discordant values between the two assays. A much lower correlation was observed between anti-thyroglobulin and anti-hTPO antibody levels ($r=0.315$; $p<0.05$). At higher serum dilutions (1/1000 and 1/10,000), at which low affinity-high capacity binding reactions will be reduced, the correlation between anti-MSA and anti-hTPO antibody values was greatly improved ($r=0.906$ and 0.902, respectively; $p<0.001$), and there were no longer widely discrepant values between the two assays.

In summary, the present study indicates that recombinant hTPO expressed in non-thyroidal cells can provide an unlimited source of hTPO of unvarying quality for anti-hTPO antibody assays. This material offers increased specificity over standard anti-MSA assays that use thyroid cell microsomes as antigen.

Résumé

Nous avons comparé la thyropéroxydase humaine exprimée par recombinaison génétique en cellules eucaryotes, avec celle contenue dans des microsomes provenant de thyroïdes de Basedow, en tant que source d'antigènes destinés à la détection immunologique des anticorps anti-microsomiaux / anti-TPO. Le dosage immuno-enzymatique (ELISA) de 51 serum, sélectionnés de manière à présenter une distribution variée de concentrations d'anticorps anti-microsomiaux (anti-MSA), dosés à la dilution 1/100, a montré une corrélation convenable entre les concentrations d'anticorps anti-microsomiaux et d'anticorps anti-TPO. ($r = 0.668$; $p<0.001$). Cependant, un certain nombre de serum, dont le taux en anti-MSA était élevé, ont présenté des valeurs nettement discordantes entre les deux dosages. Une corrélation moindre est apparue entre les taux d'anticorps anti-TPO et les taux d'anticorps anti-thyroglobuline.($r = 0.315$; $p<0.05$). Lorsque le serum a été davantage dilué (1/1000 et 1/10 000), à des dilutions qui diminuent les réactions de basse-affinité et de haute capacité, la corrélation entre les taux mesurés d'anticorps anti-MSA et anti-hTPO a augmenté (respectivement : $r = 0.906$ et 0.902), et l'on n'a plus trouvé de valeurs largement discordantes entre les 2 dosages.

En résumé, la présente étude montre que l'expression de la hTPO recombinante dans les cellules non-thyroïdiennes, pouvait produire une source illimitée de hTPO de qualité stable pour les dosages sur les anticorps anti-hTPO. Ce matériel offre une spécificité supérieure à celle des dosages standard anti-MSA qui utilisent comme antigène les microsomes des cellules thyroïdiennes.

The thyroid specific nuclear factor, TTF-1, binds to the rat thyroperoxidase promoter

H. Francis-Lang, M. Price, U. Martin and R. Di Lauro

European Molecular Biology Laboratory (EMBL), Meyerhofstrasse 1, 6900 Heidelberg, FRG

INTRODUCTION

The follicular cells of the thyroid gland function to regulate the synthesis and secretion of thyroid hormones. The formation of thyroid hormone requires the concentration of iodine from the blood stream, the iodination and coupling of specific tyrosine residues on thyroglobulin (Tg) and the break-down of thyroglobulin to release T3 and T4. These individual steps are performed and controlled by thyroid specific proteins and we have been interested to determine how these tissue-specific functions are established at the molecular level.

Genes encoding two thyroid specific proteins have been cloned in the rat. Tg, the glycoprotein precursor for thyroid hormone synthesis (Musti et al., 1986) and TPO which catalyses the iodination and coupling of tyrosine residues in Tg (Isozaki et al., 1989, RDL, MP and HF-L, unpublished). Analysis of the tissue specific expression of the rat thyroglobulin promoter previously demonstrated that a DNA fragment of 170 bp (Musti et al., 1987) contains the information for expression in the differentiated thyroid cell line, FRTL5. Subsequent analysis of this thyroglobulin promoter region revealed that it binds three different nuclear factors, TTF-1, TTF-2 and UFA (Civitareale et al., 1989). Two of these factors, TTF-1 and TTF-2 are only found in differentiated thyroid cell lines and thyroid tissue while UFA appears to be a ubiquitous factor.

TTF-1 is probably the most important factor in the thyroglobulin promoter, binding at three different sites which share a common sequence motif. Mutations in two of these sites significantly depress promoter activity *in vivo* suggesting that TTF-1 is a positive factor which is able to mediate tissue specific expression of the thyroglobulin promoter. We demonstrate here that TTF-1 also binds to several sites in the TPO promoter, suggesting that it could be a general regulator of thyroid differentiation.

MATERIALS AND METHODS

To isolate TPO cDNA and genomic clones, a thyroid cDNA library was preapared in lambda gt11. 8×10^5 plaques were screened using as a probe a porcine TPO cDNA from the 3' end of the cDNA. Isolated clones were purified and inserts subcloned and sequenced. A 0.7kb cDNA insert with homology to the human cDNA was used to screen a genomic library in lambda EMBL3, from which 20 clones were isolated. A 5.8kb segment of 5' flanking region was isolated from one of the clones after establishing the position of the initiation of transcription.

RNA isolation was carried out by the guanidium thiocyanate phenol procedure, and poly (A)+ was prepared from this by oligo dT cellulose chromatography. For RNA gel blots, 4ug of poly (A)+ RNA were electrophoresed in formaldehyde/agarose gels and transferred to Hybond-N membrane (Amersham). Hybridizations were carried out using a modification of the Church and Gilbert method (1984) with probes labelled by randomn priming. Filters were stringently washed as described by Church and Gilbert.

Cell transfection assays were carried out by calcium phosphate coprecipitation of TPO luciferase constructs with the plasmid RSV CAT, which was used as an internal control for transfection efficiency. Cell extracts were prepared 48h after transfection and assayed for luciferase (de Wet et al,1987) and CAT activity (Gorman et al,1982).

Nuclear extracts from FRTL-5 and Rat-1 cells were prepared as previously described (Civitareale et al, 1989). Footprinting analysis was performed according to Musti et al,(1987) on a restriction fragment derived from the plasmid 400TPO extending from -368 to +70.

RESULTS

Isolation of rat TPO cDNA and genomic clones

We have recently isolated a cDNA clone for rat TPO clone by hybridisation to a porcine cDNA clone (kindly provided by Basil Rapoport). This cDNA clone was subsequently used to isolate a rat genomic TPO clone in order to begin an analysis of the TPO promoter region.

A map of the rat TPO promoter is shown in Fig.1. The transcription start site was determined by primer extension and revealed a cluster of start sites. This has also been observed in the human TPO gene (Kimura et al, 1989).

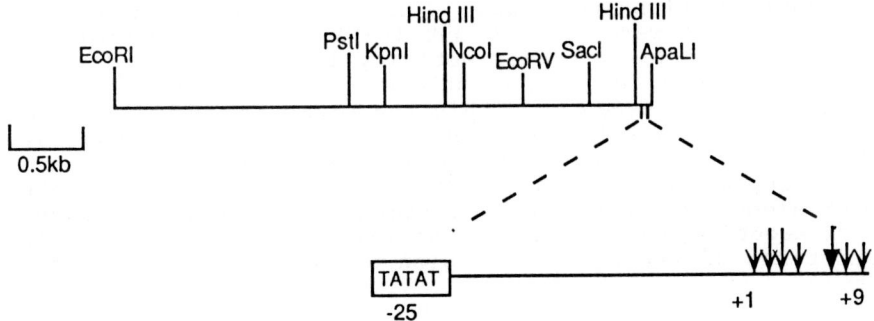

Fig.1. Map of the 5' promoter region of the rat thyroperoxidase gene. Primer extension analysis revealed the presence of two clusters of transcription start sites. Each cluster contained major and minor start points, as indicated by the arrows. By analogy with the human promoter, we have designated the most 5' site as nucleotide +1.

Expression analysis of the rat TPO promoter

In order to determine the tissue distribution of TPO mRNA, Northern blot analysis was carried out with several adult rat tissues using a 5' cDNA fragment (0.7 Kb SalI/EcoRI fragment). As shown in Fig. 2., TPO mRNA is observed only in RNA from the differentiated thyroid cell line, FRTL-5 and thyroid tissue. Two transcripts are found which may be the result of alternative splicing, as appears to be the case with the human TPO message (Kimura et al, 1987).

Fig.2. Northern hybridization analysis of the rat thyroperoxidase gene. A 0.7kb EcoRI-SalI fragment from the 5' end of the rat thyroperoxidase cDNA, was hybridized to 4ug of various poly (A)+ RNAs, obtained from 4 week old rats. Size markers, 18S and 28S ribosomal RNA are given on the side. The arrowheads denote the position of two transcripts present only in thyroid and FRTL-5 mRNA.

Transfection experiments using two constructs containing different lengths of TPO 5' flanking region linked to the reporter gene luciferase, (Fig. 3.) were carried out in FRTL5 and a control non-thyroid cell line Rat-1. Promoter activity is only observed in the differentiated thyroid cell line and not in the non-thyroid cell line, indicating that sequences within the promoter region are able to confer tissue-specificity on a heterologous reporter gene. The longer of the two constructs, TPO 3000 demonstrates a low basal promoter activity while the shorter construct, TPO 400, demonstrates a 5-10 fold higher activity. This large difference would suggest some kind of negative element within the region upstream of -400 and further deletions of the promoter region are being assayed to test this point.

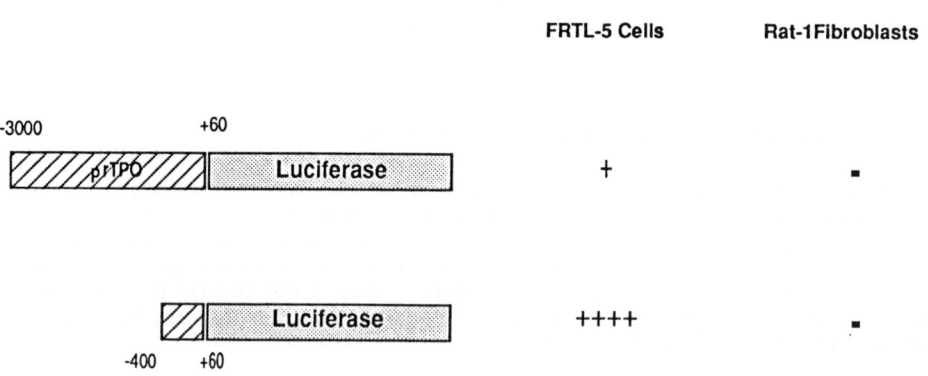

Fig.3. The rat thyroperoxidase promoter is capable of conferring cell type specific expression of a luciferase reporter gene in a cell transfection assay.

Biochemical analysis of the TPO promoter region

The results of DNAse I protection assays using a fragment of 370bp from the TPO promoter are summarised in Fig. 4. Nuclear extracts prepared from FRTL5 cells protect three areas of the TPO promoter, centered around -55bp (C), -105bp (B) and -145bp (A) upstream of the transcription start site. Comparison of protection observed using affinity purified TTF-1 from calf thyroids or TTF-1 produced from its cDNA clone in bacteria (unpublished) indicates that TTF-1 is the activity binding in the A and C regions. With the purified protein two other binding sites are observed at C' (centered at -75bp) and B (centered at -110bp). Binding of TTF-1 is not observed at the B site in the FRTL-5 crude nuclear extract since here the binding region overlaps with the binding site for a ubiquitous factor, as demonstrated by protection of this region also in the Rat-1 nuclear extract. The C' site has the weakest affinity for

TTF-1 as shown by titration analysis with the purified protein. In the A region an extension of the footprint is observed comparing FRTL5 nuclear extract with purified TTF-1. Interestingly this region in the rat exhibits a striking sequence homology with the human TPO promoter.

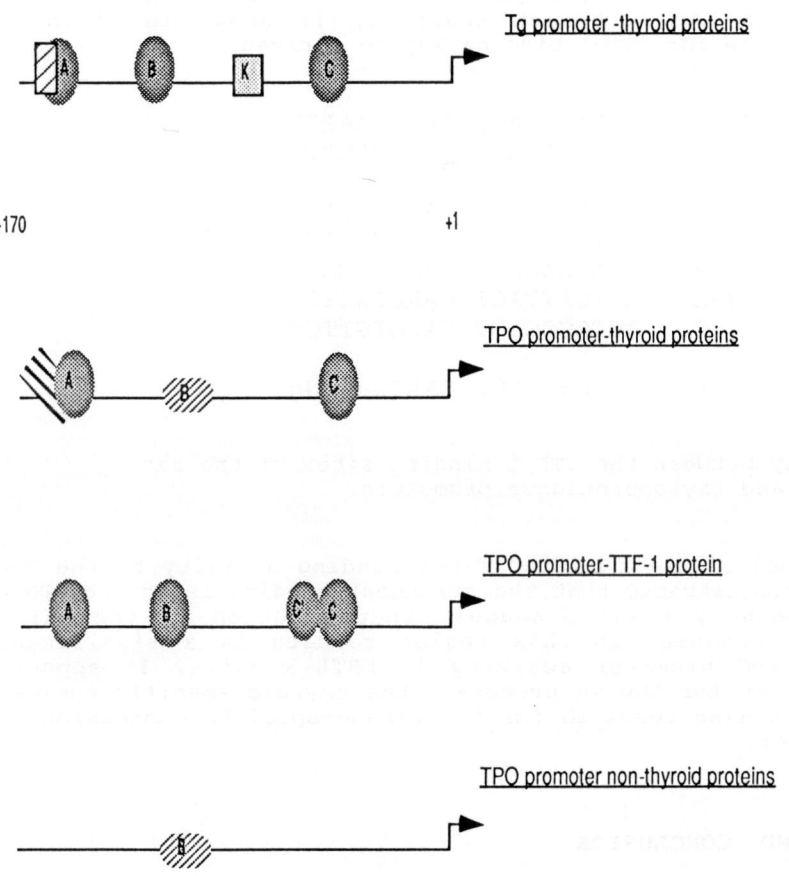

Fig.4. Schematic representation of the protein binding sites of the rat thyroglobulin and thyroperoxidase promoters. Results were obtained by DNase I protection analysis of the rat TPO promoter using nuclear extracts from rat FRTL-5 cells (thyroid proteins), Rat-1 fibroblasts (non-thyroid proteins), affinity purified TTF-1 from calf thyroids, or TTF-1 produced from its cDNA clone in bacteria. The analysis of the thyroglobulin promoter has been reported (Civitareale et al, 1989).

When the situation of binding activities to the TPO promoter is compared with that to the Tg promoter (Civitareale et al., 1989), it is apparent that they show similar features : both bind the thyroid specific nuclear factor TTF-1 more than once and at similar distances from the transcription start site. Both also bind ubiquitous factors.

A list of the TTF-1 binding sequences in both TPO and Tg promoters as derived from the footprint analysis, is shown in Fig.5. A consensus sequence for TTF-1 binding may be derived.

```
        TpoA      AGGTGCCACT  CATAGAAAGC
        TpoB      CCAGGACACA  CAAGCACTTG
        TpoC'     TGGAGCCACT  CCTGTCTAAG
        TpoC      GATGCCCACT  CAAGCTTAGA
        Tg-A'     GGTGACCACT  CCAGGACATG
        Tg-B      GGAGCAGACT  CAAGTAGAGG
        Tg-A      ACTGATTACT  CAAGTATTCT
        Tg-C      ACTGCCCAGT  CAAGTGTTCT

   CONSENSUS      PugtGNcCACT CAAGtataNg
```

Fig.5. Homology between the TTF-1 binding sites of the rat thyroglobulin and thyroperoxidase promoters.

A titration analysis of purified TTF-1 binding activity to the TPO promoter has demonstrated that the strongest binding is to the TPO C region. Preliminary results suggest that mutation of the TTF-1 binding site consensus in this region results in a significant reduction in TPO promoter activity in FRTL-5 cells. It appears therefore that as for the Tg promoter, the thyroid specific nuclear factor TTF-1 is also required for the tissue-specific expression of the TPO promoter.

DISCUSSION AND CONCLUSION

We have begun an analysis of the elements responsible for the thyroid specific expression of the TPO promoter. As in the case of the Tg promoter, binding of a thyroid specific activity is observed. The availability of purified TTF-1, allowed us to demonstrate that the thyroid specific binding activity interacting with two of the sites in the TPO promoter, is TTF-1. The fact that TTF-1 is essential for the expression of the Tg gene, coupled with our initial observations that it is required for TPO expression, suggest that this factor may be involved in the coordinate expression of genes transcribed in the thyroid. Further evidence for a role of TTF-1 in the activity of the TPO promoter comes from experiments carried out with transformed FRTL-5 cell lines. Cells transformed with Ki-ras lack TTF-1 binding activity (Avvedimento et al.,1988) and we have demonstrated that TTF-1 mRNA is absent (data not shown). These transformed cells do not have detectable TPO mRNA and the TPO promoter is inactive in cell transfection assays. To completely define the requirements for TPO gene expression, we are currently mutagenising all of the identified protein binding sites in order to establish the role of each in TPO promoter activity.

REFERENCES

Avvedimento, V.E., Musti, A.M., Fusco, A., Bonapace, M.J. and Di Lauro, R. (1988): Neoplastic transformation inactivates specific trans-acting factor(s) required for the expression of the thyroglobulin gene. *Proc. Natl. Acad. Sci. USA* 85, 1744-1748.

Church, G.M. and Gibert, W. (1984): Genomic sequencing. *Proc. Natl. Acad. Sci. USA* 81, 1991-1995.

Civitareale, D., Lonigro, R., Sinclair, A.J. and Di Lauro R. (1989): A thyroid specific nuclear protein essential for tissue specific expression of the thyroglobulin promoter *EMBO J.*, 8, 2537-2542.

de Wet, J.R., Wood, K.V., Deluca, M., Helsinki, D.R. and Subramani, S. (1987): Firefly luciferase gene : Structure and expression in mammalian cells. *Mol. Cell. Biol.*, 7, 725-737.

Gorman, C., Moffat, L.F. and Howard, B.H. (1982): Recombinant genomes which express chloramphenicol acetyltransferase in mammalian cells. *Mol. Cell. Biol.* 2, 1044-1051.

Isozaki, O., Kohn, L.D., Kozak, C.A. and Kimura, S. (1989): Thyroid Peroxidase: Chromosomal localisation in mouse and regulation of gene expression by comparison to thyroglobulin in rat FRTL-5 cells. *Mol. Endocrinol.*, 3, 1681-1691.

Kimura, S., Kotani, T., Wesley McBride, O., Umeki, K., Hirai, K., Nakayama, T. and Ohtaki,O. (1987): Human thyroid peroxidase: Complete cDNA and protein sequence, Chromosome mapping, and identification of two alternately spliced mRNAs. *Proc. Natl. Acad. Sci. USA*, 5555-5559.

Kimura, S., Hong Y-S., Kotani, T., Ohtaki S., and Kikkawa, K. (1989): Structure of the human thyroid peroxidase gene: Comparison and relationship to the human myeloperoxidase gene. *Biochemistry* 28, 4481-4489.

Musti, A.M., Avvedimento, V.E., Polistina, C. Ursini, M.V.,Obici, S. Nitsch, L., Cocozza, S. and Di Lauro, R. (1986): The complete structure of the rat thyroglobulin gene. *Proc. Natl. Acad. Sci. USA* 83, 323-327.

Musti, A.M., Ursini, M.V., Zimarino,V., Avvedimento, V.E. and Di Lauro, R. (1987): A thyroid specific nuclear protein recognises the rat thyroglobulin promoter. *Nucl. Acids Res.* 15, 8149-8166.

Résumé

L'ARN messager de la thyroperoxydase (TPO) se trouve spécifiquement localisé dans le tissu de la thyroïde et les lignées cellulaires différenciées de la thyroïde. Le clonage du gène de la TPO de rat a permis l'analyse moléculaire de son expression restreinte. Des fragments de 400 et 3000 bp de la région 5' du gène contenant le site d'initiation de transcription permettent une transcription hétérologue et ceci, uniquement dans les lignées cellulaires de thyroïde FRTL5. Ceci indique que la spécificité tissulaire de la TPO est transmise, du moins en partie, au niveau de la transcription. Cependant le fragment le plus long a une activité 5 à 10 fois plus faible, suggérant la présence d'un élément régulateur négatif. La comparaison entre les promoteurs de deux gènes spécifiques de la thyroïde, la thyroglobuline et la TPO, révèle des traits communs quant à leur organisation. Tous deux présentent plus d'un site d'association avec le facteur TTF1, spécifique de la thyroïde, ainsi qu'avec divers autres facteurs. Ces sites d'interraction sont à une distance simlaire du point d'initiation de transcription.

Hormonal regulation of iodination

B. Corvilain, C. Gerard, E. Raspe, A. Lefort, J. Mockel, J. Van Sande and J.E. Dumont

Institute of Interdiciplinary Research (IRIBHN), Université Libre de Bruxelles, School of Medicine, Route de Lennik 808, B1070 Brussels, Belgium

INTRODUCTION
The synthesis of thyroid hormones by the thyroid requires iodide and thyroglobulin as substrates and an oxidation system to iodinate tyrosyl groups in thyroglobulin and to link them into iodothyronines (Taurog et al., 1986; Nunez et al., 1982). This synthesis can therefore be limited or controlled at the level of iodide supply, by the availability of correct thyroglobulin (i.e. thyroglobulin allowing the coupling of iodotyrosines), as well as by the activity of the oxidation system. The spatial architecture of the follicle which insures concentration of iodide and thyroglobulin at the oxidation site i.e. at the periphery of the follicular lumen is also crucial for the efficiency of the synthesis. Alteration at any of these levels may impair thyroid hormone synthesis and depending on the conditions any of these steps may become limiting and therefore subject to control. In this brief review, we shall briefly summarize our knowledge of the acute and chronic control of thyroid hormone synthesis in the two species mst studied in our laboratory: dog and man.

CONSTITUENTS OF THE THYROID IODINATION SYSTEM
The constitutive elements of the thyroid iodination system are discussed at length elsewhere in this book. It is therefore only necessary here to briefly outline what is known about them. The H_2O_2 generating system is now being purified and analyzed by Pommiers's group in Paris (Virion et al., 1984). As already known from earlier studies in crude homogenates it consists of an oxidase using $NADPH_2$ as coenzyme. As the pentose phosphate shunt is the main pathway for NADP reduction in the thyroid, this pathway constitutes therefore the main $NADPH_2$ supply for the system (Dumont et al., 1971). In the apical membrane, the topology of the H_2O_2 generating system is such that it faces the cytosol on one side from which $NADPH_2$ is provided and the lumen in which the substrates of thyroperoxidase, iodide and thyroglobulin are concentrated on the other and this is also the side which thyroperoxidase faces (Virion et al., 1984; Nunez et al., 1982). Thyroperoxidase is a membrane hemoprotein whose catalytic site bathes in the lumen.

The third element of the system is thyroglobulin which provides the matrix in which the tyrosines to be iodinated are inserted and whose structure allows efficient coupling of these iodotyrosines into iodothyronines.

The same enzymatic machinery (H_2O_2 generating system, thyroglobulin, thyroperoxidase) catalyzes both iodination of the tyrosyls groups in thyroglobulin and their oxidative coupling. The generation of H_2O_2 and of oxidized iodine is toxic for the cell. The life of leucocytes in which similar systems are activated is drastically shortened. This suggests a need for compartmentation of these toxic derivatives and is one a posteriori explanation of this compartmentation. The enzymatic systems involved in detoxification of the H_2O_2 leaking back into the cell are catalase and glutathione peroxidase, which also utilizes $NADPH_2$ as coenzyme and therefore the pentose phosphate pathway as supply of $NADPH_2$ (Benard & De Groot, 1962).

CONTROL SYSTEMS IN THE THYROID
The regulation of the thyroid cell was once a classical example of the concept one hormone - one cell type - one intracellular secondary messenger with its pleiotypic effects. It should now rather be considered as a network of crosslinked regulatory steps where the extracellular and intracellular signal-molecules act on their receptors as bits of information in an electronic circuit, i.e., express on/off regulations with no definite general physiological meaning per se (Dumont et al., 1981). Such networks differ from one cell type to another and for a given cell type from one species to another. Only in a given cell type does the physiological coherence of the network emerge. In the case of the thyroid, many apparent discrepancies in the literature are explained if this is taken into acount.

In this short review we shall describe the coherent patterns of regulation in the dog and human thyroid models (Maenhaut et al., 1990). Figure I is the scheme which summarizes in a simplistic way our present knowledge of the regulation of the dog and human thyrocytes. Controls common to dog and man are indicated by straight lines; controls found only in the dog by a punctuated line and those found only in human by dashed lines. In the center, what is regulated : function, gene expression or differentiation, growth. On the left, the cyclic AMP cascade, on top, the PiP_2 Ca^{++} cascade.

In the dog thyroid, the main and best known circuit involves thyrotropin (TSH) stimulation of plasma membrane adenylate cyclase. Cyclic AMP produced by the cyclase is the intracellular signal molecule, which, by activating cAMP-dependent protein kinases, will enhance the main functions of the gland: the iodination of thyroglobulin and iodothyronine formation, i.e., the synthesis of thyroid hormones, the uptake of thyroglobulin and its hydrolysis, i.e., the secretion of thyroid hormones and the synthesis of thyroglobulin at the level of gene transcription (Dumont et al., 1981).

In the dog thyroid, the main fundamental effects of TSH are reproduced by cyclic AMP analogs and agents such as forskolin and cholera toxin which increase cyclic AMP accumulation in many

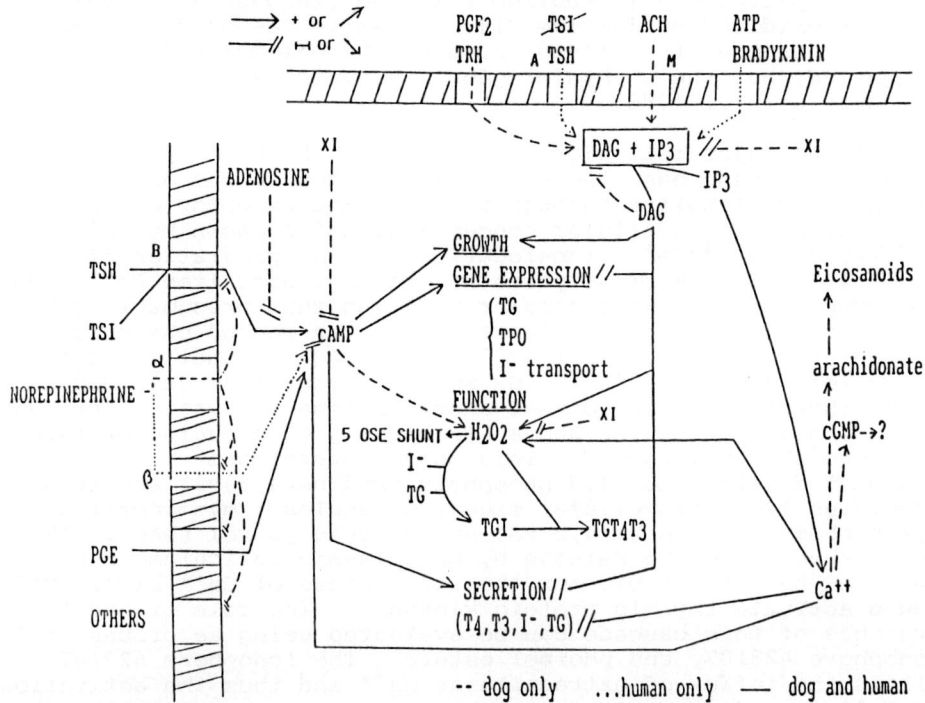

Fig. 1. Controls in the dog and human thyrocytes.
Abbreviations : Ach : acetylcholine; DAG : diacylglycerol; IP_3 : myo-inositol 1,4,5 phosphate; PG : prostaglandin; TG : thyroglobulin; TGI : iodinated thyroglobulin; TPO : thyroperoxidase; TSI : thyroid stimulating immunoglobulins; XI : unknown iodinated inhibitor; 5 OSE SHUNT : pentose phosphate pathway. Lines indicate controls : ─> positive control or stimulation; ─// negative control or inhibition.

tissues by activating adenylate cyclase and its GTP binding stimulating transducing protein Ns. They are thus mediated by cyclic AMP. By analogy with the β-receptor mediated action of norepinephrine they have been called B-effects.

Other extracellular signal molecules, prostaglandins of the E type and to a lesser extent norepinephrine through β receptors, activate thyroid adenylate cyclase and mimic the TSH effects. The abnormal thyroid stimulating immunoglobulins (TSI), which appear in the serum of patients with Graves'disease, also activate adenylate cyclase, presumably by binding to the TSH receptors. In thyroid as in other systems, adenylate cyclase is negatively regulated by receptor activated inhibitory GTP binding transducing protein Ni. In the dog thyrocyte, norepinephrine through α_2-receptors exerts this control. Adenosine directly inhibits cyclase. Negative feedback is also exerted on the TSH stimulatory pathway by the substrate of thyroid specialized metabolism : iodide (through a not yet defined oxidized derivative XI). Negative feedbacks by the thyroid hormones themselves and even thyroglobulin have been suggested, but their physiological relevance is still unknown (Pisarev et al., 1985).

The second major cell signalling system, the Ca^{++}- phosphatidyl-inositol cascade has also been demonstrated in the dog thyroid cells. Acetylcholine through a muscarinic receptor enhances free calcium intracellular concentration (as shown by Quin 2 fluorescence), $^{45}Ca^{++}$ translocation and the generation of Ins(1,4,5)P3. The first phase of intracellular free Ca^{++} rise is independent of extracellular Ca^{++} and thus presumably originates from intracellular stores. The second phase is dependent on extracellular Ca^{++} which suggests that it is caused by an influx of this Ca^{++}. By analogy with other cell models, it is therefore inferred that acetylcholine activates, through its muscarinic receptor and a GTP binding transducing protein, a membrane phospholipase C. This enzyme hydrolyses phosphatidyl-inositol 4,5 phosphate (PtdIns(4,5)P2) and thus generates two intracellular signal molecules : myo-inositol 1,4,5 phosphate (Ins(1,4,5)P3) and diacylglycerol (DAG). IP3 would then cause the release by endoplasmic reticulum of stored Ca^{++} and be responsible for the first phase of Ca^{++} rise. DAG would activate thyroid protein kinase C. The role of the two branches of this cascade can be evaluated using as probes Ca^{++} ionophore A23187, and phorbol esters. The ionophore A23187 allows the influx of extracellular Ca^{++} and thus the activation of Ca^{++} dependent systems; phorbol esters are specific long acting analogs of DAG. In the dog thyroid, all the effects of acetylcholine appear to be mediated by Ca^{++}: they are reproduced by the ionophore A23187 in the presence of extracellular Ca^{++}, or by high concentrations of extracellular Ca^{++}; they are inhibited in Ca^{++} depleted cells or by Ca^{++}-channel blockers such as Co^{++} or Mn^{++}. These effects are: the activation of protein iodination and glucose oxidation, the enhancement of cyclic GMP accumulation, the synthesis of prostaglandin and the inhibition of cyclic AMP accumulation and thyroid hormone secretion. The inhibition of cyclic AMP accumulation is caused by an activation by Ca^{++} of Ca^{++} calmodulin-dependent cyclic nucleotide phosphodiesterase . The inhibition of thyroid hormone secretion is caused both by this inhibition of cyclic AMP accumulation and by a direct effect on the secretory mechanism. The effects of the other intracellular signal generated by phospholipase C, diacylglycerol, can be inferred from the action of phorbol esters. These tumor promoters, as Ca^{++}, enhance protein iodination and inhibit thyroid hormone secretion. On the other hand, they appear to inhibit the first steps of the Ca^{++}-phosphatidylinositol cascade (IP$_3$ generation and Ca^{++} influx) and the consequent effect of the free intracellular Ca^{++} rise : the enhancement of cyclic GMP accumulation. DAG could therefore exert a negative feedback on the cascade (Maenhaut et al., 1990).

$PGF_{2\alpha}$, TRH and NaF reproduce some of the effects of acetylcholine in the dog thyrocyte. In dog thyroid cells, TSH enhances [^{32}P] phosphate and [^{3}H] inositol incorporation into phosphoinositides. It also stimulates $^{45}Ca^{++}$ efflux from prelabelled dog thyroid cells. These have been called A effects. This may suggest that TSH also activates the Ca^{++}-phosphatidylinositol cascade. However, TSH fails to enhance IP_3 generation in dog thyroid slices. Increased incorporation of ^3H inositol in IP_3, observed in some experiments, merely reflects increased incorporation in the precursors Pi, PiP and PiP_2. The meaning of the TSH A effects on dog thyrocyte Ca^{++} and phosphatidylinositol metabolism remains therefore obscure.

Iodide inhibits signal generation at the 2 major regulatory steps : cyclic AMP generation and phospholipase C. I^- must penetrate the cell and be oxidized to act. Indeed, the effect of I^- is prevented by $NaCLO_4$ which inhibits uptake and by methimazole which inhibits I^- oxidation. Quite a few other similar effects of I^- have been reported, notably by Pisarev. The identity of the postulated iodinated inhibitor(s) remains unknown. One clue may be that all these effects of iodide bear on membrane enzymes (Pisarev et al., 1985).

In the human thyrocyte a similar regulatory circuit has been demonstrated. Thyrotropin (TSH), through cyclic AMP, activates specialized functions of the tissue (transport of iodide, thyroid hormone secretion) and growth. Some of these stimulations are acute (within minutes) and require no prior protein synthesis (thyroid hormone synthesis and secetion) while others (iodide transport and growth) require just such a step. In the human thyrocytes, TSH and some neurotransmitters (ATP, bradykinin, etc) also activate the phosphatidylinositol 4-5 phosphate (PiP_2) cascade releasing $Ins(1,4,5)P_3$ and DAG in the cell. IP_3 elicits the release of calcium from endoplasmic reticulum and raises intracellular free calcium levels ($Ca^{++}i$). DAG and Ca^{++} act in parallel on function, inhibiting secretion and activating iodination and thyroid hormone synthesis. The dual action of thyrotropin may involve two different receptors as drawn on Fig. 1, or one receptor activating the GTP binding transducing proteins(G proteins) controlling the two cascades. The effect of TSH on the $PtdIns(4,5)P_2$ cascade is less sensitive to the hormone and slower than the action on cyclic AMP accumulation.
This general scheme applies to other species we have studied, except for a few important differences :
1) the action of TSH on the Pi cascade does not occur at physiological hormone levels in some species, among which dog
2) the neurotransmitters acting on the two cascades differ from one species to another. For example the PiP_2 cascade is activated by acetylcholine in dog but not in human thyrocytes. β adrenergic cyclic AMP response also varies much between species (small in dog, higher in human)

Three major pathways exert a delayed control on thyroid cell differentiation and mitogenesis in the dog thyroid.
Thyrotropin, through cyclic AMP, enhances both the expression of differentiation (iodide trapping, thyroglobulin and thyroperoxidase gene expression, etc) and mitogenesis. As shown by in situ hybridization to thyroglobulin mRNA the expression of differentiation and mitogenesis takes place in the same thyroid cells. Epidermal growth factor, which activates its EGF protein

tyrosine kinase receptor, induces cell proliferation and dedifferentiation. Serum through unknown factors and receptors acts in the same way. Phorbol esters, the long lasting analogues of diacylglycerol, through activation of protein kinase C also stimulate cell proliferation and induce dedifferentiation. All these effects on differentiation are reversible in cell culture and can be dissociated from the effects on mitogenesis by using confluent cultures (Maenhaut et al., 1990).

ACUTE CONTROL OF IODINATION AND THYROID HORMONE SYNTHESIS
Theoretically iodination could be controlled at any of the levels of the iodide-thyroglobulin iodothyronine pathway: i.e. at the supply of substrates (iodide, thyroglobulin, H_2O_2) or at the level of iodination itself. Physiologically important controls bear on the limiting step of the pathway and this may vary depending on the species, physiological or pathological condition. Thyroglobulin supply is not limiting under physiological conditions. In genetic defects of thyroglobulin, compensatory iodination on endogenous or exogenous albumin or other proteins takes place, but iodotyrosines coupling is deficient in the absence of the matrix provided by thyroglobulin to set iodotyrosines in the correct position (Nunez et al., 1982).

Under physiological conditions iodide trapping is limiting protein iodination in dog and to some extent in human thyroids. Increasing iodide supply by progressive saturation of the pump is sufficient to greatly increase protein iodination. On the other hand, stimulation of organification is not demonstrated unless increasing iodide concentration to unphysiological levels makes iodination limiting. It is interesting in this regard that autonomous nodules which synthesize and secrete thyroid hormones in excess, independently of TSH, show increased iodide trapping but normal conversion of this iodide to iodinated proteins (Van Sande et al., 1988).

As in this symposium we are mainly concerned with the iodination system per se, we shall therefore only consider the controls bearing directly on this system. Under conditions in which it is limiting, i.e. at high iodide concentrations, protein iodination is stimulated in the thyroid cells by the Ca^{++}-PiP_2 cascade in all the mammalians studied . Both ionophore A23187, which activates the Ca^{++} branch of this cascade, and phorbol esters which mimic the action of diacylglycerol on protein kinase C, stimulate, albeit with various amplitudes, protein iodination in thyroid slices. This cascade, itself is activated in different species by different neurotransmitters: in dog by acetylcholine and muscarinic receptors, in human by ATP and purinergic receptors, etc (vide supra). Protein iodination is activated by the TSH cyclic AMP cascade in the dog thyroid and in some other species. However in most species including man, cyclic AMP has little positive effect or may even decrease protein iodination. Iodide which inhibits both the TSH cyclic AMP and the Ca^{++} PiP_2 cascades also inhibits the stimulations by these cascades of its own oxidation.

The control of the iodination could bear on the H_2O_2 generating system or on thyroperoxidase. Thyroperoxidase which has been recently cloned and sequenced, does not contain in its cytoplasmic CO_2H terminal canonical target sequences for phosphorylation by cyclic AMP dependent protein kinases (Libert et al., 1987). Moreover in human thyroid slices thyroperoxidase is not phosphorylated in response to thyrotropin which activates both the cyclic AMP and the Ca^{++} PiP_2 cascades. There is therefore no indication of a posttraductional modulation of the activity of this enzyme. On the other hand, there is good indication that H_2O_2 supply is limiting the iodination process (Corvilain et al., 1988; Bjorkman et al., 1988). Addition of H_2O_2 or of a H_2O_2 generating system to thyroid slices or particulates greatly enhances protein iodination in cells and in acellular systems. Moreover in dog thyroid slices all the experimental conditions leading to enhanced iodination also cause a stimulation of H_2O_2 formation: treatment with carbamylcholine, phorbol esters, Ca^{++} ionophore (A23187), ionomycin, TSH, forskolin, dibutyryl cyclic AMP, PGF_2, TRH, NaF, alkaline pH, Mn^{++} in Ca^{++} depleted medium, etc. There is a strict parallelism between concentration action relationships for TSH, and carbamylcholine on protein iodination and H_2O_2 generation. Finally increasingly severe glucose and calcium depletion in the medium decrease H_2O_2 generation and protein iodination in parallel. Thus there is no doubt that protein iodination is mainly controlled at the level of H_2O_2 generation. Iodide which inhibits its own oxidation also inhibits H_2O_2 generation by an effect on cyclic AMP accumulation, on PiP_2 hydrolysis and also by an action downstream frm these intracellular signals on the H_2O_2 generating system. All these effects of iodide are relieved by methimazole which suggests that they are mediated by an organified form of iodine (Corvilain et al., submitted).

It is interesting to point out that H_2O_2 generation by inducing the oxidation of $NADPH_2$ and thus increasing NADP supply in the cell also controls the activity of the pentose phosphate pathway. Indeed addition of H_2O_2 and all the agents or conditions that activate the H_2O_2 generation also stimulate the activity of the pentose phosphate pathway. H_2O_2 generation "pushes" the iodination and by its consumption of $NADPH_2$ "pulls" the pentose phosphate pathway (Corvilain et al., submitted).

Similar conclusions apply to protein iodination in the human thyroid with one major exception: cyclic AMP does not activate H_2O_2 generation or iodide binding to proteins in this tissue. However, as thyrotropin also activates the Ca^{++} PiP_2 cascade in human thyroid cells, it also enhances, by this pathway, H_2O_2 generation and protein iodination.

DELAYED OR CHRONIC CONTROLS OF THYROID HORMONE SYNTHESIS

It is well known that stimulated thyroids take up and organify more iodide than controls and conversely that resting thyroids metabolize less iodide. Similarly, whatever the specialized enzyme or even house keeping enzyme studied its cell content increases under chronic stimulation and conversely. However to our knowledge no systematic quantitative study of iodide incorporated into proteins under conditions where trapping is not limited has been carried out in chronically stimulated or repressed thyroids. Delayed or chronic controls generally involve gene expression, at the transcription or at the translation level. In the case of protein iodination, only thyroperoxidase has been cloned, only for this element of the system do we have specific antibodies. Thus detailed biochemical analysis of the delayed controls have only been carried out on thyroperoxidase.

In human thyroid cells in culture, thyroperoxidase synthesis, as evaluated by 2D gel electrophoresis, is stimulated by thyrotropin, an effect which is mimicked by forskolin and thus ascribed to the TSH induced cyclic AMP signal.

In dog thyroid cells, thyroperoxidase gene transcription is also controlled by thyrotropin through cyclic AMP. Contrary to Tg, the regulation of TPO gene seems to correspond to the classical models of genes in which the promoter is regulated directly via cAMP regulatory elements: 1) the kinetics of transcriptional activation is rapid (in slices and in primay cultures); 2) the activation does not require prior or ongoing protein synthesis; it is not inhibited by cycloheximide; 3) a sequence close to the canonical cAMP responsive element has been demonstrated in the promoter... 4) the control by thyrotropin does not require insulin stimulation (Gerard et al., 1988). The details of this regulation are now delineated (see Abramowicz et al. in this volume).

REFERENCES

Benard, B. & DeGroot, L.J. (1969): The role of hydrogen peroxide and glutathione in glucose oxidation by the thyroid. Biochim. Biophys. Acta 111: 258.

Bjorkman, U. & Ekholm, R. (1988): Accelerated exocytosis and H_2O_2 generation in isolated thyroid follicles enhance protein iodination. Endocrinology 122: 488.

Corvilain, B., Van Sande, J. & DUMONT, J.E. (1988): Inhibition by iodide of iodide binding to proteins: the "Wolff-Chaikoff-effect" is caused by inhibition of H_2O_2 generation. Biochem. Biophys. Res. Commun. 154: 1287.

Dumont, J.E. (1971): The action of thyrotropin on thyroid metabolism. In Vitamins and Hormones, Academic Press (N.Y. and London), vol. 29, 287.

Dumont, J.E., Takeuchi, A., Lamy, F., Gervy-Decoster, C., Cochaux, P., Roger, P., Van Sande, J., Lecocq, R. & Mockel, J. (1981): Thyroid control: an example of a complex cell regulation network. Adv. Cyclic Nucl. Res. 14: 479.

Gerard, C.M., Lefort, A., Libert, F., Christophe, D., Dumont, J.E., Vassart, G. (1988): Transcriptional regulation of the thyroperoxydase gene by thyrotropin and forskolin. Mol. Cell. Endocrinol. 60: 239.

Libert, F., Ruel, J., Ludgate, M., Swillens, S., Alexander, N., Vassart, G., Dinsart, C. (1987): Thyroperoxidase, an auto-antigen with a mosaic structure made of nuclear and mitochondrial gene modules. EMBO J 6: 4193.

Maenhaut C., Lefort, A., Libert, F., Parmentier, M., Raspé, E., Roger, P., Corvilain, B., Laurent, E., Reuse, S., Mockel, J., Lamy, F., Van Sande J., & Dumont, J.E. (1990): Function, proliferation and differentiation of the dog and human thyrocyte. Horm. Metab. Research (in press).

Nunez, J. & Pommier, J. (1982): Formation of thyroid hormones. Vitam. Hormon. 39: 175.

Pisarev, M.A. (1985): Thyroid autoregulation. J. Endocrinol. Invest. 8: 475.

Taurog, A. (1986): Hormone synthesis : Thyroid iodine metabolism. In The Thyroid, Werner (ed), ed 5. JB Lippincott Co Philadelphia, p 53.

Van Sande, J., Lamy, F., Lecocq, R., Mirkine, N., Rocmans, P., Cochaux, P., Mockel, J., Dumont, J.E. (1988): Pathogenesis of autonomous thyroid nodules : in vitro study of iodine and adenosine 3',5'-monophosphate metabolism. J. Clin. Endocrinol. Metab. 66: 570.

Virion, A., Michot, J.L., Deme, D., Kanieuwski, J., Pommier, J. (1984): NADPH-dependent H_2O_2 generation and peroxidase activity in a thyroid particulate fraction. Mol. Cell. Endocrinol. 36: 95-105.

Regulation by TSH and thyroid stimulating antibodies of TPO expression

L. Chiovato, P. Vitti, C. Mammoli, F. Santini, M. Tonacchera, P. Lapi, P. Cucchi, P. Carayon* and A. Pinchera

*Cattedra di Endocrinologia e Medicina Costituzionale, Universita di Pisa, viale del Tirreno 64, 56018, Tirrenia-Pisa, Italy; and *INSERM U.38 Laboratoire des Hormones Protéiques, Faculté de Médecine, 27, Bd Jean Moulin, 13385, Marseille Cedex 5, France*

SUMMARY

The mechanisms responsible for the expression of the thyroid microsomal/peroxidase autoantigen (M/TPO-Ag) were studied in FRTL-5 cells and in primary cultures of human thyroid cells prepared from Graves' or nontoxic goiters. The indirect immunofluorescence (IFL) technique using human sera positive for anti-microsomal antibody (anti-MAb) was employed to detect M/TPO-Ag. Studies were performed to ascertain whether M-Ag recognized by human anti-MAb could be identified with thyroid peroxidase (TPO). Preabsorption experiments showed that, similarly to solubilized human thyroid microsomes, purified human TPO abolished the binding of anti-MAb to human thyrocytes, while no inhibition was obtained by preabsorption with control human tissues. The identity of M-Ag and TPO was also demonstrated using a double layer IFL technique which allowed a simultaneous staining of the antigen(s) recognized by human anti-MAb and by a monoclonal anti-TPO antibody. After 3-15 days of TSH withdrawal from the culture medium the M/TPO-Ag disappeared from the surface and cytoplasm of thyroid cells. Readdition of TSH (0.1-100 mU/ml) to cells lacking M/TPO-Ag elicited its reappearance within 48-72 h. This effect of TSH was prevented by actinomycin D and cycloheximide but not by methimazole. Two stimulators of the adenylate cyclase-cAMP system (cholera toxin and forskolin), a phosphodiesterase inhibitor (isobutylmethylxanthine) and 8-bromo-cAMP mimicked TSH in inducing the reappearance of M/TPO-Ag. Thyroid stimulating antibody (TSAb) of Graves' disease also reproduced the effect of TSH on M/TPO-Ag reexpression in thyroid cells. By contrast, 12-0-tetradecanoyl-phorbol 13-acetate, epidermal growth factor, estradiol or NaI were ineffective in inducing M/TPO-Ag. The present data indicate that: i) the expression of M/TPO-Ag in thyroid cells is dependent on TSH stimulation, through pathways which involve cAMP production, mRNA formation and protein synthesis, ii) TSAb reproduces this effect of TSH; iii) estradiol and NaI have no direct influence on the expression of the M/TPO-Ag.

INTRODUCTION

The thyroid microsomal autoantigen (M-Ag) is a target of the immune aggression in Hashimoto's thyroiditis, idiopathic myxedema and Graves' disease (Weetman & MacGregor, 1984; Pinchera et al., 1985). It was previously shown in our (Pinchera et al., 1980; Fenzi et al., 1982) and other (Khoury et al.,1981) laboratories that M-Ag , historically considered a cytoplasmic lipoprotein, is also represented on the thyroid cell surface at the microvillar pole, and may be involved in the complement-mediated cytotoxicity of sera from patients with autoimmune thyroid disorders (Khoury et al., 1984). Moreover, recent evidence indicates that in autoimmune thyroid glands follicular cells bearing HLA class II molecules (DR) (Hanafusa et al., 1983) can directly present their surface autoantigens to the immune system (Londei et al., 1985). The latter mechanism could initiate and/or maintain the autoimmune process against the thyroid gland (Bottazzo et al., 1983). In the last few years evidence was also provided that in human glands M-Ag can be identified with thyroid peroxidase (TPO) (Czarnocka et al., 1985; Mariotti et al., 1987; Ruf et al., 1987).

The mechanisms leading to the expression of M-Ag in follicular cells were unknown until we demonstrated that M-Ag is present on the surface of a peculiar strain of differentiated rat thyroid cells (FRTL-5) and that its expression is modulated by thyrotropin (TSH) (Chiovato et al., 1985). These results promptd us to investigate the mechanisms responsible of M-Ag expression in FRTL-5 and human thyroid cells. Furthermore, the putative identity of M-Ag and TPO was investigated in terms of antigenic properties and TSH-dependent modulation.

MATERIALS AND METHODS

Thyroid cell cultures

FRTL-5 cells and primary cultures of human thyroid cells prepared by collagenase digestion from surgical specimens of nontoxic or Graves' goiters were used. Cells were seeded onto round coverslips plated in 24-well plates and were cultured in Coon's modified Ham F-12 medium supplemenetd with 5% adult calf serum, and a 6-hormone mixture (6H medium) containing: insulin (1.6 µM), cortisol (10 nM), transferrin (62.5 nM), l-glycyl-histidyl-lysine (25 nM), somatostatin (6.25 nM) and TSH (300 µU/ml) (Chiovato et al., 1985).

Experimental procedure

Thyroid cells were cultured for 7-15 days in the above described medium deprived of TSH (5H medium). At the end of this period thyrocytes were recultured for 3-7 days in 5H medium containing TSH (0.1-100 mU/ml) or other agents: cholera toxin (10 pM), forskolin (5-50 µM), 8-bromo-cAMP (0.5mM), isobutylmethylxanthine (IBMX, 0.5 mM), IgG containing TSAb (1 mg/ml), NaI (0.1-10 mM), estradiol (3.6-73.5 nM), 12-0-tetradecanoyl-phorbol 13-acetate (TPA, 10-100 ng/ml) or epidermal growth factor (EGF,1 nM). In other experiments thyrocytes, deprived of TSH for 7-15 days were recultured in

5H medium containig the hormone (0.1-10 mU/ml) plus actinomycin D (0.5-5 µg/ml), cycloheximide (10 µM) or methimazole (MMI, 0.1-2 mM).

Sera

Sera from 5 patients with Hashimoto's thyroiditis were selected on the basis of the following antibody pattern: high titers of anti-microsomal antibody (anti-MAb); undetectable anti-thyroglobulin antibody and thyroid stimulating antibody (TSAb) (Vitti et al., 1982) or TSH-blocking antibodies (Chiovato et al., 1987). Sera from normal subjects were used as controls. TSAb-IgG was obtained by DEAE Sephadex separation from the serum of a patient with active Graves' disease.

Single and double indirect immunofluorescence (IFL)

Indirect IFL using sera containing anti-MAb was employed to detect M/TPO-Ag on thyroid cell surface and in the cytoplasm (Chiovato et al., 1985). In the double IFL procedure human thyroid cells were incubated in the sequence with: 1) an anti-TPO monoclonal antibody (Czarnocka et al., 1985) (10 ng/ml); 2) a rhodaminated goat anti-mouse Ig conjugate; 3) a human serum containing anti-MAb; 4) a fluoresceinated sheep anti-human Ig conjugate (Chiovato et al., 1989).

Preparation of human thyroglobulin (Tg), microsomal fractions and thyroid peroxidase (TPO)

Human Tg (19 S) was purified from saline extracts of nontoxic goiters as previously described (Mariotti et al., 1979). Microsomes were prepared by differential centrifugation from human thyroid, placenta, liver and spleen, and were solubilized with deoxycholate (Mariotti et al., 1979). Human TPO was purified from solubilized thyroid microsomes by affinity chromatography (Czarnocka et al. 1985), using a monoclonal antibody specifically directed to human TPO (Czarnocka et al., 1985, Ruf et al., 1987).

Preabsorption experiments

In some experiments anti-MAb positive sera were absorbed with purified TPO (10 µg), Tg (10 µg) or solubilized microsomes (1 mg) from human thyroid and control tissues. After separation at 105.000 x g, supernatants were tested in the IFL procedure (Chiovato et al., 1988).

RESULTS

Specificity of IFL for recognition of M/TPO-Ag, and identification of M-Ag with TPO

All Hashimoto's sera used in this study produced a clear staining of the surface and the cytoplasm of FRTL-5 and human thyroid cells cultured in medium containing TSH.

Negative results were obtained with normal sera. To demonstrate that the antigen stained by anti-MAb sera was M-Ag and that it could be identified with TPO, preabsorption experiments were performed on FRTL-5 and human thyroid cells. Preabsorption with thyroid microsomes and TPO abolished the staining of thyroid cells while no effect was produced by preabsorption with Tg or microsomes from control tissues (Chiovato et al., 1988). When double IFL was performed on human thyroid cells, anti-MAb positive sera and the anti-TPO monoclonal Ab produced a surface and cytoplasmic staining. The same cells were stained by the two antibodies and in no case was a dissociation of the green and red fluorescence observed. Moreover, preincubation of cells with anti-MAb positive sera abolished the subsequent binding of the anti-TPO monoclonal Ab (Chiovato et al., 1989).

Table 1
Induction of surface M/TPO-Ag in FRTL-5 cells or human thyroid cells previously deprived of TSH for 7-15 days 48 h after addition to cultures of TSH, cholera toxin, forskolin, IBMX, 8-bromo-cAMP, TSAb-IgG, estradiol or NaI.

ADDITION	FRTL-5 CELLS	HUMAN THYROID CELLS
TSH (2.5 mU/ml)	+++	+
TSH (100 mU/ml)	+++	++
Cholera toxin (10 pM)	++	+
Forskolin (50 µM)	+++	+++
IBMX (0.5 mM)	+	+
8-Br-cAMP (0.5 mM)	+	+
TSAb-IgG (1 mg/ml)	+++	++
Estradiol (73.5 nM)	-	-
NaI (10 mM)	-	-

* The scoring of surface IFL is indicated as: (-) = negative; (+) = 10-30% positive cells; (++) = 30-80% positive cells; (+++) => 80% strongly positive cells.

Modulation of M/TPO-Ag expression in thyroid cells

When TSH was added to the culture medium, M/TPO-Ag was always present in the cytoplasm and on the surface of FRTL-5 cells and could be identified for at least 30 days in human thyroid cells. Withdrawal of TSH from the culture medium for 3-15 days produced a progressive disappearance of M/TPO-Ag from surface and cytoplasm of FRTL-5 cells and human thyroid cells. The time of TSH deprivation required for M/TPO-Ag disappearance was shorter in FRTL-5 cells than in human thyroid cells, moreover longer periods of TSH starvation were required in primary cultures from Graves' goiters with respect to cells prepared from nontoxic glands. In 3 primary cultures from Graves' goiters a limited percentage of cells (1-5%) retained their positivity for M/TPO-Ag even after 30 days of incubation in medium deprived of TSH (Chiovato et al., 1989).

Reexposure to TSH (0.1-100 mU/ml) of thyroid cells lacking M/TPO-Ag led to the reappearance of this antigen on the surface and in the cytoplasm. The effect of TSH was dose and time dependent in the range of 24-72 h. The minimal concentration of TSH able to restore M/TPO-Ag was lower in FRTL-5 cells and varied in primary cultures obtained from different goiters. While 100% of FRTL-5 cells recovered M/TPO-Ag after TSH readdition, the maximal percentage of human thyroid cells recovering their positivity for this antigen ranged from 30% to 70%.

To investigate whether this phenomenon was mediated by cAMP, TSH was substituted for by cholera toxin, forskolin, 8-bromo-cAMP or IBMX. All these substances induced the surface and cytoplasmic M/TPO-Ag in FRTL-5 cells and human thyroid cells (Table 1). In the majority of human thyroid cell cultures the percentage of positive cells recruited after addition of the highest dose of forskolin was greater (70-80%) than that obtained with the superoptimal concentration of TSH. Reappearance of M/TPO-Ag was also produced when TSAb-IgG was added to 5H medium. EGF stimulated the growth of human thyroid cells but was unable to reexpress M/TPO-Ag. Similarly TPA, although producing a mitotic effect, failed to induce the reappearance of the M/TPO-Ag in FRTL-5 cells (Table 2). No effect on the reappearance of M/TPO-Ag was observed in cultures incubated with estradiol or NaI without TSH.

In some experiments FRTL-5 and human thyroid cells lacking M/TPO-Ag after TSH deprivation were challenged with the hormone in the presence of actinomycin D, cycloheximide or MMI. Both actinomycin D and cycloheximide prevented the reappearance of the surface and cytoplasmic M/TPO-Ag induced by TSH. By contrast, the addition of MMI to the medium containing TSH did not prevent the reappearance of M/TPO-Ag produced by the hormone.

Table 2
Effect of EGF and TPA on surface M/TPO-Ag expression and cell growth in thyroid cells previously maintained in medium deprived of TSH for 12 days. The action of TSH on parellel cultures is shown for comparison.

Addition	HUMAN THYROID CELLS		FRTL-5 CELLS	
	IFL*	Cell number**	IFL*	Cell number**
None	Negative	3.5 ± 0.8	Negative	1.9 ± 0.07
EGF (1 nM)	Negative	10.2 ± 2.5	--	--
TPA (100 ng/ml)	--	--	Negative	3.5 ± 0.37
TSH (0.3 mU/ml)	Positive	4.3 ± 1.2	Positive	8.0 ± 0.72

* IFL on thyroid cells was performed using an anti-MAb positive serum after 48 h, 72 h and 7 days of incubation.
** Cells were counted after 7 days of culture in medium containing EGF, TPA or TSH. Results are expressed as mean $\pm$ S.D.(x 100.000).

DISCUSSION

The mechanisms involved in the expression of M/TPO-Ag were investigated in FRTL-5 cells and in primary cultures of human thyroid cells prepared from Graves' and nontoxic goiters. Studies were also performed to ascertain whether M-Ag stained by IFL in thyroid cells could be identified with TPO. Preabsorption experiments showed that, similarly to solubilized human thyroid microsomes, TPO abolished the binding of anti-MAb to thyroid cells, while no inhibition was obtained by preabsorption with control human tissues or Tg. Moreover, using double IFL, the pattern of fluorescence produced on human thyrocytes by a monoclonal anti-TPO Ab was undistinguishable from that obtained with anti-MAb positive sera (Chiovato et al., 1989). These data indicate that the antigen recognized by anti-MAb in human thyroid cells is indeed TPO.

Withdrawal of TSH from the culture medium induced a disappearance of M/TPO-Ag from surface and cytoplasm of FRTL-5 and human thyroid cells. The time of TSH deprivation required for the disappearance of M/TPO-Ag was longer in primary cultures obtained from Graves' goiters than in those derived from nontoxic goiters. TSAb bound in vivo to follicular cells could explain the delayed disappearance of M/TPO-Ag from primary cultures of Graves' goiters. At variance with FRTL-5 cells, a limited percentage (1-5%) of human thyroid cells from some Graves' goiters retained M/TPO-Ag despite prolonged starvation from TSH. This phenomenon can be explained by the presence in the original goiter of autonomous follicles already independent from TSH control in vivo (Studer, 1986). Following readdition of TSH, M/TPO-Ag reappeared in 100% of FRTL-5 cells and in up to 30%-70% of human thyroid cells. Failure to completely recover M/TPO-Ag in primary cultures can be attributed to a progressive reduction of TSH receptors in cultured human thyrocytes (Bidey et al., 1981). In agreement with this hypothesis, in our experiments forskolin was able to recruit a number of M/TPO-Ag positive cells (up to 80%) greater than that obtained with any dose of TSH (Chiovato et al., 1989). TSH action on thyroid cells is mediated by cAMP dependent and cAMP independent pathways. Indeed in our experiments several agents known to increase cAMP content in thyroid cells: cholera toxin, forskolin, 8-bromo-cAMP, IBMX, and TSAb mimicked TSH in the induction of M/TPO-Ag. On the contrary, activation of cAMP-independent pathways by EGF in human thyroid cells and by TPA in FRTL-5 cells did not produce a reexpression of M/TPO-Ag. These data support the hypothesis that the adenylate cyclase cAMP system is the main pathway involved in the expression of M/TPO-Ag in thyroid cells. Actinomycin D, an inhibitor of DNA replication and mRNA formation, or cycloheximide, an inhibitor of protein synthesis at the polyribosome level were able to prevent the reappearance of M/TPO-Ag induced by TSH, indicating that mRNA formation and subsequent protein synthesis must be operating. Methimazole, a drug blocking the enzymatic activity of TPO, was also tested as a putative inhibitor of M/TPO-Ag expression (Marcocci et al., 1982). However, this drug was unable to interfere with the expression of M/TPO-Ag.

Autoimmune thyroid disorders are more common in females than in men, but the reason for this remains unknown. Among different explanations, an influence of estrogens was supposed. The question could be raised whether these steroids might influence the "antigenicity" of follicular cells. However, estradiol was unable to restore the expression of M/TPO-Ag in human thyroid cells, indicating that these steroids do not exert a direct effect in terms of thyroid autoantigen expression. Epidemiological observations in man and experimental findings in autoimmune thyroiditis of genetically susceptible chicken and rats have suggested an association between iodide intake and the occurrence of autoimmune thyroiditis in man (Safran et al., 1987). The possibility that iodide could influence the expression of M/TPO-Ag was checked in our cultures, but NaI in the absence of TSH did not induce M/TPO-Ag.

The following conclusions can be drawn from our studies: i) the expression of M/TPO-Ag in thyroid cells is dependent on TSH stimulation, through pathways which involve cAMP production, mRNA formation and protein synthesis; ii) TSAb reproduces the effect of TSH, thus explaining why M/TPO-Ag is so abundant in Graves' goiters; iii) the modulation of M/TPO-Ag by TSH acquires particular relevance in view of previous findings indicating that this hormone enhances the expression of HLA-DR induced by interferon-gamma in human thyroid cells (Todd et al., 1987), taken together these data explain the decrease of circulating anti-MAb observed during L-thyroxine therapy in hypothyroid patients with Hashimoto's thyroiditis (Chiovato et al., 1986); iv) other agents, such as MMI, NaI and estradiol, that are supposed to play a role in autoimmune thyroid disorders, do not interfere with or stimulate the expression of M/TPO-Ag.

REFERENCES

Bidey, S.P., Marshall, N.J. & Ekins R.P. (1981): Characterisation of the cyclic AMP response to thyrotrophin in monolayer cultures of normal human thyroid cells. *Acta Endocrinol.* 98, 370-375.

Bottazzo, G.F., Pujol-Borrell, R., Hanafusa, T. & Feldmann, M. (1983): Hypothesis: role of aberrant HLA-DR expression and antigen presentation in the induction of endocrine autoimmunity. *Lancet* 2, 1115-1119.

Chiovato, L., Marcocci, C., Mariotti, S., Mori, A. & Pinchera, A. (1986): L-thyroxine therapy induces a fall of thyroid microsomal and thyroglobulin antibodies in idiopathic myxedema and in hypothyroid, but not in euthyroid Hashimoto's thyroiditis. *J. Endocrinol. Invest.* 9, 299-305.

Chiovato, L., Vitti, P., Cucchi, P., Mammoli, C., Carayon, P. & Pinchera, A. (1989): The expression of the microsomal/peroxidase autoantigen in human thyroid cells is thyrotrophin-dependent. *Clin. Exp. Immunol.* 76, 47-53.

Chiovato, L., Vitti, P., Lombardi, A., Ceccarelli, P., Cucchi, P., Marcocci, C., Carayon, P. & Pinchera, A. (1988): Studies on the mechanism responsible for thyrotropin-induced expression of microsomal/peroxidase antigen in FRTL-5 cells. *J. Clin. Endocrinol. Metab.* 123, 1140-1146.

Chiovato, L., Vitti, P., Lombardi, A., Kohn, L.D. & Pinchera, A. (1985): Expression of the microsomal antigen on the surface of continuously cultured rat thyroid cells is modulated by thyrotropin. *J. Clin. Endocrinol. Metab.* 61, 12-16.

Chiovato, L., Vitti, P., Lombardi, A., Lopez, G., Santini, F., Macchia, E., Fenzi, G.F., Mammoli, C., Battiato, S. & Pinchera, A. (1987): Detection and characterization of autoantibodies blocking the TSH-dependent cAMP production in FRTL-5 cells *J. Endocrinol. Invest.* 10, 383-390.

Czarnocka, B., Ruf, J., Ferrand, M., Carayon, P. & Lissitzky, S. (1985): Purification of the human thyroid peroxidase and its identification as the microsomal antigen involved in autoimmune thyroid diseases. *FEBS Lett.* 190, 147-152.

Fenzi, G.F., Bartalena, L., Chiovato, L., Marcocci, C., Rotella, C. M., Zonefrati, R., Toccafondi, R. & Pinchera, A. (1982): Studies on thyroid cell surface antigens using cultured human cells. Clin . Exp . Immunol . 47, 336-344.

Hanafusa, T., Pujol-Borrell, R., Chiovato, L., Russell, R.C.G., Doniach, D. & Bottazzo G.F. (1983): Aberrant expression of HLA-DR antigen on thyrocytes in Graves' disease: relevance for autoimmunity. Lancet 2, 1111-1115.

Khoury, E.L., Bottazzo, G.F. & Roitt, I.M. (1984): The thyroid microsomal antibody revisited: its paradoxical binding in vivo to the apical surface of the follicular epithelium. J . Exp . Med. 159, 577-591.

Khoury, E.L., Hammond, L., Bottazzo, G.F. & Doniach, D. (1981): Presence of organ specific microsomal autoantigen on the surface of human thyroid cells in culture: its involvement in complement mediated cytotoxicity. Clin. Exp. Immunol. 45, 316-325.

Londei, M., Bottazzo, G.F. & Feldmann, M. (1985): Human T cell clones from autoimmune thyroid glands: specific recognition of autologous thyroid cells. Science 228, 85-87.

Marcocci, C., Chiovato, L. , Mariotti, S. & Pinchera, A. (1982): Changes of circulating thyroid autoantibody levels during and after therapy with methimazole in patients with Graves' disease. J. Endocrinol. Invest. 5, 13-19.

Mariotti, S., Pinchera, A., Marcocci, C., Vitti, P., Urbano, C., Chiovato, L., Tosi, M. & Baschieri, L. (1979): Solubilization of human thyroid microsomal antigen. J. Clin. Endocrinol. Metab. 48, 207-212.

Mariotti, S., Anelli, S., Ruf, J., Bechi, R., Czarnocka, B., Lombardi, A., Carayon, P. & Pinchera, A. (1987): Comparison of serum thyroid microsomal and thyroid peroxidase autoantibodies in thyroid diseases. J. Clin. Endocrinol. Metab. 65, 987-993.

Studer, H. (1986): Growth control and follicular cell neoplasia. In Frontiers in Thyroidology, eds. G. Medeiros-Neto & E. Gaitan, pp. 131-138. New York: Plenum Press.

Pinchera, A., Fenzi, G.F., Bartalena, L., Chiovato, L., Marcocci, C., Toccafondi, R., Rotella, C.M., Aterini, S. & Zonefrati, R. (1980): Thyroid cell surface and thyroid stimulating antibodies in patients with thyroid autoimmune disorders. In Thyroid Research VIII, eds. J.R. Stockigt & S. Nagataki, pp. 707-709. Canberra: Australian Academy of Science.

Pinchera, A., Fenzi, G.F., Vitti, P., Chiovato, L., Bartalena, L., Macchia, E. & Mariotti, S. (1985): Significance of thyroid autoantibodies in autoimmune thyroid diseases. In Autoimmunity and the Thyroid, eds. P.G. Walfish , J.R. Wall & R. Volpe, pp. 139. Toronto: Academic Press.

Ruf, J., Czarnocka, B., De Micco, C., Dutoit, C., Ferrand, M. & Carayon, P. (1987): Thyroid peroxidase is the organ-specific 'microsomal' autoantigen involved in thyroid autoimmunity. Acta Endocrinol. 1115 (Suppl 281), 49-55.

Todd, I., Pujol-Borrell, R., Hammond, L.J., McNally, J.M., Feldmann, M. & Bottazzo, G.F. (1987) Enhancement of thyrocyte HLA class II expression by thyroid stimulating hormone. Clin. Exp. Immunol. 69, 524-530.

Vitti, P., Valente, W.A., Ambesi-Impiombato, F.S., Fenzi, G.F., Pinchera, A. & Kohn, L.D. (1982): Graves' IgG stimulation of continuously cultured rat thyroid cells: a sensitive and potentially useful clinical assay. J. Endocrinol. Invest. 5,179-182.

Weetman, A.P. & McGregor, A.M. (1984): Autoimmune thyroid disease: Development in our understanding. Endocr. Rev. 5, 309-320.

Résumé

Les mécanismes responsables de l'expression des antigènes microsomiaux/thyropéroxydase, ont été étudiés dans les cellules FRTL-5 et dans des cultures primaires de cellules thyroïdiennes préparées à partir de goitres sains ou de goitres de Basedow. Les antigènes microsomiaux/thyropéroxydase ont été détectés en utilisant la technique d'immunofluorescence indirecte (IFL) à l'aide d'anticorps microsomiaux du serum positif humain. L'étude visait à confirmer que les antigènes microsomiaux reconnus par les anticorps anti-microsomiaux humains pouvaient être identifiés à la thyropéroxydase. Les expériences de préabsorption ont montré que, d'une façon identique aux microsomes thyroïdiens humains en solution, la TPO humaine purifiée inhibait la liaison des anticorps anti-microsomiaux aux thyrocytes humains, alors qu'on n'obtenait aucune inhibition après préabsorption avec des tissus humains de contrôle. L'identité entre l'antigène microsomial et la TPO a également été démontrée par une technique de double marquage par fluorescence indirecte qui permet la coloration simultanée de l'antigène reconnu par un anticorps anti-microsomial humain et par un anticorps monoclonal anti-TPO. Après 3 à 15 jours d'une culture en l'absence de TSH, les antigènes microsomiaux/TPO disparaissent de la surface et du cytoplasme des cellules. L'addition de la TSH (0.1-100 mU/ml) à des cellules dépourvues de M/TPO-Ag entraîne sa réapparition dans un délai de 48 à 72 H. Cette action de la TSH est inhibée par l'actinomycine D et la cycloheximide, mais non par le méthimazole. Deux stimulateurs du système adénylate cyclase-cAMP (la toxine du choléra et la forskoline), un inhibiteur de la phosphodiétérase (l'isobutylméthylxanthine) et le 8-bromo-cAMP, induisent eux aussi, comme la TSH, la réapparition des antigènes M/TPO. Les anticorps thyro-stimulants de la maladie de Basedow reproduisent eux aussi l'effet de la TSH sur la réexpression de l'antigène M/TPO dans les cellules thyroïdiennes. Par contre, ni le 12-O-tetradecanoyl-phorbol 13 acetate, l'EGF, ni l'estradiol ni le NaI n'ont réussi à induire les antigènes M/TPO. Les présents résultats montrent que:
1) L'expression des antigènes M/TPO dans les cellules thyroïdiennes dépend de la stimulation de la TSH par l'intermédiaire de la production de cAMP, la formation d'ARN messager, et la synthèse protéique.
2) Les anticorps thyro-stimulants reproduisent l'effet de la TSH.
3) Ni l'estradiol ni le NaI n'ont d'effet direct sur l'expression de l'antigène M/TPO.

Thyroglobulin, thyroid peroxidase and iodide carrier display different sensitivities to hormonal induction and to neoplastic transformation

R. Zarrilli[1], S. Formisano[1][2] and B. Di Jeso[1]

[1] *Dipartimento di Biologia e Patologia Cellulare e Molecolare and Centro di Endocrinologia ed Oncologia Sperimentale del CNR, II Facoltà di Medicina e Chirurgia, Napoli, Italy.* [2] *Istituto di Biologia, Facoltà di Medicina, Udine, Italy*

In this study we compared the expression of three molecules, characteristic of the thyroid differentiated state, in response to hormones and to neoplastic transformation by oncogenes.

The sensitivity of these molecules to hormones was studied on FRTL-5 cells, a continuous rat thyroid cell line, the sensitivity to neoplastic transformation in a close correlated cell line, the PC thyroid cells. Thyroglobulin (TG) and Thyroid Peroxidase (TPO) mRNA levels were evaluated by northern blot analysis and normalized on beta-actin mRNA levels; iodide (I^-) carrier expression was studied by measuring the I^- uptake (pmoles of I^- / μg of DNA).

TG and TPO mRNA levels are induced by TSH and by Insulin/IGF-I. The TSH concentrations effective on TPO ($10^{-10}/10^{-8}$ M) are also effective on TG and the same is true for Insulin/IGF-I (0.01-0.1 μg/ml IGF-I). Forskolin (5 μM) mimics TSH induction on both genes. Also, the time course of induction of TG and TPO by TSH and by Insulin/IGF-I (maximal effect at 30 hours) show a great similarity. However, the maximal levels of induction are different between TG and TPO genes. TG is equally sensitive to Insulin/IGF-I and to TSH (3-4 fold induction). TPO is more sensitive to TSH (5-6 fold induction) than to Insulin/IGF-I (2-3 fold increase only). I^- carrier is exclusively and to a great extent (15 fold) responsive to TSH, Insulin/IGF-I being without effect in a 10^3 fold concentration range.

When the PC thyroid cells are transfected with the human c-myc oncogene TG and TPO mRNA levels are not decreased, while the maximum velocity (V_{max}) of I^- uptake is decreased of 30%. The PC cells infected with the Polyoma Murine Leukemia virus, which carries the polyomavirus middle-T-antigen gene, show only a slight decrease of TG mRNA levels, a total extinction of the TPO gene and a 70% decrease in V_{max} of the I^- uptake. The PC cells transfected with both, c-myc and middle-T-antigen, display a complete extinction of TG, TPO and I^- carrier functions.

In conclusion, I^- carrier, TPO and TG display a differential sensitivity to TSH induction (I^- carrier > TPO > TG) and the same scalar sensitivity to oncogene transformation. This suggests that oncogene transformation could interfere with the TSH action on thyroid cells.

The thyroid peroxidase gene : accurate localisation by non-isotopic *in situ* hybridisation to chromosome 2p13

P.S. Barnett, B. Bhatt*, A. Pagliuca*, G. Mulfti*, A.M. McGregor and J.P. Banga

Departments of Medicine and Haematology*, King's College School of Medicine, Bessemer Road, London SE5 9PJ, UK

Although the gene for thyroid peroxidase (TPO) has been mapped to the short arm of chromosome 2 (2pter-p12) by somatic cell hybridisation, its precise localisation remains to be determined.

TPO plays a pivotal role in the biosynthesis of thyroid hormones from thyroglobulin and is also the target autoantigen in thyroid autoimmune disease. TPO shows a high degree of sequence homology to other related peroxidases such as myeloperoxidase and eosinophil peroxidase. Two alternatively spliced forms of TPO cDNA which are thought to be derived from the same gene transcript have been identified and fully sequenced.

A biotinylated 2Kb TPO cDNA probe (representing TP0-1) derived from a Graves' thyroid cDNA library was hybridised to metaphase chromosomes. The biotin label was detected by immunocytochemistry and the signals amplified by silver precipitation which results in a black silver dot at the gene locus.

We now demonstrate the accurate localisation of the TPO gene to chromosome 2p13 (see diagram below). The peak at 17q22-q23 represents cross hybridisation with the gene for myeloperoxidase which is known to map to this region. Interestingly, the smaller peak of silver dots observed at 2p23-p24 possibly represents cross hybridisation of the TPO cDNA probe to another related peroxidase.

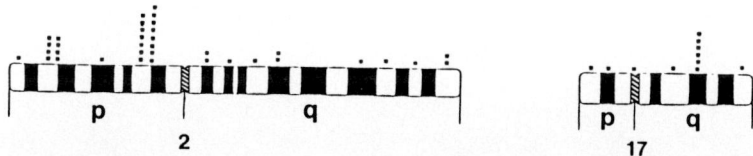

The idiogram above shows the sum of silver dots counted on chromosomes 2 and 17 from 50 metaphase spreads.

Structure and function

Structure et fonction

Immunochemical properties of hTPO

B. Czarnocka*, J. Ruf**, M. Ferrand** and P. Carayon**

* Department of Biochemistry, Medical Center of Postgraduate Education, Warsaw, Poland and ** Laboratoire de Biochimie Médicale, INSERM U.38, Faculté de Médecine, Marseille, France

INTRODUCTION

Human thyroid peroxidase is a glycosylated hemoprotein firmly bound to membranes of the thyroid cell, and involved in the biosynthesis of thyroid hormones. The enzyme catalyzes both the iodination and the coupling of tyrosines in thyroglobulin to yield T3 and T4 (DeGroot & Niepomniszcze, 1977 ; Nunez, 1980). The integral membrane protein nature of the TPO resulted in several difficulties in isolation and purification of the enzyme. For a while, the most successful procedure was limited proteolysis in combination with detergents (Alexander, 1979 ; Rawitch et al., 1979). Very recently, human TPO (hTPO) was purified in its native state by monoclonal antibody (mAb) assisted chromatography (Czarnocka et al., 1985a ; Ohtaki et al., 1986). hTPO has been shown to be the "microsomal antigen", a target antigen for circulating autoantibodies (aAb) present in serum of most of the patients with autoimmune thyroid diseases (Czarnocka et al., 1985a, 1985b, 1986, 1987 ; Ruf et al., 1987 ; Mariotti et al., 1987). Although the primary structure of the hTPO was determined (Libert et al., 1987 ; Kimura et al., 1987 ; Magnusson et al., 1987), there is still limited information on the higher order structure of hTPO and on the relationship between its biochemical and immunological properties. The availability of highly purified hTPO in native form and the production of mAb gave possibilities to examine the immunochemical properties of hTPO.

BIOCHEMICAL PROPERTIES OF hTPO

hTPO was purified from surgical specimens of thyroid glands by mAb assisted chromatography (Czarnocka et al., 1985a). The purification process (Table 1) yielded hTPO preparation of very high specific activity. The absorption spectra of highly purified enzyme exhibited a peak in the Soret region which shifted from 411 nm to 422 nm by reducing agents (Ruf et al., 1987). More complex analysis of absorption spectra of the hTPO were performed by Ohtaki et al. (1985, 1986) and provided information on the nature of prosthetic group, which is presumably protohem IX. The specific adsorption of hTPO to Concanavalin A and the reaction with Schiff's reagent indicate its glycoproteic nature. The enzymatic activity of hTPO is very sensitive to disulphide bridge reducing agents and completely abolished by as low as $5.10^{-5}M$ concentration of dithioeritritol. The molecular composition of the affinity purified hTPO analyzed by SDS-PAGE revealed two bands at 95 and 105 kDa in the presence of 5 % 2-mercaptoethanol Fig.1, left panel ; in non-reducing conditions the enzyme resolved in one large band migrating in the same region (Fig.1, right panel) . The RZ value has been used as an index of purity of the enzyme. The preparation of hTPO obtained by us (Czarnocka et al.,

Table 1 - Activity of thyroid peroxidase at various stages of purification.

Stage of purification	Total protein (mg)	Total units	Specific activity (U/mg)	Purification factor
Microsomes	791	915	1.1	1
Solubilisate	383	861	2.2	2
Affinity chromatography	1.6	610	381	331

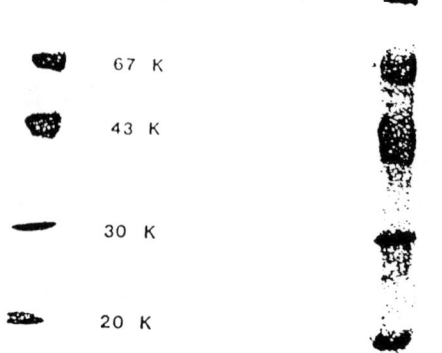

Fig.1 - Polyacrylamide gel electrophoresis of affinity purified hTPO in reducing (left panel) and non-reducing (right panel) conditions.

1985a), as well as preparation obtained by Ohtaki et al. (1986), characterized low RZ value (0.25-0.26), although their purities based on SDS-PAGE were greater than 90 %. The discrepancies beween A411 nm/A280 nm ratio and electrophoretic purity could be due to overestimation of the protein concentration (Ohtaki et al. 1986). Moreover, Kimura et al. (1987), showed two forms of hTPO cDNAs, encoding for polypeptides of 97 and 103 kDa, suggesting that two proteins might be generated through alternate splicing of the same gene. Independently carried out works of others groups revealed, that the microsomal antigen existed as a duplex of peptides migrating in the 100 kDa region on SDS-PAGE (DeGroot et al., 1987).

IMMUNOLOGICAL PROPERTIES OF hTPO

aAb reacting with highly purified hTPO were detected in serum of patients with autoimmune thyroid diseases (AIDT) containing anti-microsomal aAb, regardless of the presence or absence of anti-thyroglobulin aAb (Czarnocka et al., 1985a, 1985b, 1986 ; Ruf et al., 1987). Interaction between hTPO and anti-microsomal aAb was observed in several experimental conditions using individual, as well as pooled sera or purified IgG. Anti-microsomal aAb bound to hTPO (Fig.2) , inhibited anti-hTPO mAb binding to hTPO (Fig.3) and immunoprecipitated hTPO (Fig.4) . The identity of both anti-microsomal and anti-TPO aAb was shown by their co-purification on the hTPO-assisted chromatography (Czarnocka et al., 1987). This identity was also strongly supported by correlation analyzis of anti-hTPO and anti-microsomal aAb titers in a large series of patients with AITD (Mariotti et al., 1987). The presence of circulating anti-hTPO aAb in patients with AITD was also identified by others (Portman et al., 1985 ; Kotani et al., 1986).

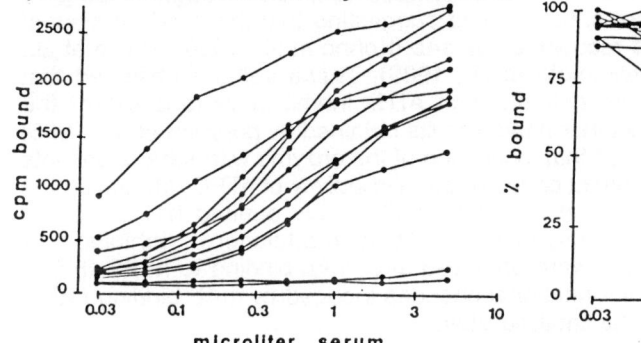
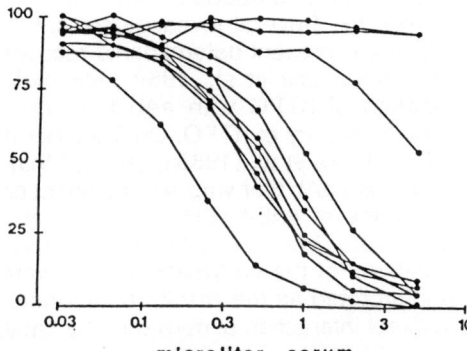

Fig.2 - Dose response curves of binding to coated hTPO of autoantibodies in sera from 2 normal subjects (2 lower curves) and 10 patients with autoimmune thyroid diseases.

Fig.3 - Dose response curves of inhibition of anti-TPO monoclonal Ab binding to coated hTPO by sera from 2 normal subjects (2 upper curves) and 10 patients with autoimmune thyroid diseases.

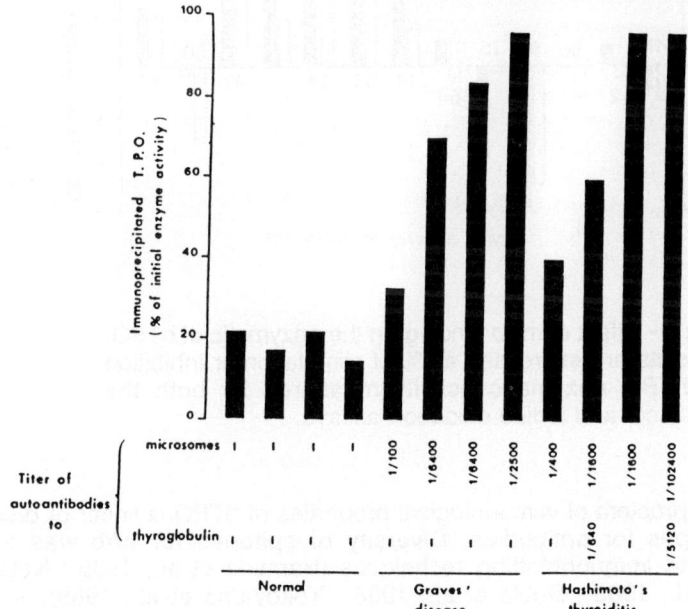

Fig.4 - Human thyroid peroxidase activity after precipitation by various sera from a patients with Hashimoto's and Graves' disease and normal sera. Each bar represents individual serum.

It is well accepted (Pommier et al., 1973 ; Nunez & Pommier, 1982), that TPO has two catalytic sites , one for tyrosyl residue in thyroglobulin or aromatic donor molecule such as guaiacol and the other for iodide. This raised the possibility that interaction between the hTPO and antibodies might affect the enzymatic function through binding to catalyticsites. Several investigators obtained data suggesting that the catalytic sites of hTPO would present determinants recognized by aAb (Kohno et al., 1986 ; Doble et al., 1988 ; Yokoyama et al., 1989 ; Okamoto et al., 1989). These authors observed that incubation of hTPO with aAb from patients with AITD inhibit in various extent the enzymatic activity of hTPO. On the other hand, results obtained by portman et al. (1985) and Czarnocka et al. (1985a) showed that incubation of the enzyme with sera of patients with different aAb titer was without effect on the enzymatic activity of hTPO; Moreover, the interference of anti-hTPO mAb (Ruf et al., 1989) with highly purified hTPO did not demonstrate the antigenicity of catalytic sites. Some modulation (inhibition or stimulation) of the enzymatic activity were observed after mAb binding to hTPO (Fig.5) and interpreted as the result of conformational changes induced by mAb binding rather than direct interaction of mAb with the catalytic sites.

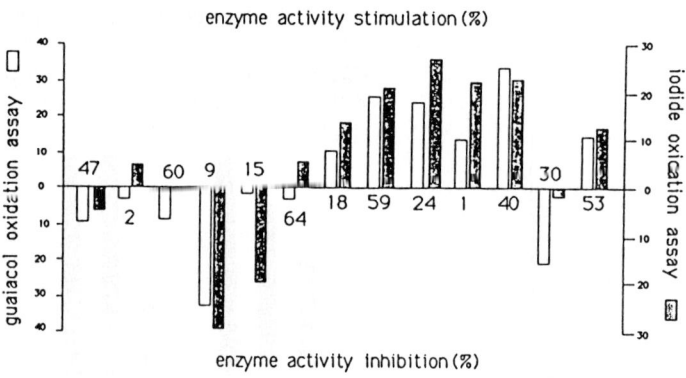

Fig.5 - Effect of mAb binding on the enzymatic of hTPO. Results are expressed as % of stimulation or inhibition of hTPO enzymatic activity measured by both the guaiacol and iodide oxidation assays.

Another important problem of immunological properties of hTPO is linear or discontinous structure of epitopes for antibodies. Diversity of epitopes for aAb was shown by electrophoresis and immunoblotting techniques (Hamada et al., 1985 ; Kotani et al., 1986 ; Kohno et al., 1986 ; Doble et al., 1988 ; Yokoyama et al., 1989). It was also demonstrated that electrophoresis under reducing conditions diminished dramatically the immunological reactivity of hTPO/microsomal antigen (Banga et al., 1984, 1985 ; Hamada et al., 1987 ; Kotani et al., 1986 ; Doble et al., 1988). The disulphide bridge reducing agents were also found to be strong inhibitors of the reaction between hTPO and aAb (Gardas et al., 1990) as well as mAb (Ruf et al., 1989). This inhibition was especially pronounced at alkaline pH. However, hTPO/microsomal antigen cross-linking with glutaraldehyde or formation of antigen-antibody complexes induce resistance to reducing agents (Gardas & Domek, 1989), thus pointing out, that disulphide bridges are not directly involved in antibody binding. Adverse evidence was brought by Yokoyama et al. (1989). These authors were able to show preserved immunoreactivity of hTPO autoantigenic properties after treatment with reducing agents. However, the aAb titer of the sera tested was higher than 1/100000 which could be an important point in interpretation of the observed results. The discrepancy concerning the effect of reduction on the hTPO/microsomal antigen could be first of all due to the conditions in which chemical alterations of the antigen are carried out . The binding activity remaining after reduction of the hTPO/microsomal antigen observed with mAb (Fig.6), as well as aAb could be explained by the interaction of antibodies with partially denatured epitopes or some sequential epitope(s) (Ruf et al., 1989 ; Gardas et al., 1990). Taking into account the diversity of data on autoantigenic epitopes and data for mAb epitopes, the importance of the three-dimensional structure of hTPO in the immunological activity should be stressed. Thus, the loss of this structure resulted in dramatically diminished binding of both aAb and mAb, implying the discontinuous structure of most of the hTPO epitopes. The remaining binding activity observed for few mAb and some aAb preparation may be accounted for by sequential epitope(s).

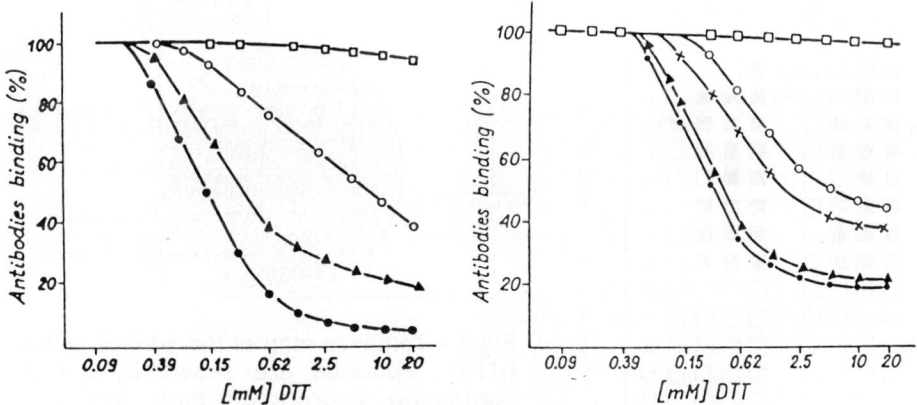

Fig.6 - Destruction of mAb and aAb epitopes of hTPO by dithioeritritol in solid - phase bound hTPO. Results are expressed % of antibody binding. □────□ mAb 47 ; ▲────▲ mAb 53 ; ●────● mAb 64 ; O────O polyclonal anti-hTPO Ab ; X────X pooled patients serum.

The cross-reactivity of anti-hTPO with human myeloperoxidase, bovine lactoperoxidase and horseradish peroxidase showed epitopes common to all enzymes tested, despite of their various origins (Ruf et al., 1989). Although, the tissue specific expression pattern and physiological roles of the tested enzymes are quite different, this finding suggested that common epitopes recognized by mAbs are phylogenetically conserved through evolution. The molecular biology techniques demonstrated striking homology between hTPO and human myeloperosidase, showing that they are related members of the same gene family, evolved from a common ancestral gene (Libert et al., 1987 ; Kimura & Ikeda-Sato, 1988 ; Kimura et al., 1989).

It has been proposed, that only a part of the hTPO molecule presents antigenic activity for aAb (Libert et al., 1987). Information on the distribution of epitopes on the surface of hTPO could extended our understanding of the enzymatic and antigenic function of the hTPO in AITD. It must be pointed out, however, that for this type of study the polyclonal nature of autoantibodies have some limits. Development of several mAb to hTPO give a chance to obtain more revelant results especially if large panel of mAb is used to map important part of hTPO. More recently, the criss-cross experiments revealed (Ruf et al., 1989) the existence of at least four antigenic domains on the hTPO molecule. Polyclonal aAb from patients with AITD reacted strongly with two domains Fig.7, identified by mAb, while binding with the two others was much weaker (Ruf et al., 1989). This suggest, that, only a part of the whole hTPO molecule is strongly involved in the autoimmun process.

Fig.7 - Schematic representation of the inhibition of mAb binding to coated hTPO by pools of human sera. A pool of normal human sera served as the blank control.
Inhibition level: ■ strong ▨ medium ☐ slight

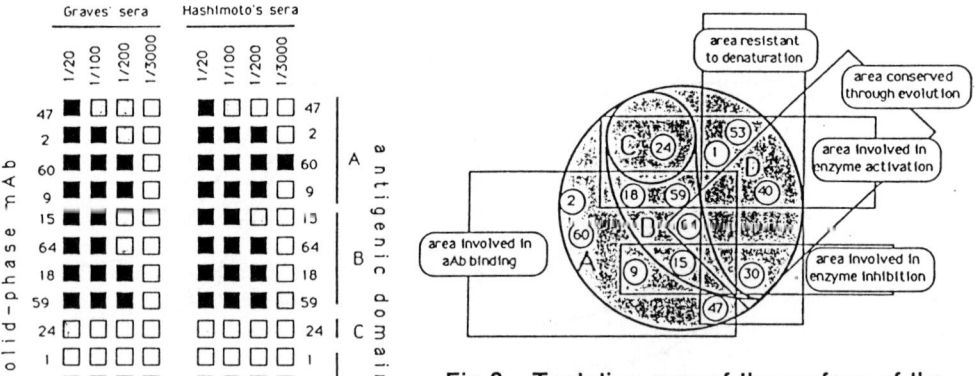

Fig.8 - Tentative map of the surface of the hTPO. Epitopes are shown by a disc containing appropriate mAb and are localized on the relevant antigenic domains. They also localize various areas according to biochemical properties.

CONCLUSION

The investigation performed during the past years extended our knowledge of the biochemical and immunological properties of hTPO. These properties may be summarized by a schema Fig.8, that we already proposed (Ruf et al., 1989). Although the nature of hTPO as the microsomal antigen is known since 1985, there are still several problems which remained to be clarified due to the complexity of both immune reaction between hTPO and antibodies and autoimmune processes. One of the most important factor awaiting to be solved is the interaction between hTPO and thyroglobulin and the common contribution of this two autoantigens to the autoimmune processes leading to autoimmune thyroid diseases.

REFERENCES

Alexander, N.M. (1977) : Purification of bovine thyroid peroxidase. Endocrinology 100, 1610-1620.

Banga, J.P., Pryce, G., Hammond, L. & Roitt, I.M. (1984) : Characterization of the human thyroid microsomal antigen involved in thyroid autoimmunity. Biochem. Soc. Trans. 12, 1118-1119.

Banga, J.P., Pryce, G., Hammond, L. & Roitt, I.M. (1985) : Structural features of the autoantigens involved in thyroid autoimmune disease : the thyroid microsomal/microvillar antigen. Mol. Immun. 22, 629-642.

Czarnocka, B., Ruf, J., Ferrand, M., Carayon, P. & Lissitzky, S. (1985a) : Purification of the human thyroid peroxidase and its identification as the microsomal antigen involved in autoimmune thyroid diseases. FEBS Lett. 190, 147-152.

Czarnocka, B. Ruf, J., Ferrand, M. & Carayon, P. (1985b) : Antigenic relationship between thyroid peroxidase and the microsomal antigen involved in thyroid autoimmune diseases... Acad. Sci. (D), (Paris) 300-577-580.

Czarnocka, B., Ruf, J., Ferrand, M., Lissitzky, S. & Carayon, P. (1986) : Interaction on of highly purified thyroid peroxidase with anti-microsomal antibodies in autoimmune thyroid diseases. J. Endocrinol. Invest. 9, 135-138.

Czarnocka, B., Ruf, J., Alquier, C., Toubert, M.E., Dutoit, C., Ferrand, M. & Carayon, P. (1987) : Further evidence that thyroid peroxidase and the "microsomal antigen" are the same entity. In Thyroid Autoimmunity, eds. A. Pinchera, S.H. Ingbar, J. McKenzie & G. F. Fenzi, pp. 285-288. New York and London : Plenum Press.

DeGroot, L.J., Portman, L. & Hamada, N. (1987) : Progress in understanding the thyroid microsomal antigen. In Thyroid Autoimmunity, eds. A. Pinchera, S.H. Ingbar, J. McKenzie & G.F. Fenzi, pp. 27-34. New York and London : Plenum Press.

Doble, N.D., Banga, J.P., Pope, R., Lalor, E., Kilduff, P. & McGregor, A.M. (1988) : Autoantibodies to the thyroid microsomal/thyroid peroxidase antigen are polyclonal and directed to several distinct antigenic sites. Immunology 64, 23-29.

Gardas, A. & Domek, H. (1988) : The effect of sulphydryl reagents on the human thyroid microsomal antigen. J. Endocrinol. Invest. 11, 335-388.

Gardas, A., Domek, H. & Czarnocka, B. (1990) : The effect of dithiotreitol on thyroid peroxidase and microsomal antigen epitopes recognized by auto and monoclonal antibodies. Autoimmunity (accepted for publication).

Hamada, N., Grimm, C., Mori, H. & DeGroot, L.J. (1985) : Identification of a thyroid microsomal antigen by Western blot and immunoprecipitation. J. Endocrinol. Metab. 61, 120-128.

Hamada, N., Portman, L. & DeGroot, L.J. (1987) : Characterization and isolation of thyroid microsomal antigen. J. Clin. Invest. 79, 819-825.

Kimura, S., Kotani, T., McBride, O.W., Umeki, K., Kirai, K., Nakayama, T. & Ohtaki, S. (1987) : Human thyroid peroxidase : Complete cDNA and protein sequence, chromosome mapping, and identification of two alternately spliced mRNAs. Proc. Natl. Acad. Sci. USA 84, 5555-5559.

Kimura, S. & Ikeda-Sato, M. (1988) : Human myeloperoxidase and thyroid peroxidase, two enzymes with separate and distinct physiological functions, are evolutionarily related members of the same gene family. Proteins : Struc., Funct., Genet. 3, 113-120.

Kimura, S., Hong, Y.-S., Kotani, T., Ohtaki, S. & Kikkawa, F. (1989) : Structure of the human thyroid peroxidase gene : comparison and relationship to the human myeloperoxidase gene. Biochemistry 28, 4481-4489.

Kohno, Y., Hiyama, Y., Shimojo, N., Niimi, H., Nakajima, H. & Hosoya, T. (1986) : Autoantibodies to thyroid peroxidase in patients with chronic thyroiditis : effect of antibody on enzyme activities. Clin. Exp. Immunol. 65, 534-541.

Kotani, T., Umeki, K.., Matsunaga, S., Kato, E. & Ohtaki, S. (1986) : Detection of autoantibodies to thyroid peroxidase in autoimmune thyroid disease by micro-ELISA and immunoblotting. J. Clin. Endocrinol. Metab. 61, 928-933.

Libert, F., Ruel, J., Ludgate, M., Swillens, S., Alexander, N., Vassart, G. & Dinsart, C. (1987) : Thyroperoxidase, an auto-antigen with a mosaic structure made of nuclear and mitochondrial gene modules. Embo J. 6, 4193-4196.

Magnusson, P., Chazenbalk, G.D., Gestautas, J., Seto, P., Filetti, P., DeGroot, J.L. & Rapoport, B. (1987) : Molecular cloning of the complementary deoxyribonucleic acid from human thyroid peroxidase. Mol. Endocrinol. 1, 856-861.

Mariotti, S., Anelli, S., Ruf, J., Bechi, K., Czarnocka, B., Lombardi, A., Carayon, P. & Pinchera, A. (1987) : Comparison of serum thyroid microsomal and thyroid peroxidase autoantibodies in thyroid diseases. J. Clin. Endocrinol. Metab. 65, 987-993.

Nunez, J., (1980) : Iodination and thyroid hormone synthesis. In The Thyroid Gland, ed. M. De Visscher, pp. 39-59. New York : Raven Press.

Nunez, J. & Pommier, J. (1982) : Formation of thyroid hormones. Vitam. Horm. 39, 175-229.

Ohtaki, S., Kotani, T. & Nakamura, Y. (1986) : Characterization of human thyroid peroxidase purified by monoclonal antibody-assisted chromatography. J. Clin. Endocrinol. Metab. 63, 570-576.

Okamoto, Y., Hamada, N., Saito, H., Ohno, M., Noh, J., Ito, K. & Mori, H. (1989) : Thyroid peroxidase activity-inhibiting immunoglobulins in patients with autoimmune thyriod disease. J. Clin. Endocrinol. Metab. 68, 730-734.

Pommier, J., Deme, & Nunez, J. (1973) : Effect of iodide concentration on thyroxine synthesis catalyzed by thyroid peroxidase. Eur. J. Biochem. 37, 406-414.

Portman,L., Hamada, N., Heinrich, G. & DeGroot, L.J. (1985) : Anti-thyroid peroxidase antibody in patients with autoimmune thyroid disease : possible identity with anti-microsomal antibody. J. Clin. Endocrinol. Metab. 61, 1001-1003.

Rawitchn, A.B., Taurog, A., Chernoff, S.B. & Dorris, M.L. (1979) : Hog thyroid peroxidase ; physical, chemical, and catalytical properties of the highly purified enzyme. Arch. Biochem. Biophys. 194- 244-257.

Ruf, J., Czarnocka, B. De Micco, C., Ferrand, M. & Carayon, P. (1987) : Thyroid peroxidase is the organ-specific "microsomal" autoantigen involved in thyroid autoimmunity. Acta Endocrinol. Suppl. 281 (Copenh) 115,49-56.

Ruf, J., Toubert, M.E., Czarnocka, B., Durand-Gorde, J.M., Ferrand, M. & Carayon, P. (1989) : Relationship between immunological structure and biochemical properties of human thyroid peroxidase. Endocrinology. 125, 1211-1218.

Yokoyama, N., Taurog, A. & Klee, G. (1989) : Thyroid peroxidase and thyriod microsomal autoantibodies. J. Clin. Endocrinol. Metab. 68, 766-773.

Résumé

La peroxydase thyroïdienne humaine (hTPO) est une hémoprotéine glycosylée fermement attachée aux membranes des cellules thyroïdiennes. Cette enzyme est impliquée dans la formation des hormones thyroïdiennes (T3, T4).

Récemment, la hTPO a pu être immuno-purifiée sous sa forme native à partir de microsomes, grâce à l'utilisation d'un anticorps monoclonal (mAb). La hTPO pure possède une activité enzymatique spécifique 330 fois plus importante que celle détectée dans les microsomes. Cette activité peut être neutralisée par l'emploi d'agents réducteurs. La hTPO absorbe dans la région de Soret, se fixe à la Concanavaline A et réagit positivement au réactif de Schiff. Son poids moléculaire apparent est de 100 KDa.

L'étude de la réactivité immunologique de la hTPO vis à vis d'autoanticorps (aAc) sériques provenant de patients atteints de maladies thyroïdiennes auto-immunes a permis d'identifier cette enzyme à l'antigène microsomal, un auto-antigène majeur de la thyroïde.

L'immuno-structure de la hTPO a pu être abordée grâce à la production d'une batterie de mAb. Ces mAb reconnaissent divers sites antigéniques de la hTPO ; certains d'entre-eux reconnaissent aussi des sites présents sur d'autres peroxydases. La hTPO possède au moins 4 régions antigéniques parmi lesquelles 2 sont reconnues par les aAc. Ces diverses régions antigéniques contiennent des épitopes pouvant être de nature séquentielle ou conformationnelle. Les aAc semblent être dirigés en majorité contre des sites conformationnels impliquant l'intégrité des ponts disulfures de la hTPO. Les mAb et les aAb interfèrent peu ou pas du tout dans l'activité enzymatique de la hTPO.

L'ensemble de ces données a permis d'aborder l'étude de la structure biochimique et immunologique de la hTPO. Le rôle de la hTPO et des aAc qui lui sont spécifiques dans l'auto-immunité thyroïdienne reste cependant à clarifier.

The location and nature of the N-linked oligosaccharide units in porcine thyroid peroxidase : studies on the tryptic glycopeptides

A.B. Rawitch, G. Pollock, S.X. Yang and A. Taurog*

*Department of Biochemistry and Molecular Biology, University of Kansas Medical Center, Kansas City, KS 66103 and * Department of Pharmacology, University of Texas Southwestern Medical Center, Dallas, TX 75235, USA*

Thyroid Peroxidase (TPO) is a heme-containing glycoprotein associated with the apical membrane of the secretory epithelial cells surrounding the thyroid follicles. This enzyme has been shown to be responsible for the catalysis of both the iodination of tyrosine residues within thyroglobulin and the subsequent coupling of selected iodotyrosines to form thyroxine and triiodothyronine (Taurog, 1986). Thus TPO is essential for the biosynthesis of thyroid hormones. In addition, TPO has recently been shown to be the principal component of the microsomal antigen that elicits the production of the serum microsomal autoantibodies associated with autoimmune thyroid disease (Czarnoka et.al., 1985, Portmann et.al., 1985 and Kotani et.al., 1986).

The predicted amino acid sequences of porcine (Magnusson et.al., 1987) and human (Kimura et.al., 1987) thyroid peroxidase have been recently determined from cloned cDNA. In the case of the porcine enzyme (Magnusson et.al,1987) the predicted amino acid sequence contains 926 amino acid residues with a molecular weight of 100,400 and five putative N-linked glycosylation sites. The location and nature of the N-oligosaccharides in porcine TPO can not, however, be established from such data.

In an earlier report (Rawitch et.al., 1979), the basic chemical and physical properties of a highly purified trypsin/detergent solubilized TPO preparation were described. This highly stable preparation retained virtually all of the enzymatic activity associated with the native or unmodified TPO, but contained two polypeptide fractions cross-linked by disulfide bonds and appeared to be derived from a larger precursor through tryptic cleavage. Composition analysis of the TPO indicated close to 10% carbohydrate with multiple residues of mannose, glucosamine and glucose, two residues of galactose and single residues of fucose and xylose.

The data reported here address the question of the location of the glycosylation sites within the primary sequence of TPO as well as the nature of the oligosaccharides at each location.

MATERIALS AND METHODS

TPO preparation - Highly purified, trypsin/detergent solubilized

TPO preparation TPO XII was prepared as previously described (Rawitch et.al., 1979) with only minor modifications. The trypsin concentration used in this purification was increased to 280 mg/liter. In addition, 1% Triton X-100 was present during the extraction along with deoxycholate and the pH of the extract was adjusted to pH 8.0 and the salt concentration to 0.15 M in KCl. This preparation had a 410 nm / 280 nm ratio of 0.433 and a specific enzymatic activity in iodide oxidation, guaiacol oxidation, iodination and coupling assays comparable to preparations previously reported (Rawitch et.al., 1979). Protein concentrations were determined by the method of Lowry (Lowry et.al., 1951)

Reduction and Alkylation and Tryptic Digestion - Approximately 10 mg of TPO XII was dialyzed extensively against 0.1% ammonium bicarbonate in 3500 MW cutoff small diameter dialysis tubing and then lyophilized. The resulting material was dissolved in a Tris.HCl buffer containing 8M urea and reduced and alkylated as previously described (Gregg et.al., 1988). Following the reduction and alkylation, the material was re-dialyzed against 0.1% ammonium bicarbonate for 48 hours and then against 1.0% ammonium bicarbonate for an additional 24 hours. The dialyzed protein was digested with TPCK treated-trypsin at 37 degrees for 4 hours. Equal amounts (0.22 mg) of trypsin were added initially and after two hours of digestion. The digestion was terminated by freezing and the digest lyophilized for 72 hours to remove the volatile buffer. The lyophilized digest was then stored at -20 degrees until the HPLC fractionation.

HPLC Fractionation - A three mg sample of the tryptic digest was applied to a Vydac semi-preparative C18 reversed phase HPLC column (1 x 25 cm) in 0.05M ammonium acetate, pH 6.0. Gradient elution carried out using a linear acetonitrile gradient from 0 to 50% over 100 minutes at a flow rate of 5 ml/min. One minute (5 ml) fractions were collected and stored at 4 degrees. The total tryptic digest was fractionated in three chromatographic runs. Twenty percent of the volume of each fraction was concentrated to dryness in a vacuum evaporation apparatus and assayed for neutral sugar content. The corresponding regions containing significant neutral sugar were pooled from the three runs, concentrated and further fractionated in a second HPLC system using the same column but equilibrated with 0.1% trifluoroacetic acid. In this case, the flow rate was adjusted to 4 ml/min and shallow, linear gradients of acetonitrile changing at a rate of 1% per 4 minutes were employed to further purify neutral sugar containing peptides. Each peak in the re-chromatography was collected by hand, concentrated and subjected to amino acid analysis and those with glucosamine were further subjected to neutral sugar analysis and gas- phase peptide sequencing.

Carbohydrate Analysis - Aliquots of fractions from HPLC runs were screened for neutral sugar using the orcinol-sulfuric acid procedure (Rawitch et.al., 1968). Fractions were compared to a standard curve using mannose as a reference. Specific sugar compositions were established on samples of TPO or isolated glycopeptide fractions following hydrolysis in 2 M trifluoroacetic acid (TFA) at 100 degrees for 6 hours. The hydrolysates were taken to dryness in a vacuum concentrator and the samples then dissolved in water and applied to a Dionex CarboPac PA1 strong anion ion exchange column equilibrated with 15 mM NaOH. The chromatography was carried out isocratically at a flow rate of 1 ml per minute and sugars were detected using a Dionex PAD (pulsed amperometric detector) (Hardy et.al., 1988). An internal standard of 2-deoxyglucose was employed to correct for handling losses and detector response variability. In some cases, samples were also hydrolyzed in 6 N HCl at 100 degrees for 4 hours to increase the recovery of glucosamine.

Amino Acid Analysis and Peptide Sequencing - Samples for amino acid analysis were dissolved in 200 microliters of 3X distilled constant boiling HCl with addition of a crystal of solid phenol. The samples were sealed in evacuated tubes and hydrolyzed 20 h at 105 degrees. The hydrolyzed samples were then brought to dryness in an evacuated desiccator over NaOH pellets. The dry hydrolyzed samples were reconstituted in 0.2 N sodium citrate buffer, pH 2.2, and analyzed using a Beckman 121MB amino acid analyzer. The amino acid analyzer was equipped with an automatic sample injector and a 2.8mm x 190mm column containing Beckman AA-10 cation exchange resin. Elution was performed in a three step gradient using buffers obtained from Beckman Instruments. Calculation of data was performed by a Beckman Model 126 Data System to determine amino acid concentrations of each sample injected. Data was further manually reduced to obtain total protein content, percentage of each amino acid present and residues of each amino acid per molecule.

Amino terminal sequences were determined on 2 nmole samples of intact peptides, using a gas phase instrument (Applied Biosystems Model 470A) and the ABS 03CPTH program. Liberated PTH-amino acids were identified by HPLC on a Waters instrument. Solvent A was 4.5 mM sodium acetate, pH 4.32, in a mixture of 5 parts buffer to 1 part acetonitrile. Solvent B was 60% isopropanol in water. Elution consisted of 100% A for 1 min. A gradient over 4.25 min, ending at 65% A, 35% B was applied followed by isocratic elution continued for 3.5 min. A second linear gradient to 50% A, 50% B in 30 s was then applied and isocratic elution then maintained for 2 min. The system was then re-equilibrated with 100% A. The repetitive yield for the sequenator was periodically checked and averaged near 93%. The placement of each glycopeptide within the linear structure of porcine TPO was based on both amino terminal sequence and amino acid composition data and was facilitated by reference to the known cDNA structure for the protein (Magnusson et.al., 1987)

RESULTS

Carbohydrate Analysis of Intact TPO - The neutral and amino sugar contents of the trypsin solubilized TPO are shown in Table I. The data are compared with those obtained in an earlier study (Rawitch et.al., 1979) of TPO preparation VII by gas-liquid chromatography of alditol acetate derivatives.

TABLE I

Sugar Residue	Residues/Mole GLC-alditol acetate [a]	Residues/Mole Ion Exchange
Fucose	1	1.7
Xylose	1	-
Mannose	27	28.3
Galactose	2	0.6
Glucose	8	1.7
N-acetyl glucosamine	12	14.3

[a] (Rawitch et.al., 1979)

HPLC Separation of Tryptic Peptides and Glycopeptides - The primary HPLC separation of a tryptic digest of porcine TPO in the 0.05 M ammonium acetate / acetonitrile system at pH 6.0 is shown in Figure 1.

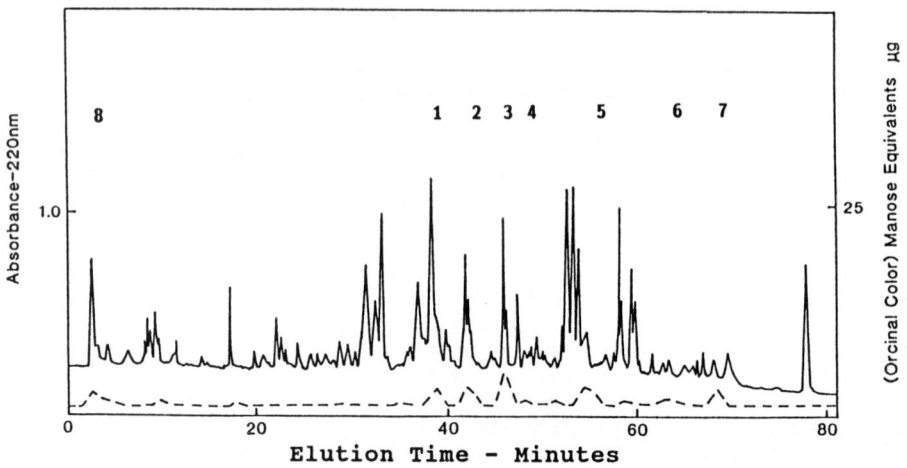

Figure 1 - HPLC of a tryptic digest of reduced and alkylated TPO. The numbers above the profile designate the carbohydrate positive fractions C18-1 through C18-8 which were pooled for further chromatography and glycopeptide purification.

TABLE II

HPLC Fraction No.	Glycosylated Asparagine Residue Position	Oligosaccharide Composition
C18-1	342	$Man_{7.1}NAG_{2.6}$
C18-2	*342	$Man_{7.3}NAG_{2.5}$
C18-3	*307	$Man_{4.0}NAG_{1.7}$
C18-4	---	---------
C18-5	*277	$Man_{5.4}NAG_{2.0}$
C18-6	---	---------
C18-7	*129	$Man_{7.3}NAG_{2.5}$
C18-8	---	---------

Abbreviations: Man - mannose, NAG - N-acetylglucosamine, Glu - glucose, Gal - galactose, Fuc - fucose. The asterisk indicates that two forms of the glycopeptide with the same glycosylated sequence were isolated from the same initial HPLC fraction in subsequent chromatography. Dashed line indicates no pure glycopeptide was obtained from the fraction.

Fractions (5 ml) were collected from the semi-preparative HPLC runs and an aliquot was taken from each fraction for neutral sugar analysis. The elution profile contained a total of approximately 60 peaks and 8 areas which contained neutral sugar as measured in a micro-orcinol assay. Each of the carbohydrate containing regions was pooled, taken to dryness by lyophilization, and re-chromatographed in a complementary HPLC solvent system (0.1% TFA in water) to obtain chromatographically homogeneous peaks. Each of the purified glycopeptide fractions was then subjected to amino acid analysis, peptide sequencing and sugar analysis. The results are summarized in Table II along with the placement of the glycosylated asparagine residue within the predicted amino acid sequence of porcine TPO (Magnusson et.al., 1987).

DISCUSSION

In an earlier report (Rawitch et.al., 1979), the basic chemical and physical properties of trypsin / detergent solubilized porcine thyroid peroxidase were described and the glycoprotein nature of the enzyme noted. With the cloning and sequencing of a complete cDNA, the predicted amino acid sequence of the unmodified enzyme became available (Magnusson et.al., 1987) and the relationship of the trypsin / detergent solubilized active derivative to the intact or native enzyme could be defined (Yokoyama and Taurog, 1988). The predicted cDNA sequence contains a total of five putative sites for N-linked glycosylation. Since it is impossible to tell from the cDNA data alone, which of these putative sites for N-linked glycosylation is actually modified with carbohydrate, the current study was initiated in order to define which of the five putative sites in TPO actually carries an oligosaccharide.

HPLC of a tryptic digest of reduced and alkylated TPO yielded a pattern containing approximately 60 peaks and 5 major and 3 minor peaks or areas of neutral sugar. Each of the areas containing carbohydrate was pooled and subjected to additional HPLC chromatography in order to obtain homogeneous peaks. While a total of 9 carbohydrate containing peptides were obtained, only four discrete glycosylated sites were defined, with multiple forms of each glycosylated peptide being detected. It is assumed that the multiple forms of the same glycosylated sequence which were observed in this study were due to a combination of oligosaccharide micro-heterogeneity and at least in one case (the tryptic peptides related to residue 342) alternate tryptic cleavage. These findings are summarized in Figure 2 below.

While four of the five putative sites for N-linked glycosylation were confirmed as glycosylated, a single putative site at residue 265 was not found in a glycosylated form. While the intact TPO showed a carbohydrate composition which contained mannose and N-acetyl glucosamine as the predominant sugars, small amounts of fucose and galactose were also observed along with several residues of glucose. Analysis of the carbohydrate composition of each of the confirmed glycopeptides, however, indicated compositions consistent with only "high mannose" type oligosaccharides (mannose and glucosamine only). The small amounts of galactose, fucose and glucose observed in the starting TPO preparations may be attributed to either a minor carbohydrate containing contaminant in the initial TPO samples or to an alternate glycosylation variant not detected in these experiments. It should be noted that all of the putative sites and confirmed glycosylation sites in porcine TPO are located in the N-terminal third of the predicted TPO sequence between residues 129 and 342 in what is believed to be the extracellular domain of TPO.

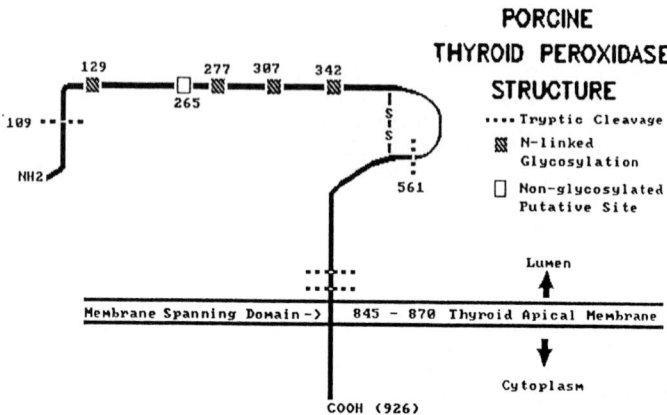

Figure 2. - A model of thyroid peroxidase showing the pattern of glycosylation and the proposed tryptic cleavages occurring during trypsin/detergent solubilization (Yokoyama and Taurog, 1988)

REFERENCES

Czarnocka B. , Ruf, J., Fernand, M. Carayon, P. and Lissitzky, S. (1985) Purification of the human thyroid peroxidase and its identification as the microsomal antigen involved in autoimmune thyroid. *FEBS Lett.* 190, 147-52.

Gregg, J. Dziadik-Turner, C., Rouse, J, Hamilton, J. and Rawitch, A. (1988) A comparison of 30-kDa and 10-kDa hormone-containing fragments of bovine thyroglobulin. *J. Biol. Chem.* 263, 5190-96.

Hardy, M., Townsend, R. and Lee, Y.C. (1988) Monosaccharide analysis of glycoconjugates by anion exchange chromatography with pulsed amperometric detection. *Anal. Biochem.* 170, 54-62.

Kimura, S., Kotani, T., McBride, O., Umeki, K., Hirai, K., Nakayama, T. and Ohtaki, S. (1987) Human thyroid peroxidase: complete cDNA and protein sequence, chromosome mapping, and identification of two alternatively spliced mRNAs. *Proc. Natl. Acad. Sci. USA* 84, 5555-59.

Kotani, T., Umeki, K., Matsunaga, S., Kato, E. and Ohtaki, S. (1986) Detection of autoantibodies to thyroid peroxidase in autoimmune thyroid disease by micro-ELISA and immunoblotting. *J. Clin. Endo. Metab.* 61, 928-33.

Lowry, O., Rosebrough, N., Farr, A. and Randall, R. (1951) A sensitive method for the measurement of protein concentrations. *J. Biol. Chem.* 193,265-75.

Magnusson, R., Gestautas, J., Taurog, A. and Rappaport, B. (1987) Molecular cloning of the structural gene for porcine thyroid peroxidase. *J. Biol. Chem.* 262, 13885-88.

Portmann, L., Hamada, N., Heinrich, G. and DeGroot, L. (1985) Anti-thyroid peroxidase antibody in patients with autoimmune disease: Possible identity with antimicrosomal antibody. J.Clin. Endo. and Metab. 61, 1001-3.

Rawitch, A., Liao, T. and Pierce, J. (1968) The amino acid sequence of a tryptic glycopeptide from human thyroglobulin. *Biochimica et Biophysica Acta* 160, 360-67.

Rawitch, A., Taurog, A., Chernoff, S. and Dorris, M. (1979) Hog thyroid peroxidase: physical, chemical and catalytic properties of the highly purified enzyme. *Arch. Biochem. Biophys.* 194, 244-57.

Taurog, A. (1986) Hormone synthesis: Thyroid Iodine Metabolism. in *Werner's The Thyroid,* eds.S.H. Ingbar and L.E. Braverman, pp. 53-97. Philadelphia: J.B. Lippincott.

Yokoyama, N. and Taurog, A. (1988) Porcine thyroid peroxidase: relationship between the native enzyme and an active, highly purified tryptic fragment. *Molecular Endocrinology* 2, 838-44.

Résumé

Des séquences amino-acides de thyropéroxydase humaine et porcine ont été récemment déterminées à partir de clones d'ADN complémentaire. Dans le cas de l'enzyme porcin, la séquence aminoacide contient 926 acides aminés et présente un poids moléculaire de 100.400, et 5 sites possibles de glycosylation. La localisation et la nature des N-glycanes de la thyropéroxydase porcine, ne peut cependant être extrapolée à partir de tels résultats. Dans un précédent article (Rawitch et.al.Biochim. Biophys. Acta 160, 360-67 (1979)), nous avons décrit les propriétés chimiques et physiques d'une préparation hautement purifiée de TPO préparée par solubilisation et action de la trypsine. La TPO contenait 2 fractions polypeptiques reliées par un pont disulfure et apparaissait dériver d'un précurseur de taille plus importante par clivage tryptique. L'analyse de la composition de la TPO indiquait qu'elle contenait près de 10% d'oligosaccharides avec de multiples résidus de mannose et de glucosamine, plusieurs résidus de glucose, 2 résidus de galactose et un seul résidu de fucose et de xylose. La présente étude visait à définir lequel des 5 sites possibles de la TPO portait un résidu N-glycanique. La séparation par HPLC d'une TPO réduite et alkylée, et traitée par la trypsine fournissait un profil montrant approximativement 60 pics dont 5 pics majeurs et 3 mineurs contenant des sucres neutres. Chacun des pics des oligosaccharides a été soumis à une chromatographie par HPLC, afin d'obtenir des pics homogènes. Alors que 9 peptides contenant des oligosaccharides ont été obtenus, 4 sites de glycosylation seulement ont été définis, avec chaque fois des peptides glycosylés de forme différente. Il a été supposé que les séquences amino-acides glycosylées présentaient des formes variées d'oligosaccharides dues en général à une micro-hétérogénéité des résidus oligosaccharidiques, et au moins dans un cas (le peptide obtenu par trypsilisation à proximité du résidu 342), à un clivage tryptique alternatif. 4 des 45 sites possibles de N-glycosylation se sont avérés effectivement glycosylés. Un seul site possible, situé au résidu 265 ne se présentait pas sous une forme glycosylée. Et si la TPO intacte présentait une composition oligosaccharidique contenant du mannose et de la N-acétyl glucosamine comme sucres prédominants, on pouvait également observer de petites quantités de fucose et de galactose mêlés à plusieurs résidus de glucose. L'analyse de la composition en sucres de chacun des glycopeptides montrait des compositions conformes au type "riche en mannose" (mannose et glucosamine exclusivement). La proportion de mannose et de glucosamine variait fortement selon les différents types de glycopeptides isolés. Les petites quantités de galactose, fucose, et glucose observées au début des préparations de TPO peuvent être dues soit à un contaminant faiblement glycosylé, présent dans la préparation initiale, soit à une glycosylation présentant une forme différente, et non détectée dans ces expériences.

Thyroperoxidase selects either one- or two-electron oxidations of iodotyrosine and thyroglobulin, depending on their iodine contents

M. Nakamura, I. Yamazaki* and S. Ohtaki **

*Biophysics Division, Research Institute of Applied Electricity, Hokkaido University, Sapporo 060 and ** Central Laboratory of Clinical Investigation, Medical College Hospital, Miyazaki Medical College, Kiyotake, Miyazaki 889-16, Japan, * Present address : Dept. of Chemistry and Biochemistry, Utah State University, Logan, UT 84322-0300, USA*

Introduction

Thyroperoxidase catalyzes iodination of tyrosine and oxidative coupling of two diiodotyrosine residues in thyroglobulin to form thyroxine(Taurog, 1986). It has been confirmed that the primary reaction catalyzed by the enzyme is iodination of tyrosine. Since the iodination itself takes place in two steps from tyrosine to diiodotyrosine via monoiodotyrosine, the iodine distribution in thyroglobulin has been analyzed at different stages of its enzymatic iodination. We have recently found that a curious fact that thyroperoxidase catalyzes one-electron oxidation of diiodotyrosine and two-electron oxidation of monoiodotyrosine and tyrosine(Ohtaki et al., 1982; Nakamura et al., 1985). Much attention has been paid to the regulation of thyroid hormone synthesis by thyroperoxidase. Since most of the kinetic experiments have been carried out on the reaction of thyroperoxidase with free tyrosine and iodotyrosines, question will arise as to whether the same mechanism can be applied to thyroxine synthesis in thyroglobulin. In this paper we will report results of the reaction of thyroperoxidase with thyroglobulin from patients with Graves' disease and its more iodinated one in comparison with reactions of free tyrosine and diiodotyrosine.

Materials and Methods

Thyroperoxidase used in this experiments was purified from hog thyroid microsomes by immunoaffinity chromatography(Nakagawa et al., 1985).

Spectrophotometric measurements were performed using a Union Giken Rapid Reaction Analyzer RA 1300 for rapid reactions. ESR spectra were recorded on a Varian E 109B spectrometer equipped with a stopped flow apparatus. The reactions were carried out in 0.1 M potassium phosphate (pH 7.4), at $20^{\circ}C$.

Results

In general, peroxidase reactions are formulated as follows.

$$\text{peroxidase} + H_2O_2 \xrightarrow{k_1} \text{Compound I (EO)} \quad (1)$$

$$\text{Compound I} + AH_2 \xrightarrow{k_2} \text{Compound II (EOH)} + AH^{\cdot} \quad (2)$$

$$\text{Compound II} + AH_2 \xrightarrow{k_3} \text{peroxidase} + AH^{\cdot} \quad (3)$$

In most cases, the catalytic intermediate observed in the steady state is Compound II, since Reaction 1 is fast and $K_2 > 10\ k_3$ (Chance, 1952). When the electron donor is a phenolic compound, it is believed to be oxidized by way of one-electron transfer. If peroxidase is present as Compound II in the steady state of the reaction, Reaction 3 is rate-limiting, and the oxidation of AH_2 occurs by way of one-electron transfer(Yamazaki, 1971). This conclusion can be derived from the analysis of stopped flow traces at two wavelengths isosbestic between any pair of the three enzyme forms involved in the catalytic cycle. Figure 1 shows the spectral changes of thyroperoxidase after reaction with H_2O_2. The formation of the primary intermediate (Compound I) was followed by its spontaneous conversion to the secondary intermediate that was identified to be Compound II. The spectra exhibited that 430 nm was an isosbestic wavelength between ferric and Compound I, and 420 nm was between ferric and Compound II. Kinetic results on the oxidations of L- and D-tyrosines, monoiodotyrosine and diiodotyrosine, in the presence of horseradish peroxidase and lactoperoxidase led us to conclude that these reactions occurred by way of one-electron transfer. The reaction catalyzed by thyroperoxidase was not simple. The kinetic traces obtained in the oxidation of L-and D-tyrosine, monoiodotyrosine, and diiodotyrosine were grouped into two categories. There was no essential difference among the three peroxidases in the mechanism of diiodotyrosine oxidation(Ohtaki et al., 1982; Nakamura et al., 1985). The enzyme intermediate of thyroperoxidase observed in the steady state of diiodotyrosine oxidation was compound II, and the rate constant for Reaction 3 was calculated from the stopped flow trace to be $6.5 \times 10^4\ M^{-1}S^{-1}$ according to Chance's equation(Chance, 1952). In contrast, the intermediate of thyroperoxidase appearing in the steady state of oxidations of L-tyrosine, and monoiodotyrosine was Compound I instead(Fig.2).

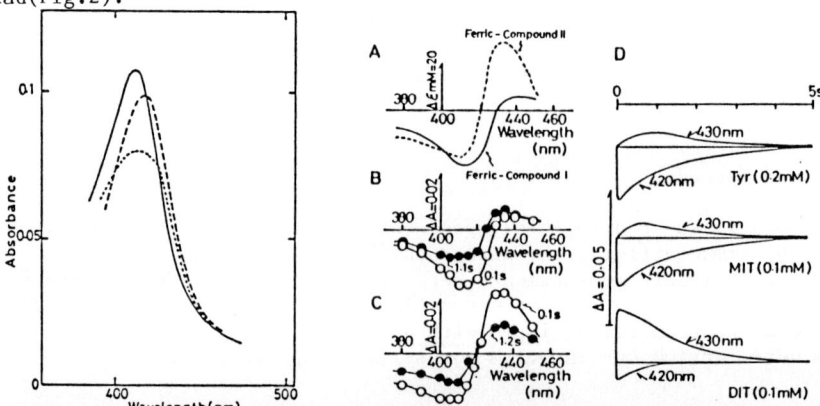

Fig.1(left) Spectral changes of thyroperoxidase after reaction with hydrogen peroxide. The reaction was carried out at pH 7.4 in the presence of 0.9 μM thyroperoxidase and 11 μM H_2O_2. Compounds I (dotted line) and II (broken line) were obtained at 60 ms and 8 s after the reaction was started.

Fig.2(right) Difference spectra of thyroperoxidase observed during the oxidation of tyrosine and diiodotyrosine. The difference spectra were plotted from stopped flow traces at varying wavelengths. Reaction mixtures contained 0.95 μM enzyme, 8 μM H_2O_2 and an electron donor. A, typical difference spectra for the formation of Compounds I and II from the ferric enzyme: B and C, difference spectra observed during the oxidations of 0.2 mM tyrosine (B) and 0.1 mM diiodotyrosine (C). The reaction time is indicated. D, stopped flow traces at two wavelengths for 0.2 mM tyrosine, 0.1 mM monoiodotyrosine (MIT), and 0.1 mM diiodotyrosine (DIT).

The rate constant for Reaction 3 could be measured directly from the reaction of Compound II with electron donors(Ohtaki et al., 1982). The observed first order rate constant was proportional to the concentration of added donors, and the second order rate constants thus calculated are listed in Table I. Here, Reaction 2' is formulated as follows.

$$\text{Compound I} + AH_2 \xrightarrow{k_2'} \text{peroxidase} + A \qquad (2')$$

In order to conclude that the mechanism is a two-electron oxidation, it is necessary to confirm not only that the enzyme intermediate is Compound I, but also that Reaction 3 is slower than Reaction 2(or 2'). In case of tyrosine and monoiodotyrosine, Reaction 2' is much faster than Reaction 3(Ohtaki et al., 1982). Since horseradish and milk peroxidases both catalyze one-electron oxidation of all phenols, it might be said that the catalytic property of thyroperoxidase is peculiar. We tentatively assume that the substitution at 2- and 6-positions of phenol with bulky or heavy atoms and groups changes the oxidation mechanism from a two-electron to a one-electron type (Nakamura et al., 1985). Questions will arise as to whether the same mechanism can be applied to oxidation mechanism of thyroglobulins, having different iodine contents. The enzyme intermediate in the steady state of oxidation of 0.2 % iodine thyroglobulin was Compound I, whereas Compound II appeared in the oxidation of 0.7% iodine thyroglobulin (Fig.3). Figure 3 also shows kinetic traces of these intermediates. The results suggest that the enzyme catalyzed two-electron oxidation of 0.2% iodine thyroglobulin and one-electron oxidation of 0.7% iodine thyroglobulin. The kinetic confirmation that thyroperoxidase caused the two-electron oxidation of 0.2% iodine thyroglobulin was made by comparison between rate constants for reactions of the thyroglobulin with Compounds I and II of the enzyme(Fig.4). The rate constants thus obtained are also listed in Table I.

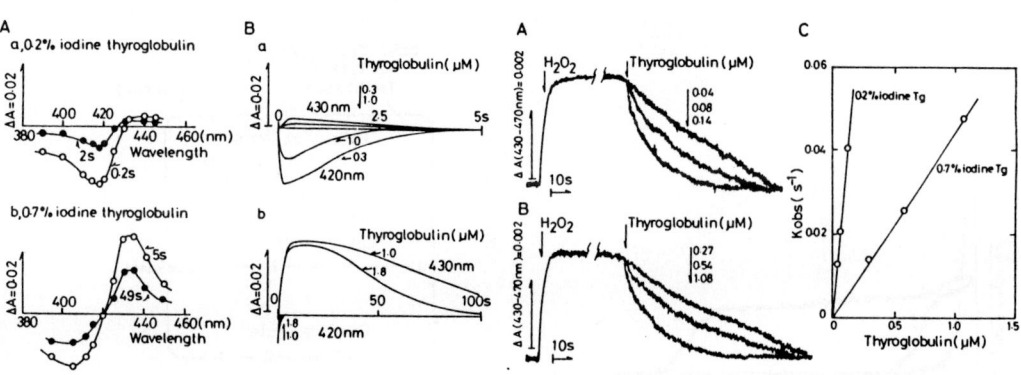

Fig.3(left) Difference spectra of thyroperoxidase observed during the oxidation of 0.2 and 0.7 % iodine thyroglobulins. Reaction mixtures contained 1.0 μM enzyme, 8 μM H_2O_2, and 0.3 μM 0.2% (a) or 1.8 μM 0.7% (b) iodine thyroglobulin. A, difference spectra : B, stopped flow traces.

Fig.4(right) Direct observation of the reaction of Compound II with 0.2% (A) and 0.7%(B) iodine thyroglobulins. Thyroglobulin (Tg) was added 1.0 min after 1.5 μM H_2O_2 was added to 0.1 μM thyroperoxidase. The observed first order rate constants are plotted against the concentration of thyroglobulin (c).

Table I.

Rate constants ($M^{-1}s^{-1}$) and peroxidase intermediates in the rate-determining step. The intermediate was either Compound I or II, which is denoted in parentheses. The rate constant for A was obtained from stopped flow kinetics. The value for B were obtained from reactions of thyroperoxidase Compound II with electron donors.

	Lactoperoxidase A	Thyroid peroxidase A	B
		$M^{-1}s^{-1}$	
0.2% Iodine thyroglobulin	<1 × 10² (II)	4.7 × 10⁷ (I)	2.8 × 10⁶
0.7% Iodine thyroglobulin	<1 × 10² (II)	9.8 × 10⁴ (II)	4.3 × 10⁴
L-Tyrosine	9.8 × 10³ (II)	4.5 × 10⁴ (I)	9.5 × 10
Diiodotyrosine	2.1 × 10³ (II)	6.5 × 10⁴ (II)	2.5 × 10⁴

The table shows that 0.2% iodine thyroglobulin reduced Compound II by 2 orders of magnitude slower than Compound I. The rate constant for the reaction of 0.7% iodine thyroglobulin with Compound II obtained from two independent experiments are consistent. Therefore, we can conclude that Compound I is directly reduced back to the ferric form by 0.2% iodine thyroglobulin and in two steps via Compound II by 0.7% iodine thyroglobulin. ESR detection of radicals in thyroglobulin is not successful. However, reduction and acceleration of ascorbate radical formation by 0.2 and 0.7% iodine thyroglobulins, respectively, have been observed (Fig.5). The results indicate that diiodotyrosine residues are mainly oxidized to react with ascorbate in 0.7% iodine thyroglobulin (Nakamura et al., 1989). Among the resulting diiodotyrosine radicals, hormonogenic residues undergo coupling to form thyroxine.

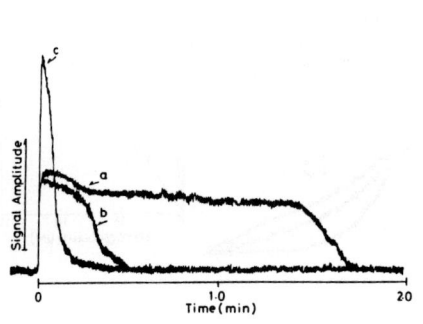

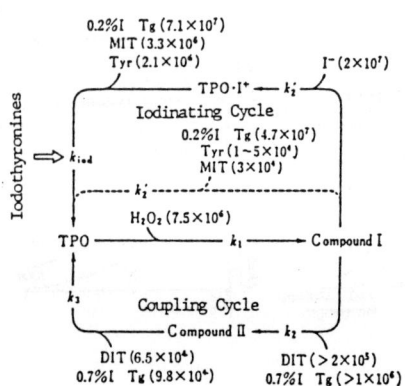

Fig.5(left) Effect of thyroglobulin upon the steady state concentration of ascorbate radical in the reaction of thyroperoxidase. The final concentrations in the stopped flow cell were; 50 μM ascorbate, 25 μM H_2O_2, and 0.4 μM thyroperoxidase for the control (a). To a, 6 μM 0.2 % or 5 μM 0.7 % iodine thyroglobulin was added for b and c, respectively.

Fig.6(right) Mechanism of reaction catalyzed by thyroperoxidase. Values in parentheses denote second order rate constants($M^{-1}s^{-1}$).

Discussion

Thyroperoxidase plays two catalytic roles in the biosynthesis of thyroxine. The primary step catalyzed by the enzyme is iodination of tyrosine. The stopped flow kinetics with thyroperoxidase have led us to conclude that iodide is oxidized by Compound I by way of two-electron transfer with a rate constant of 2 x $10^7 M^{-1}s^{-1}$. The rate is so fast that the iodinating cycle proceeds predominantly in the presence of limited amount of hydrogen peroxide, iodide or tyrosine residues of thyroglobulin (Fig.6)

The sites of thyroxine synthesis are located near the amino and carboxyl ends of the thyroglobulin monomer(Malthiery and Lissitzky, 1987). A relationship between iodine content and the numbers of iodothyronine and iodotyrosine has been reported. The fact that thyroxine is formed at an early stage of iodination has suggested that the native structure of thyroglobulin plays an important role in "preferential formation of thyroxine"(Gavaret et al., 1977). However, little evidence has been reported that how thyroperoxidase switches the activity from iodination to oxidative coupling. The inhibition of the iodinating activity of thyroperoxidase by diiodotyrosine has been explained in terms of accumulation of Compound II during the reaction. The number of diiodotyrosine residues in thyroglobulin changes from 1.1 to 8.7 as the iodine content is increased from 0.2 to 0.7%(Sorimachi and Ui, 1974). Therefore, the present results support the idea that the increase of diiodotyrosine residue in thyroglobulin inhibits further iodination by switching the catalytic cycle from the two-electron to one-electron catalytic cycle(Fig.6).

No significant oxidation of thyroglobulin by lactoperoxidase was observed. It seems therefore, unlike iodination, that the oxidation of thyroglobulin occurs through more specific interaction with thyroperoxidase. This might be a physiologically important difference in the catalytic activity of lactoperoxidase and thyroperoxidase.

Conclusion

Thyroperoxidase catalyzed the two-electron oxidation of tyrosine and monoiodotyrosine, and one-electron oxidation of diiodotyrosine. This difference in the reaction with tyrosine and diiodotyrosine was also observed in the reaction of thyroperoxidase with 0.2 and 0.7% iodine human thyroglobulins. The result supports the hypothesis that the increase in the diiodotyrosine residue inhibits further iodination by changing the catalytic cycle of thyroperoxidase from the two-electron to the one-electron catalytic cycle.

References

Chance,B. (1952):The kinetics and stoichiometry of the transition from the primary to the secondary peroxidase peroxide complexes. Arch.Biochem.Biophys. pp.416-424

Gavaret,J.M., Deme,D., Nunez,J. and Salvatore,G. (1977):Sequential reactivity of tyrosyl residues of thyroglobulin upon iodination catalyzed by thyroid peroxidase. J.Biol.Chem. 252 pp.3281-3285

Malthiery,Y. and Lissitzky,S. (1987):Primary structure of human thyroglobulin deduced from the sequence of its 8448-base complementary DNA. Eur.J.Biochem. 165 pp.491-498

Nakagawa,H., Kotani,T., Ohtaki,S., Nakamura,M. and Yamazaki,I. (1985):Rapid isolation of the native form of thyroid peroxidase by monoclonal antibody-assisted immunoaffinity chromatography. Biochem.Biophys.Res.Commun. 127 pp.8-14

Nakamura,M., Yamazaki,I.,Nakagawa,H. and Ohtaki,S. (1983):Steady state kinetics and regulation of thyroid peroxidase-catalyzed iodination. J.Biol.Chem. 258 pp.3837-3842

Nakamura,M., Yamazaki,I., Kotani,T. and Ohtaki,S. (1985):Thyroid peroxidase selects the mechanism of either 1- or 2-electron oxidation of phenols, depending on their substituents. J.Biol.Chem. 260 pp.13549-13552

Nakamura,M., Yamazaki,I., Kotani,T. and Ohtaki,S. (1989):Thyroglobulin-mediated one- and two-electron oxidations of glutathione and ascorbate in thyroid peroxidase systems. J.Biol.Chem. 246 pp.12909-12913

Sorimachi,K. and Ui,N. (1974):An improved chromatographic method for the analysis of iodoamino acids in thyroglobulin. J.Biochem. 76 pp.39-45

Taurog,A. (1986).Hormone synthesis:Thyroid iodine metabolism in the Thyroid, eds. Ingbar,S. and Braverman,L.E., J.B.Lippincott Co, Philadelphia pp.53-79.

Ohtaki,S., Nakagawa,H., Kimura,S. and Yamazaki,I. (1981):Analysis of catalytic intermediates of hog thyroid peroxidase during its iodinating reation. J.Biol.Chem. 256 pp.805-810

Ohtaki,S., Nakagawa,H., Nakamura,M. and Yamazaki,I. (1982):One- and two-electron oxidations of tyrosine, monoiodotyrosine, and diiodotyrosine catalyzed by hog thyroid peroxidase. J.Biol.Chem 257 pp.13398-13403

Yamazaki,I. (1971):One-electron and two-electron transfer processes in the enzymic oxidation and reduction. Adv.Biophys. 2 pp.33-76

Abstract

We examined the reaction of thyroperoxidase with tyrosine derivatives and thyroglobulin by the use of stopped flow kinetics, together with ESR and compared with that of lactoperoxidase. Lactoperoxidase catalyzed exclusively one-electron oxidation of tyrosine derivatives. However, thyroperoxidase did two-electron oxidation of tyrosine and monoiodotyrosine and one-electron oxidation of diiodotyrosine. This difference in the reaction of thyroperoxidase with tyrosine and diiodotyrosine was also observed in the reaction of the enzyme with 0.2 and 0.7% iodine thyroglobulins, respectively. Iodinating activity of thyroperoxidase was inhibited when the reaction was carried out in the presence of diiodotyrosine. From these results, we concluded that the changing of the mechanism from the two-electron to the one-electron type with the increase in the iodine content in thyroglobulin is a kind of regulation so that the enzyme synthesizes preferentially thyroxine at the expense of limited amount of substrates.

Résumé

Nous avons étudié la réaction de la TPO aux dérivés de tyrosine et de thyroglobuline, au moyen du stopped flow associé à l'ESR, et nous l'avons comparée à celle de la lactopéroxydase. La lactopéroxydase a catalysé les dérivés de tyrosine par une oxydation à un électron, exclusivement, tandis que la TPO effectuait une oxydation de tyrosine et de monoiodotyrosine à 2 électrons et une oxydation de diiodotyrosine à un électron. Cette différence de réaction de la TPO envers la tyrosine et la diiodotyrosine a également été observée dans la réaction de l'enzyme avec les thryroglobulines contenant respectivement 0.2 et 0.7 d'iode. L'activité d'iodation de la TPO a été inhibée lorsque la réaction s'est faite en présence de diiodotyrosine. De ces résultats, nous pouvons conclure que le passage du mécanisme de type 2-électrons au type 1-électron lorsqu'augmente le taux d'iode, est une sorte de régulation qui permet à l'enzyme de synthétiser de façon préférentielle la tyrosine, en utilisant une quantité limitée de substrats.

Thyroid peroxidase as the target for the mechanism of action of the thioureylene antithyroid drugs

A. Taurog

Department of Pharmacology, University of Texas Southwestern Medical Center, 5323 Harry Hines Blvd., Dallas, TX 75235-9041, USA

The antithyroid drugs most commonly used for the treatment of Graves' disease are 6-propylthiouracil (PTU), 1-methyl-2-mercaptoimidazole (MMI, methimazole), and carbimazole (3-carbethoxymethimazole). The latter is rapidly converted to methimazole after administration to animals (Nakashima and Taurog, 1979). These compounds are referred to as thioureylene drugs because they share the active thioureylene grouping.*

The first biochemical demonstration of peroxidase activity in the thyroid was reported by Alexander (1959). He showed that rat thyroid homogenates catalyzed the iodination of tyrosine in the presence of the H_2O_2 generating system, glucose-glucose oxidase. He also demonstrated that the reaction was inhibited by various antithyroid compounds. Subsequent studies by Hager and coworkers with highly purified chloroperoxidase, a mold enzyme that catalyzes iodination of tyrosine at acid pH's, showed that drugs related to thiouracil act as competitive inhibitors of iodination (Morris et al., 1962; Morris and Hager, 1966). The studies in Hager's laboratory provided the first demonstration of biological halogenation with a purified enzyme system and provided a model for investigators interested in biological iodination.

Early attempts to demonstrate peroxidase activity in thyroid extracts were unsuccessful, probably because, as we now know, the enzyme is membrane-bound. Isolation and purification of porcine thyroid peroxidase was first achieved after solubilization of the enzyme by treatment of the particulate fraction with trypsin and detergent (Hosoya and Morrison, 1967; Coval and Taurog, 1967; Pommier et al., 1972). Improvements in the purification procedure were subsequently reported in the author's laboratory (Taurog et al., 1970; Rawitch et al., 1979). Studies with purified TPO indicated that the same enzyme catalyzes both iodination and coupling. Availability of highly purified TPO made it possible to set up model systems for studying the mechanism of action of antithyroid drugs. Most of the data presented here are based on such studies. Some in vivo results, obtained with rats, are also included.

METHODS AND MATERIALS

Thyroid peroxidase

Porcine thyroid peroxidase was purified essentially as previously described (Rawitch et al., 1979).

^{35}S-labeled MMI and PTU

These drugs were purchased from Amersham. Specific activities were 144 mCi/mmol for ^{35}S-MMI and 132 or 212 mCi/mmol for ^{35}S-PTU (2 different preparations).

Measurement of TPO-catalyzed iodination

The model TPO incubation system contained 5µg/ml TPO, 1.5µM goiter thyroglobulin or 0.5 mg/ml BSA, 100 or 500 µM ^{131}I-iodide, 1mg/ml glucose and 0.5 µg/ml glucose oxidase, in 67 mM phosphate buffer, pH 7.0, at 37°C. MMI and PTU concentrations varied as indicated. For further methodological details see Engler et al. (1983).

Metabolism of ^{35}S-MMI and ^{35}S-PTU in vitro and in vivo, determined by HPLC

The model TPO system contained 5µg/ml TPO, 100 µM I$^-$, 25 or 50 µM ^{35}S-MMI, 100 or 150 µM ^{35}S-PTU, 1mg/ml glucose, and 0.5µg/ml glucose oxidase in 67 mM phosphate buffer, pH 7.0, at 37°C. The protein acceptor was omitted. Analysis by HPLC was performed using a reverse phase C_{18} ultrasphere column, as previously described (Taurog and Dorris, 1988).

In vivo experiments with rats

Rats weighing approximately 200g were injected ip with 1µmol/100g ^{35}S-MMI or ^{35}S-PTU. Animals were sacrificed by exsanguination under ether anesthesia, at intervals ranging from 1 to 18 hr. Thyroids were homogenized, centifuged, deproteinized, and analyzed by HPLC as previously described (Taurog et al., 1989a; Taurog and Dorris, 1989).

RESULTS AND DISCUSSION

Time course of inhibition of TPO-catalyzed iodination

Fig. 1 shows the time course of inhibition of TPO-catalyzed iodination of goiter thyroglobulin by graded doses of MMI and PTU in the model iodination system.

At all but the highest drug concentration the inhibition of iodination was transient. After a variable lag period, the duration of which depended on the drug concentration, there was escape of the iodination from inhibition. Under these conditions inhibition of iodination was reversible. However, when the drug concentration was sufficiently high, iodination was irreversibly inhibited. It is apparent from the results in Fig 1 that conclusions regarding the inhibitory effects of thioureylene drugs on TPO-catalyzed iodination are very much dependent on incubation time, as well as on drug concentration. Consider, for example, the effect of 30µM MMI on iodination. If the effect of the drug were studied within the first 10 min, it would be concluded that iodination is completely inhibited. On the other hand, if the reaction were studied at 60 min, it would appear that there had been very little inhibition of iodination.

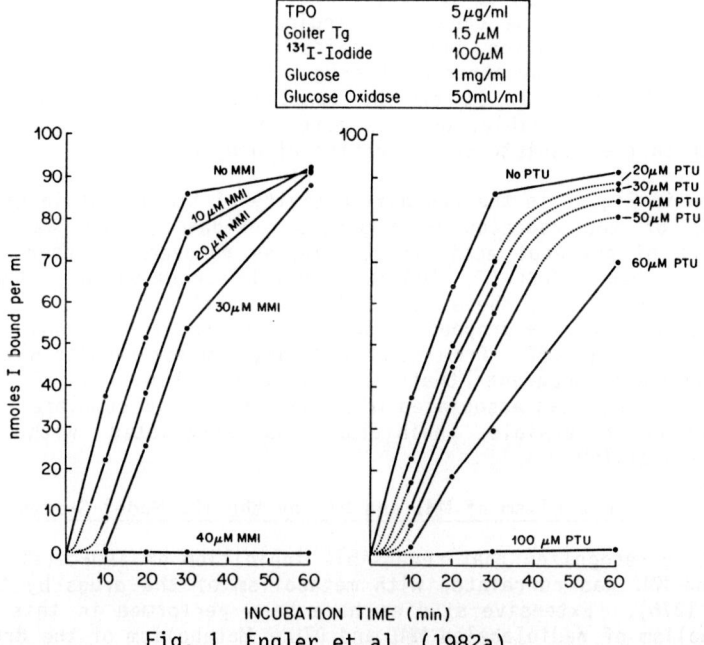

Fig. 1 Engler et al. (1982a)

Effect of iodide concentration; relationship to inactivation of TPO by MMI

Another factor that plays an important role in determining whether inhibition of iodination is reversible or irreversible is the iodide concentration. This is illustrated in Fig 2. When the incubation mixture contained 50μM MMI and 100 μM I⁻, iodination was irreversibly inhibited. However, when the iodide

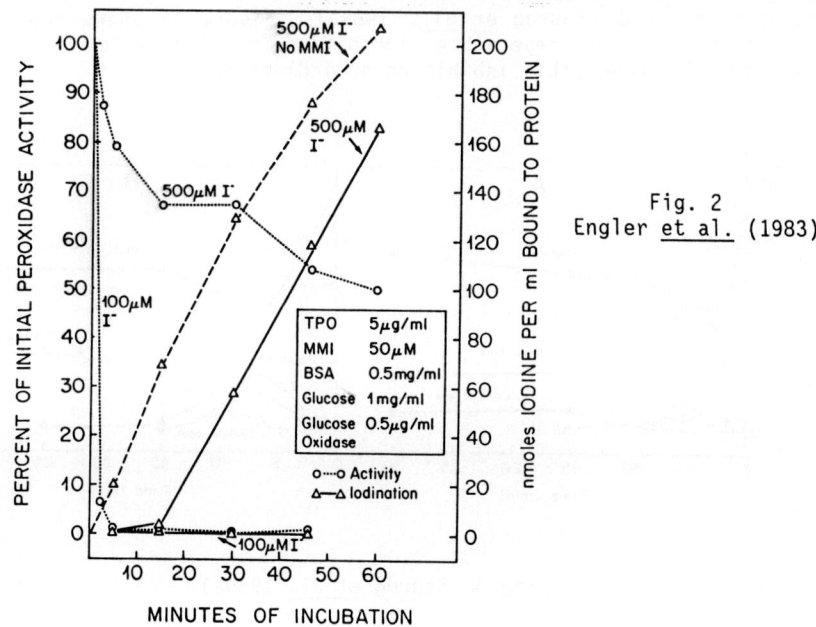

Fig. 2 Engler et al. (1983)

concentration was raised to 500 µM, inhibition of iodination by 50µM MMI became reversible. Under these conditions iodination was inhibited only during the first 15 min of incubation, but thereafter iodination proceeded at a rate close to that observed in the absence of drug. From these and many similar results with both MMI and PTU, it can be concluded that the type of inhibition, reversible or irreversible, depends more on the drug to iodide concentration ratio than on the absolute concentration of drug or iodide.

Also shown in Fig. 2 is the residual activity of the TPO at intervals after the initiation of the reaction with glucose oxidase. This was determined by measurement of guaiacol activity on samples removed at intervals. When the system contained 100µM I^-, TPO was rapidly inactivated. However, in the presence of 500 µM I^-, there was much less inactivation of TPO. Under these conditions TPO activity dropped to about 67% of the initial value in 15 min and then began to level off. From these and many similar results with both MMI and PTU, it became apparent that irreversible inhibition of iodination by thioureylene drugs was associated with very rapid and complete inactivation of TPO, whereas reversible inhibition was associated with only partial inactivation of TPO.

Metabolism of MMI and PTU by the TPO Model System

It was early recognized that reversible inhibition of TPO-catalyzed iodination by PTU and MMI was correlated with metabolism of the drugs by the TPO system (Taurog, 1976). Extensive studies have been performed in this laboratory on the metabolism of radiolabeled MMI and PTU. Metabolism of the drugs by the TPO system is largely iodide-dependent. Earlier studies were performed using paper chromatography, but more recently HPLC procedures have been developed for the separation and identification of thioureylene drug metabolites (Taurog and Dorris, 1988).

^{35}S-MMI metabolism

Fig 3 shows the time course of metabolism of ^{35}S-MMI by the TPO model system, determined by HPLC (Taurog et al., 1989a). Figure 3A shows results obtained under conditions of reversible inhibition of iodination, Fig. 3B under conditions of irreversible inhibition of iodination.

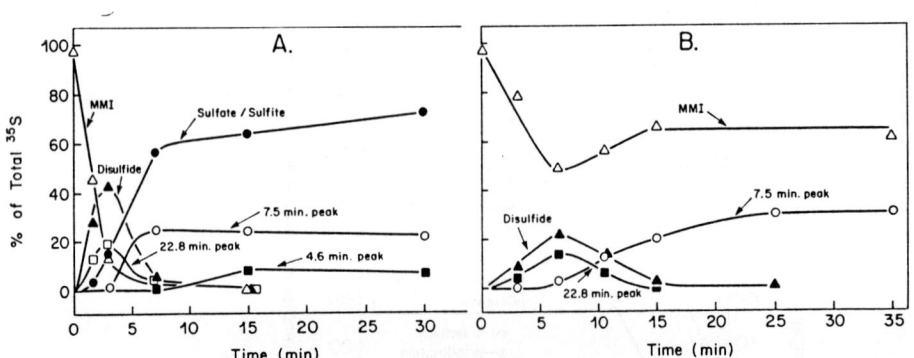

Fig 3. Taurog et al. 1989a)

Under conditions of reversible inhibition of iodination (Fig. 3A), ^{35}S-MMI disappeared rapidly, falling to 13% of the initial value in 2.5 min and to undetectable levels in 15 min. The major early ^{35}S-labeled metabolite coeluted with MMI disulfide and reached its peak (43% of total ^{35}S) in about 2.5 min. Thereafter, the level of ^{35}S- disulfide rapidly declined and was undetectable at 15 min. An unidentified, less prominent early metabolite (22.8 min) was also observed. It eluted very close to the disulfide and showed a similar rise and fall. It may represent the sulfoxide or sulfone of the disulfide. The major ^{35}S-labeled metabolite was a front running, highly polar metabolite, representing either inorganic sulfate or sulfite, or possibly a mixture of the two. Its formation started more slowly than that of the disulfide, but after a few min it began to increase steadily, and at 30 min it comprised 71% of the total ^{35}S. A second major metabolite eluted at 7.5 min and became detectable somewhat later than sulfate/sulfite. It attained a value of 25% of the total ^{35}S. The identity of this product has not been established, but we suspect that it represents MMI sulfinate (Taurog et al., 1989a).

Under conditions of irreversible inhibition of iodination (Fig. 3B), the metabolic pattern was strikingly different from that in Fig. 3A. ^{35}S-MMI disappeared more slowly and only partially, with formation of the disulfide and of the 22.8 min peak. The most notable differences compared to Fig. 3A were: 1) there was no formation of sulfate/sulfite, and 2) after reaching its minimum level at 6-7 min, MMI was partially reformed.

Metabolism of ^{35}S-PTU by the TPO model system (not shown) was similar to that of ^{35}S-MMI, but with the following differences: 1) PTU was less rapidly metabolized, 2) a much smaller percentage of the ^{35}S was metabolized to sulfate/sulfite, and 3) intermediate oxidation products between the disulfide and sulfate/sulfite were more prominent, and included PTU sulfonate (major product) as well as PTU sulfinate (Taurog et al., 1989b).

<u>Scheme to explain reversible and irreversible inhibition of iodination</u>

A scheme to explain reversible and irreversible inhibition of iodination by MMI is shown in Fig. 4 (Taurog et al., 1989a).

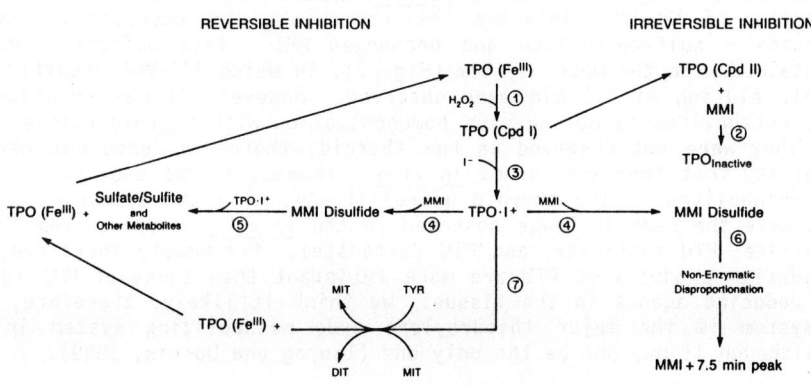

Fig. 4

The reactions associated with reversible inhibition are shown in the left half of the diagram, and those with irreversible inhibition in the right half. Reaction 1 shows the oxidation of resting TPO (ferric enzyme) by H_2O_2 to Compound I, which is rapidly transformed to TPO Compound II. As shown in reaction 2, TPO can be inactivated by MMI. The inactivation occurs with TPO Compound II (Ohtaki et al., 1982), probably via a "suicide" mechanism, involving a reaction between the heme group and an oxidized form of MMI (Engler et al., 1982b, Doerge, 1986).

TPO Compound I oxidizes I^- to I^+, which is both an iodinating agent toward tyrosine and an oxidizing agent toward MMI. Drug oxidation is the preferred reaction, and inhibition of iodination occurs only during the interval required to reduce the drug concentration to a low level. Thereafter, iodination may occur at a rate close to that observed in the absence of drug (Fig. 1). Reversible inhibition depends on the competition between MMI and tyrosine for I^+. Irreversible inhibition, on the other hand, depends on the rapid inactivation of TPO by MMI.

The earliest detectable ^{35}S-metabolite is MMI disulfide, under conditions of both reversible and irreversible inhibition of iodination (reaction 4). Under reversible conditions, the disulfide is further oxidized by I^+, and sulfate/sulfite is the major ^{35}S-metabolite (reaction 5). Under irreversible conditions, TPO is rapidly inactivated (reaction 2), and only a fraction of the MMI is oxidized, only to the stage of the disulfide and its sulfone or sulfoxide. The further transformation of these metabolites is nonenzymatic, and reformation of MMI is observed, probably through a disproportionation reaction (Taurog et al., 1988a).

A high concentration of I^- relative to MMI favors reaction 3 over reaction 2, thus leading to reversible inhibition of iodination.

The same general scheme may be used to explain reversible and irreversible inhibition of iodination by PTU.

In vivo experiments with rats injected with ^{35}S-PTU or ^{35}S-MMI
--

For examination of ^{35}S-metabolites in rat thyroids in vivo, it was first necessary to homogenize the tissue and then to deproteinize the sample before it could be analyzed by HPLC (Taurog et al., 1989a; Taurog and Dorris, 1989). After injection of ^{35}S-MMI, only two ^{35}S- components were observed in thyroid ultrafiltrates - sulfate/sulfite and unchanged MMI. This differs from the results obtained with the model system (Fig. 3), in which ^{35}S-MMI disulfide and a metabolite eluting at 7.5 min were observed. However, it was demonstrated that these metabolites do not survive homogenization with thyroid tissue. The fact that they were not observed in the thyroid, therefore, does not exclude the possibility that they are formed in vivo. Indeed, in the case of ^{35}S-PTU, the major metabolites in the thyroid ultrafiltrate, with the exception of the disulfide, were the same as those observed in the in vitro model system (i.e., sulfate/sulfite, PTU sulfinate, and PTU sulfonate). Presumably therefore, the higher oxidation products of PTU are more resistant than those of MMI to the action of reducing agents in the tissue. We think it likely, therefore, that the TPO system is the major thioureylene drug metabolizing system in the thyroid, although it may not be the only one (Taurog and Dorris, 1989).

Iodination in the thyroids of rats remains markedly inhibited 18h after the injection of a relatively small dose of PTU, and it was originally proposed that this prolonged inhibitory effect might involve inactivation of TPO (Shiroozu et al., 1983). However, subsequent studies employing HPLC procedures demonstrated that sufficient unchanged PTU remained in the gland even after this long interval to explain inhibition by a competitive reversible mechanism (Taurog et al., 1989).

CONCLUSION

In a model iodinating system containing purified TPO, inhibition of iodination by MMI and PTU may be reversible or irreversible, depending primarily on the relative concentrations of drug and iodide, and also on the enzyme concentration. Reversible inhibition involves competition between drug and tyrosyl residues for oxidized iodine (I^+) and is favored by a high concentration of iodide relative to drug. Under these conditions, there is extensive drug oxidation, and higher oxidation products such as the sulfinate, sulfonate, and inorganic sulfate/sulfite are formed. Irreversible inhibition, on the other hand, involves rapid and complete inactivation of the enzyme. Under these conditions only limited drug oxidation occurs, and the drug is enzymatically oxidized primarily to the disulfide and its sulfone or sulfoxide before the enzyme is completely inactivated. Inactivation of the TPO probably involves a reaction between the heme and an oxidized form of the drug. In vivo, it appears that inhibition occurs via the reversible mechanism, as extensive drug oxidation is observed in the thyroids of rats injected with ^{35}S-MMI or ^{35}S-PTU. In both cases ^{35}S-sulfate/sulfite is a major intrathyroidal metabolite.

REFERENCES

Coval, M.L., and Taurog, A. (1967): Purification and iodinating activity of hog thyroid peroxidase. J. Biol. Chem. 242: 5510-5523.

Doerge, D.R. (1986): Mechanism-based inhibition of lactoperoxidase by thiocarbamide goitrogens. Biochemistry. 25: 4724-4728.

Engler, H., Taurog, A., and Dorris, M.L. (1982a): Preferential inhibition of thyroxine and 3, 5, 3'-triiodothyronine formation by propylthiouracil and methylmercaptoimidazole in throid peroxidase-catalyzed iodination of thyroblobulin. Endocrinol. 122: 592-601.

Engler, H., Taurog, A., and Nakashima, T. (1982b): Mechanism of inactivation of thyroid peroxidase by thioureylene drugs. Biochem. Pharmacol. 31: 3801-3806.

Engler, H., Taurog, A., Luthy, C., and Dorris, M.L. (1983): Reversible and irreversible inhibition of thyroid peroxidase-catalyzed iodination by thioureylene drugs. Endocrinol. 112: 86-95.

Hosoya, T., and Morrison, M. (1967): The isolation and purification of thyroid peroxidase. J. Biol. Chem. 242: 2828-2836.

Morris, D., Eberwein, H., and Hager, L.P. (1962): On the mechanism of enzymatic halogenation by antithyroid agents. Life Sci. 7: 321-325.

Morris, D.R., and Hager, L.P. (1966): Mechanism of the inhibition of halogenation by antithyroid agents. J. Biol. Chem. 241: 3582-3589.

Nakashima, T., and Taurog, A. (1979): Rapid conversion of carbimazole to methimazole in serum; evidence for an enzymatic mechanism. Clin. Endocrinol. 10: 637-648.

Ohtaki, S., Nakagawa, H., Nakamura, M., and Yamazaki, I. (1982): Reactions of purified hog thyroid peroxidase with H_2O_2, tyrosine, and methylmercaptoimidazole (goitrogen) in comparison with bovine lactoperoxidase. J. Biol. Chem. 257: 761-766.

Pommier, J., De Prailaune, S., and Nunez, J. (1972): Peroxidase particulaire thyroidienne. Biochemie. 54: 483-492.

Rawitch, A.B., Taurog, A., Chernoff, S.B., and Dorris, M.L. (1979): Hog thyroid peroxidase: physical, chemical and catalytic properties of the highly purified enzyme. Arch. Biochem. Biophys. 194: 244-257.

Shiroozu, A., Taurog, A., Engler, H., and Dorris, M.L. (1983): Mechanism of action of thioureylene antithyroid drugs in the rat: possible inactivation of thyroid peroxidase by propylthiouracil. Endocrinol. 113: 362-370.

Taurog, A., Lothrop, M.L., and Estabrook, R.W. (1970): Improvements in the isolation procedure for thyroid peroxidase: nature of the heme prosthetic group. Arch. Biochem. Biophys. 139: 221-229.

Taurog, A. (1976): The mechanism of action of the thioureylene antithyroid drugs. Endocrinol. 98: 1031-1046.

Taurog, A, and Dorris, M.L. (1988): Propylthiouracil and methimazole display contrasting pathways of peripheral metabolism in both rat and human. Endocrinol. 122: 592-601.

Taurog, A., Dorris, M.L., and Guziec, F.S., Jr. (1989a): Metabolism of ^{35}S- and ^{14}C-labeled 1-methyl-2-mercaptoimidazole in vitro and in vivo. Endocrinol. 124: 30-39.

Taurog, A., Dorris, M.L., Guziec, F.S., Jr., and Uetrecht, J.P. (1989b): Metabolism of ^{35}S- and ^{14}C-labeled propylthiouracil in a model in vivo system containing thyroid peroxidase. Endocrinol. 124: 3030-3037.

Taurog, A., and Dorris, M.L. (1989): A reexamination of the proposed inactivation of thyroid peroxidase in the rat thyroid by propylthiouracil. Endocrinol. 124: 3038-3042.

Résumé

Dans un système d'iodation contenant de la TPO purifiée, l'inhibition de l'iodation par MMI et PTU peut-être réversible ou irréversible en fonction surtout des concentrations relatives en drogue et iode, mais également de la concentration en enzymes. L'inhibition réversible implique une compétition entre la drogue et les résidus tyrosyl pour l'iode oxydée (I+), et est favorisée par une concentration élevée en iode, par rapport à celle de la drogue. Dans ces conditions, il existe une oxydation importante de la drogue, et il se forme des produits comme le sulfinate, le sulfonate, le sulfate/sulfite inorganique. L'inhibition irréversible, quant à elle, entraîne une inactivation complète et rapide de l'enzyme. Dans ces conditions, seule une oxydation limitée de la drogue se produit, et cette drogue est oxydée enzymatiquement en disulfide, sulfone et sulfoxide, avant l'inactivation complète de l'enzyme. L'inactivation de la TPO entraîne probablement une réaction entre l'hème et une forme oxydée de la drogue. In vivo, il apparaît que l'inhibition se produit via le mécanisme réversible, puisqu'une oxydation importante de la drogue est observée dans les thyroïdes de rats auxquelles on a injecté du 35S-MMI ou du 35S-PTU. Dans les 2 cas, le 35S-sulfate/sulfite est un métabolite intrathyroïdien majeur.

Thyroid NADPH-dependent H_2O_2 generating system : mechanism of H_2O_2 formation and regulation by Ca^{2+}

C. Dupuy, A. Virion, J. Kaniewski, D. Dème and J. Pommier

INSERM U.96, Unité de Recherche sur la Glande Thyroïde et la Régulation Hormonale. 78, rue du Général Leclerc, 94275 Le Kremlin-Bicêtre Cedex, France

Introduction

Thyroid hormone biosynthesis takes place on the apical surface of the follicular cells during or after fusion of exocytosis vesicles with the apical membrane. The final two reactions, iodination of tyrosyl residues and coupling into the hormonal form, are catalyzed by thyroid peroxidase in the presence of H2O2. It has been shown that the H2O2 level controls the relative rates of the two reactions (Virion et al, 1985) and that H2O2 generation in intact cells is controlled by thyrotropin (Ahn and Rosenberg, 1970 ; Lippes and Spaulding, 1986). Several enzyme systems have been proposed as candidates for generation of H2O2, such as NADPH cytochrome c reductase, NADH cytochrome b5 reductase, monoamine oxidase and xanthine oxidase. However, histochemical studies indicate that NADPH-dependent H2O2 formation occurs on the apical surface of the follicular cells and that the rate of H2O2 generation increases when the Ca^{2+} ionophore A23187 is added to a Ca^{2+}-containing medium (Bjorkman et al., 1981). Studies carried out, in our laboratory, showed that a porcine thyroid particulate fraction contains an NADPH dependent H2O2 generating system regulated by micromolar concentration of Ca^{2+} (Virion et al, 1984, Dème et al., 1985). We proposed that the reversible activation of the NADPH-dependent H2O2 generation by Ca^{2+} is controlled by a Ca^{2+}-dependent inhibitor protein (Dupuy et al., 1988). Nakamura et al (1987) confirmed the presence of a high specific activity NADPH-dependent H2O2 generator in a thyroid plasma membrane preparation. A Ca^{2+}-independent, not inhibited by superoxide dismutase (SOD), cytochrome c reductase activity was associated with their preparation. They, then, concluded that H2O2 is not produced by the intermediary formation of O_2^-. Subsequently, (Nakamura et al, 1989) used diacetyl deutero heme-substituted HRP to detect O_2^- formation ; they reported that the superoxide anion generation occurred as the intermediary step in H2O2 formation. Recent studies, in our laboratory using electron scavengers to examine H2O2 generation in the thyroid plasma membrane provided indirect evidence that cytochrome c reductase activity is not catalyzed by the NADPH-dependent H2O2 generator and that the H2O2 generating system does not liberate O_2^- (Dupuy et al, 1989).

The present report provides a brief summary of the general characteristics of thyroid NADPH oxidase previously described and supplies new data showing that : 1) in contrast to the leukocyte NADPH oxidase, the thyroid H2O2 generator does not release O_2^- ; 2) Ca^{2+} controls the first step (i.e NADPH oxidation) of H2O2 generation via a calcium-dependent protein associated with the NADPH oxidase.

Material and Methods

NADPH oxidation, H2O2 generation, O2 consumption and cytochrome c reduction were measured as previously described (Dupuy et al, 1989). Thyroid particulate fraction was prepared as previously described (Dème et al., 1985). The preparation of plasma membrane was adapted from Nakamura et al., (1987). The procedures for preparing diacetyl deutero heme-substituted horseradish peroxidase has been described (Makino and Yamazaki, 1972). Details of other procedures are given in Figure Legends.

Results

Characteristics of the thyroid H2O2 generator.

H2O2 generation is catalyzed by NADPH oxidase according to the following reaction :
NADPH + O2 + H+ → NADP+ + H2O2
Fig. 1 shows that thyroid NADPH oxidase from plasma membrane preparation catalyzes NADPH oxidation, O2 consumption and H2O2 formation in a Ca^{2+}-dependent manner.

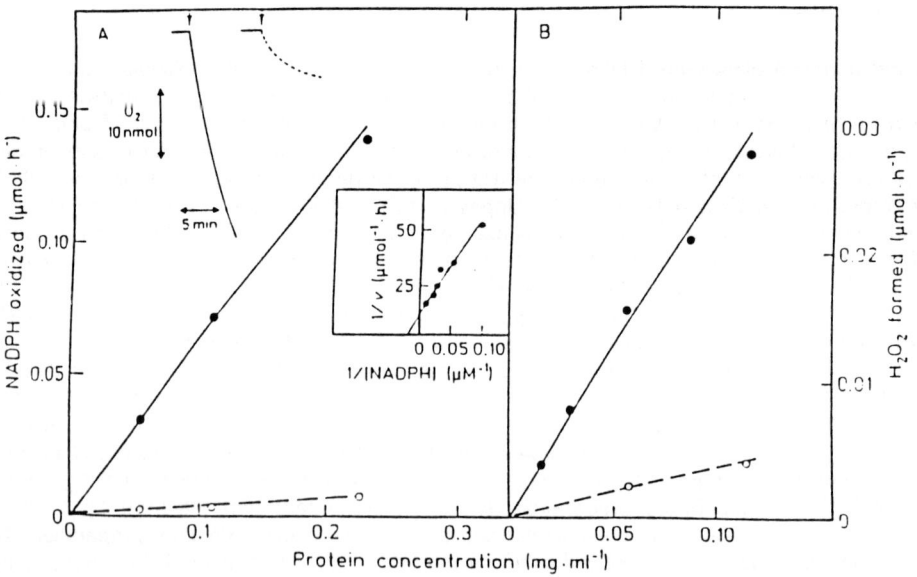

Fig. 1 : Effect of Ca^{2+} on the rate of NADPH oxidation (A) H2O2 formation (B) and oxygen consumption (inset) catalyzed by thyroid plasma membranes. Increasing amounts of membrane protein were incubated with 0.1 mM NADPH and 0.4 mM EGTA in the presence (———) or absence (- - -) of 0.5 mM CaCl2 at 30°C in 1 ml 50 mM sodium phosphate buffer pH 7.2 containing 1 mM azide.

The reversible Ca^{2+} effect occurs at micromolar concentrations (Dupuy et al., 1985 ; Nakamura et al., 1987). Ca^{2+} could be replaced by other cations, such as Cd^{2+} or Zn^{2+}, but not by Mg^{2+}.

Table 1 shows the characteristics of the different enzyme preparations.

	*H_2O_2 formation: Spec. Activity with:		Km NADPH µM	Km NADH µM	H_2O_2/NADPH	Ref.
	NADPH	NADH				
Part. Fraction	20-30	3-6	13	8	0.4	Dupuy et al 1988
Membranes Fraction	300-540	190	35	430	0.9	Nakamura et al. 1987
Membranes Fraction	300-400	-	50	-	0.6	Dupuy et al. 1989

* IU = nmoles/h/mg protein

NADPH was found to be the specific substrate for H2O2 generation. The NADPH oxidase activity was enhanced by phosphate ions at low concentrations, inhibited by Mg^{2+} at high concentration (> 2 mM) (unpublished) and increased by 5 mM ATP (Nakamura et al., 1987).

Mechanism of H2O2 generation

When an H2O2 generating system forms O_2^-, such as in granulocytes, O_2^- is usually measured by testing the reduction of a Known O_2^- scavenger, ferricytochrome c, in the presence and absence of SOD. Nakamura et al., (1987) found that thyroid plasma membranes contained an NADPH cytochrome c reductase activity. However, the cytochrome c reductase activity was : not Ca^{2+} dependent, in contrast to the other reactions (of NADPH oxydation and H2O2 formation) not SOD-inhibitable, and cytochrome c did not inhibit the O2 consumption. There was a contradiction between these observations and recent results obtained by Nakamura et al., (1989). These authors used a modified peroxidase, diacetyl deuteroheme-substituted HRP to show the formation of a compound III, a known O_2^- adduct of the peroxidase, when diacetylheme peroxidase was incubated with NADPH and thyroid plasma membrane.
We have attempted to resolve these conflicting results. using the diacetylheme peroxidase and thyroid plasma membrane. As previously found by Nakamura et al (1989), we observed the formation of compound III with peaks at 550, 585 nm and 435 nm. However, compound III formation was completely inhibited by catalase (Fig. 2) indicating that the first product would be H2O2. In addition, the NADPH oxidation rate increased as a function of the diacetyl heme-peroxidase concentration (Fig. 2 inset). The increased NADPH oxidation rate was also inhibited by catalase and enhanced by SOD. Similar results were obtained using the glucose oxidase H2O2 generator, which is known not to produce O_2^-. It was concluded that O_2^- really occurs, in the presence of an H2O2 generator, diacetyl heme peorxidase and NADPH, but is not the primary product of the H2O2 generator. O_2^- results from the oxidation of NADPH catalysed by the compound I of diacetyl heme peroxidase producing NADP° which in turn reacts with O2 to give O_2^-: NADP° + O2 → $NADP^+$ + O_2^-.
This is also, indirect evidence from our laboratory (Dupuy et al., 1989) that cytochrome c reduction is not catalyzed by the NADPH-H2O2 generating system. We have recently, been able to specifically extract the NADPH cytochrom c reductase from the thyroid plasma membrane. The thyroid plasma membranes were washed with 12 mM Chaps at 4°, which does not extract NADPH oxidase, and centrifuged. NADPH oxidase and cytochrome c reductase activities were measured in

the pellet and in the supernatant. Fig. 3 shows that the cytochrome c reductase activity was completely recovered in the supernatant fraction, while the NADPH-dependent H2O2 generating system remained in the membrane fraction.

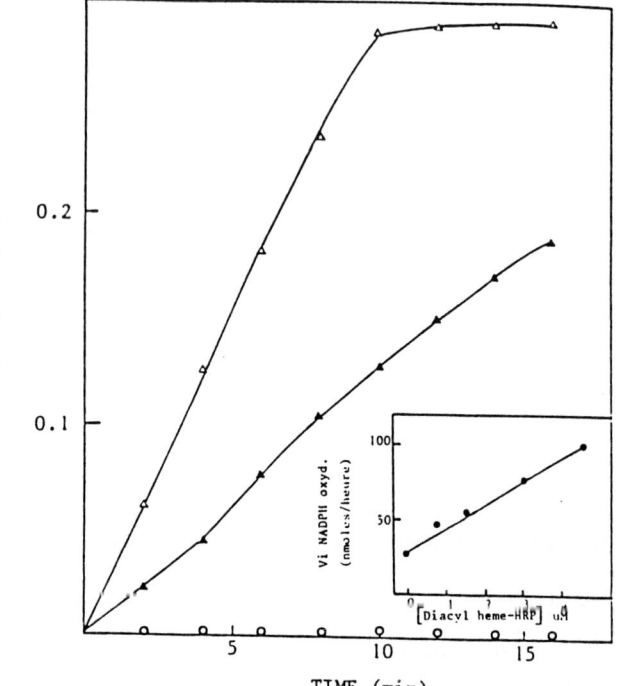

Fig. 2 : Kinetics of Compound III formation, obtained by incubating 9 µM diacetyl heme peroxidase with thyroid plasma membrane and 0.1 mM NADPH. Experiments were performed in 1 ml, 20 mM Mops buffer pH 7.2 containing 5 mM ATP, 1 mM EGTA and 1.2 mM NaCl2, at 20°C in the presence (o) or absence (Δ) of 10 µM catalase (5 x 10^4 U/mg). In the presence of 40 µg SOD (▲) Compound II was formed which could not be distinguished from Compound III at 435 nm.
Inset : the initial rate of NADPH oxidation, measured in the same conditions, as a function of diacetyl heme peroxidase concentration.

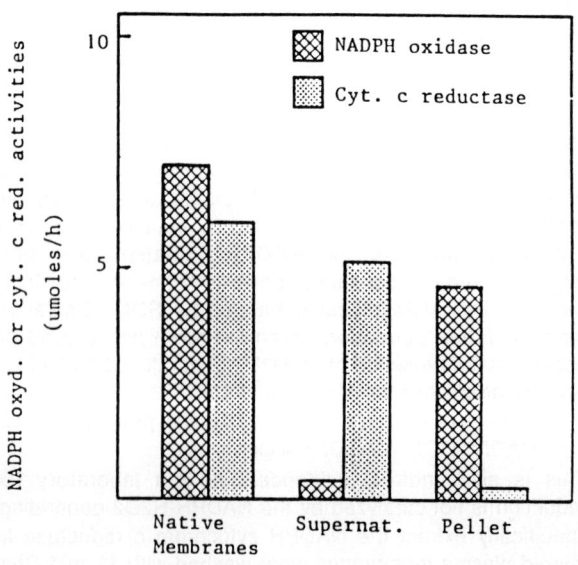

Fig. 3 : Comparison of the NADPH oxidation and cytochrome c reductase activities in the native thyroid plasma membrane and in the supernatant and pellet of the membranes washed with 12 mM Chaps at 4°C.

Ca²⁺ regulation of thyroid NADPH-dependent H2O2 generation.

We previously showed (Dupuy et al., 1988) that the activation of the NADPH-H2O2 generator by Ca^{2+} was modulated by a calcium-releasable inhibitor protein, and we found two entities of 69 and 33 kDa. In these experiments, the inhibitor protein was released by treating the particulate material with 2 mM Ca^{2+}. However, the yeild of releasable inhibitor varied greatly depending on the origin of the thyroid gland.

Other conditions were tested to obtain a more reproducible completely Ca^{2+}-independent NADPH-H2O2 generating system. Chymotrypsin hydrolyse and zinc chloride treatment of the particulate fraction both produced such an effect. Fig. 4 shows that alpha-chymotrypsin treatment of particulate preparation in the presence of 10 mM Chaps made the H2O2 generator completely insensitive to Ca^{2+} without modifying the specific activity of NADPH-dependent H2O2 generation. Similar results were obtained when the particulate fraction was treated with zinc chloride. Fig. 5 shows that desensitization is dependent on the zinc chloride concentration and temperature (inset).

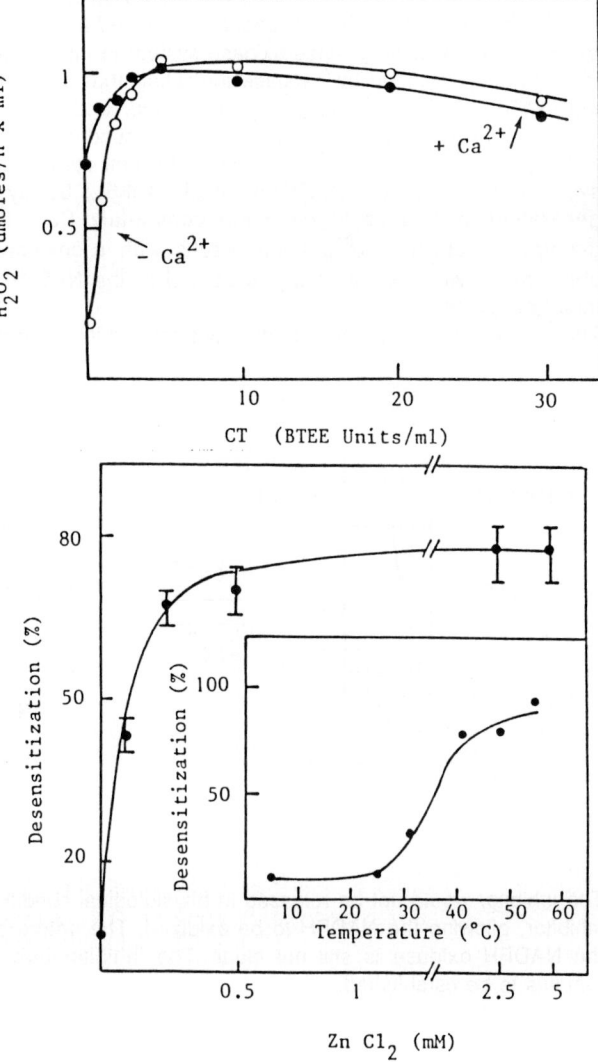

Fig. 4: Desensitization of NADPH-dependent H2O2 generation to calcium by treating the particulate fraction with α-chymotrypsin. Particulate fraction 20 mg protein/ml was incubated for 15 min at 30°C with 2 mM CaCl2, 1 mM MgCl2, 10 mM Chaps, 0.1 mg/ml DNase I (PMSF treated) and increasing amounts of TLCK treated α-chymotrypsin in 20 mM Tris/HCl) buffer pH 8.0. The reaction was stopped by adding 0.1 mM PMSF. H2O2 generation was measured as in Fig. 1 in the presence or absence of Ca^{2+}.

Fig. 5: Ca^{2+} desensitization of the NADPH-dependent H2O2 generator to Ca^{2+} by ZnCl2 treatment of the particulate fraction, as a function of the ZnCl2 concentration. Inset: the temperature-dependence of desensitization.
Activity was measured in treated, washed particulate material in the presence and absence of Ca^{2+}.

Discussion-Conclusion

It is now clearly established (Dème et al., 1985 ; Nakamura et al., 1987) that the NADPH oxidation, H2O2 formation and O2 consumption of thyroid plasma membranes are completely Ca^{2+} dependent reactions, and specific for the substrate NADPH, the results of Nakamura et al., (1987) agree with ours own observations on the presence of an associated plasma membranes cytochrome c reductase activity which is not inhibed by SOD and is not Ca^{2+}-dependent. They suggested that the reductase activity is catalyzed by the H2O2 generating system and that Ca^{2+} acts beyond the NADPH ocidation step. However, these observations do not agree with their more recent results (Nakamura et al., 1989) showing that the superoxide anion is the initial product in hydrogen peroxide formation. Our present results clearly show that the NADPH-dependent H2O2 generating system does not catalyzed superoxide anion formation for several reasons. First, the cytochrome c reductase activity is not a component of the NADPH H2O2 generator, since it can be released by washing with Chaps, without affected the H2O2 generation activity. Second, the use of diacetyldeutero-heme substituted HRP is no suitable for detecting O_2^- when NADPH is present in the medium. Indeed, the O_2^- adduct compound (compound III) is formed under these conditions, even with the glucose-glucose oxidase system in the presence of NADPH. Compound III formation is completely inhibited by catalase indicating that the initial product is H2O2. It was also shown that NADPH oxidation was greatly increased, and that the O_2^- formation would result from the oxidation of NADPH by the H2O2 adduct compound of diacetylheme peroxidase (compound I).

However, Ca^{2+} does appear to control the first step (NADPH oxidation of the H2O2 generating system). Previous results (Dème et al., 1985 ; Dupuy et al., 1988) showed that the H2O2 generation system could be made completely Ca^{2+}-insensitive without affected the H2O2 generating activity. The present results with α-chymotrypsin or Zn treatment confirm these observations and indicate that the control of the NADPH H2O2 generator by Ca^{2+} involves an inhibitor protein.

The conclusions of ours results are summarized in the following scheme.

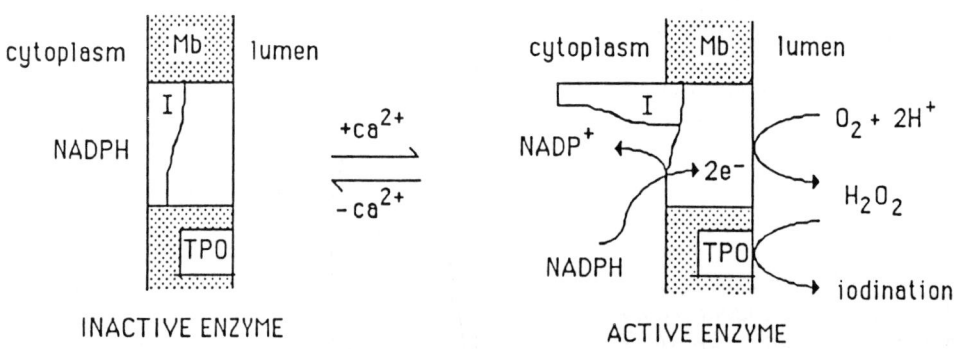

INACTIVE ENZYME   ACTIVE ENZYME

The inhibitor would not be released in physiological conditions, but Ca^{2+} would act to displace the inhibitor, allowing the NADPH to be oxidized. The nature of the linkage between the inhibitor and the NADPH oxidase is still not clear. The inhibitor may be a calcium-binding protein, but this remains to be established.

References

Ahn, C.C., and Rosenberg, I.N. (1970): Iodine metabolism in thyroid slices. Effects of TSH, dibutyryl cyclic 3',5'-AMP, NaF and prostaglandin E1. Endocrinology 86:390-405.

Bjorkman, U., Ekholm, R., and Denef, J.F. (1981): Cytochemical localisation of hydrogen peroxide in isolated thyroid follicles. J. Ultrastruct. Res. 75:105-115.

Dème, D., Virion, A., Ait Hammou, N., and Pommier, J. (1985). NADPH-dependent generation of H_2O_2 in a thyroid particulate fraction requires Ca^{2+}. FEBS Lett., 186:107-110.

Dupuy, C., Dème, D., Kaniewski, j., Pommier, J., and Virion, A. (1988). Ca^{2+} regulation of thyroid NADPH-dependent H_2O_2 generation.

Dupuy, C., Kaniewski, J., Dème, D., Pommier, J., and Virion, A. (1989). NADPH-dependent H_2O_2 generation catalyzed by thyroid plasma membranes Studies with electron scavengers. Eur. J. Biochem. 185:597-603.

Lippes, H.A., and Spaulding, S.W; (1986): Peroxide formation and glucose oxidation in calf thyroid slices : regulation by protein kinase c and cytosolic free calcium. Endocrinology, 118, 1306-1311.

Makino, R., and Yamazaki, I. (1972). Effects of 2,4 substituents of denterohemin upon peroxidase fonctions. I. Preparation and some properties of artifical enzymes. J. Biochem. 72, 655-664.

Nakamura, Y., Ogihara, S., and Ohtaki, S. (1987). Activation by ATP of calcium-dependent NADPH-oxidase-generating hydrogen peroxide in thyroid plasma mebranes. J. Biochem., 102:1121-1132.

Nakamura, Y., Ohtaki, R.M., Tanaka, T. and Ishimura, Y. (1989). Superoxide anion is the initial product in the hydrogen peroxide formation catalyzed by NADPH oxidase in porcine thyroid plasma membrane. J. Biol. Chem., 264:4759-4761.

Virion, A., Courtin, F., Dème, D., Michot, J.L., Kaniewski, JH. and Pommier, J. (1985). Spectral characteristics and catalytic properties of thyroid peroxidase compounds in the iodination and coupling reactions. Arch. Biochem. Biophys., 242:41-47.

Virion, A., Michot, J.L., Dème, D., Kaniewski, J. and Pommier, J. (1984): NADPH-dependent H_2O_2 generation and peroxidase activity in thyroid particulate fraction. Mol. Cell. Endocrinol. 36:95-105.

Résumé

Les deux dernières étapes de la synthèse des hormones thyroidiennes sont catalysées par une peroxydase fonctionnant en présence d'H2O2. Des études histochimiques ont montré que la formation de H2O2 à la surface apical de follicules thyroidiens était dépendante de NADPH et sensible au Ca^{2+}. Une NADPH oxydase produisant H2O2 et régulée par des concentrations micromolaires de Ca^{2+} a ensuite été caractérisée dans les fractions particulaires de thyroide (Virion et al., 1984) puis obtenue avec une haute activité spécifique dans une préparation de membranes plasmiques thyroidiennes (Nakamura et al., 1987). Ces auteurs montraient la présence dans leur préparation d'une activité cytochrome c réductase associée à la fraction membranaire. L'activité de la cytochrome c réductase n'était pas inhibée par la superoxide dismutase (SOD) ni dépendante du Ca^{2+}. De plus, utilisant un dérivé de la peroxydase (le diacetyl deutero heme) pour étudier le mécanisme de formation de H2O2, ils montraient la formation d'anion superoxide O_2^-. Le travail présenté ici, a pour but d'une part d'expliquer ces résultats contradictoires, et d'autres part de confirmer l'existence d'une protéine inhibitrice de la NADPH oxidase, responsable de la régulation par le Ca^{2+}. Les résultats montrent que la NADPH oxydase ne catalyse pas la formation d'anion superoxide pour plusieurs raisons.

1) La cytochrome c réductase peut être spécifiquement extraite de la fraction membranaire sans affecter le système générateur de H2O2 ; 2) l'utilisation du diacetyl deutero heme (HRP) n'est pas valable pour détecter O_2^- quand NADPH est présent (le système glucose-glucose oxydase donne des résultats identiques en présence de NADPH) : O_2^- est bien produit mais il résulte de l'oxydation de NADPH par le complexe I de la peroxydase modifiée avec la production de $NADP°$ qui réagit avec O_2 pour produire O_2^-. Cette production de O_2^- est complètement inhibée par la catalase indiquant que le premier produit formé est H_2O_2.

D'autre part, il est montré que la NADPH oxydase peut être obtenue de façon complètement désensibilisée au Ca^{2+}, soit par hydrolyse ménagée à l'α-chymotrypsin, soit par traitement au Cl2Zn du matériel particulaire. La désensibilisation par la chlorure de zinc est dépendante de la température et de la concentration en Cl2Zn.

<u>Conclusion.</u> 1) contrairement à la NADPH oxydase des leukocytes, la NADPH oxydase thyroidienne ne produit par de O_2^- ; 2) la régulation par le Ca^{2+} de la NADPH oxydase se fait par l'intermédiaire d'une protéine inhibitrice dépendante du Ca^{2+}.

Effect of deglycosylation on human and porcine thyroperoxidase activity

Y. Long, J.L. Franc and A. Giraud

INSERM U.38, Faculté de Médecine, 27 Bd Jean-Moulin, 13385 Marseille Cedex 5, France

Thyroid peroxidase (TPO) is a membrane bound glycoprotein responsible for thyroglobulin iodination in the thyroid gland. Porcine TPO (pTPO) has five putative N-linked glycosylation sites, four of which are glycosylated : Asn 129, 277, 307 and 342 (1). Human TPO (hTPO) has five putative N-linked glycosylation sites : Asn 129, 307, 342, 478 and 569, but it is not yet known which ones are glycosylated (2). To determine whether N-glycan moieties play a role in the catalytic activity of the enzymes, we examined the effect of deglycosylation on different TPO preparations.

Deglycosylation was performed with N-glycanase which cleaves most Asn-linked glycans regardless of oligosaccharide type, or with Endo H, an endoglycosidase specific for oligomannosidic type oligosaccharides.

The enzymatic activity of TPO was determined by guaiacol assay.

Three different TPOs were used :
- two were obtained by detergent extraction from thyroid microsomes and are probably full-length molecules : a porcine one, partly purified by gel filtration on Bio-Gel A5m, DEAE cellulose and affinity chromatography on concanavalin A-Ultrogel, and a human one (kind gift of Dr J. Ruf), highly purified by affinity chromatography on anti TPO monoclonal antibody.
- the third one, a porcine TPO, (kind gift of Dr J. Pommier) was obtained by a trypsin, digitonin-extraction method (3) and although it displayed full catalytic activity, it probably lacks some peptide fragments.

Deglycosylation by endo H or by N-glycanase had little or no effect on enzymatic activity of detergent-extracted hTPO and of trypsin, digitonin-extracted pTPO. But it markedly decreased (inhibition ≥ 68 %) the activity of detergent-extracted pTPO, although 1 % Triton was present in these assays to prevent aggregation and the loss of solubility that may follow deglycosylation.

Whether this effect is a direct one, species-specific and observable only with a full-length pTPO molecule, or an indirect one that would disappear on highly purified preparations of pTPO is currently under investigation.

1. Rawitch A., Pollock G., and Taurog A. (1989) Ann. Endocrinol., 50, 164 (18th Annual Meeting of ETA).

2. Libert F., Ruel J., Ludgate M., Swillers S., Alexander N., Vassart G. and Dinsart C. (1987) EMBO J. 6, 4193-4196.

3. Pommier J., De Prailauné S. and Nunez J. (1972) Biochimie 54, 483-492.

Localization and traffic

Localisation et transport

Intracellular transport and cell surface expression of thyroperoxidase

L.E. Ericson, V. Johanson, J. Mölne, M. Nilsson and T. Öfverholm

Department of Anatomy, University of Göteborg, S400 33 Göteborg, Sweden

INTRODUCTION

A basic, important feature of thyroid follicle cells is their morphological and functional polarity. The plasma membrane of the follicle cell has an apical domain which serves thyroid hormone synthesis and thyroglobulin release and uptake to and from the follicle lumen and a basolateral domain which forms the receptor-side of the cell. The specific constituents of the two plasma membrane domains are segregated by tight junctions. Thyroperoxidase (TPO) is selectively expressed in the apical plasma membrane (Nilsson et al., 1987) facing the follicle lumen where iodination of thyroglobulin takes place (Ekholm, 1990). In the present article we will discuss the polarized transfer of TPO to and from the apical plasma membrane as well as observations linking TPO to the synthesis, transport and release of thyroid hormones. In addition, we will present findings with bearings on TPO as an autoantigen.

OBSERVATIONS AND COMMENTS

Subcellular distribution of peroxidase activity
The subcellular location of peroxidase activity in thyroid follicle cells has been studied extensively using electron microscopic cytochemical technique based on the oxidation of diaminobenzidine (DAB) in the presence of hydrogen peroxide. These studies show that peroxidase activity, generally assumed to mainly represent that of TPO, is to a large extent present in intracellular compartments (Fig. 1a) and only a minor fraction is located at the apical cell surface. The dense reaction product in general fills the interior of the membrane-limited compartments, for instance exocytotic vesicles (Fig. 1b), and also forms a gradient from the outer surface of the apical plasma membrane into the colloid (Fig. 1c). This appearance of the reaction product is due to a diffusion artifact and does not indicate that the enzyme is located in the colloid, outside the membrane (Öfverholm and Ericson, 1984). In different species the intracellular

enzyme activity and that at the apical plasma membrane often have different sensitivities to the inhibitory effect of fixatives (Öfverholm and Ericson, 1984). The biochemical basis for this different fixation susceptibility is unknown.

The intracellular distribution of cytochemical peroxidase activity in thyroid follicle cells seems to follow the same pattern in all vertebrates. A similar distribution is also found in "protothyroid" cells in those chordates lacking a thyroid gland (larval lamprey, protochordates) (Fig. 1d). The protothyroid cells are surface epithelial cells located in the endostyle, a longitudinal groove in the pharyngeal floor. As in the thyroid, iodination in the endostyle is mainly an extracellular process which takes place in the pharyngeal lumen at the peroxidase-containing apical plasma membrane (Fredriksson et al., 1985; Fredriksson et al., 1988). Dunn (1980) solubilized and partly purified a membrane-bound peroxidase complex with a MW around 340 kD and with a pH optimum around 7.5. Application of methods of molecular biology on protochordate tissues appears to be an interesting possibility to explore evolutionary aspects on TPO.

Transfer of thyroperoxidase to the apical plasma membrane

On the basis of cytochemical observations, Novikoff et al. (1974) suggested that thyroglobulin and TPO were transferred to the apical cell surface of rat thyroid follicle cells in different types of vesicles. Small vesicles were supposed to contain TPO and large vesicles thyroglobulin. However, observations with cell fractionation technique (Björkman et al., 1976) as well as electron microscopic immunocytochemistry (Ring and Johanson, 1987) clearly show that typical exocytotic vesicles (diameter 150 nm) which contain peroxidase activity (Fig. 1b) also contain thyroglobulin, indicating a co-transport of thyroglobulin and TPO to the apical plasma membrane. However, this clear-cut situation in thyroid follicle cells in normal rats, in which only a single type of thyroglobulin-containing vesicles exists in the apical cytoplasm, is complicated by observations in thyroids from T_4-treated rats. In such glands an additional type of vesicles appears in the apical cytoplasm (Fig. 2a-c). These vesicles have a larger diameter (200-500 nm) than conventional exocytotic vesicles (Fig. 2c) and are morphologically similar to those supposed by Novikoff et al. to transport thyroglobulin. In fact, electron microscopic immunocytochemistry shows that these large vesicles also contain thyroglobulin (Fig. 2b) but are, in contrast to typical thyroglobulin-containing exocytotic vesicles, peroxidase-negative. In conclusion, the general rule in rat thyroid follicle cells seems to be a co-transport of thyroglobulin and peroxidase to the apical cell surface. In T_4-blocked thyroids thyroglobulin is in addition transferred to the apical surface in larger vesicles which are absent of cytochemical peroxidase activity. The exclusion of TPO from this type of vesicles suggests that selective sorting mechanisms for membrane and secretory proteins exist in the follicle cell.

Thyroperoxidase in the apical plasma membrane

When freshly isolated open human thyroid follicles are incubated with patient sera containing high titres of anti-TPO antibodies (microsomal antibodies), a

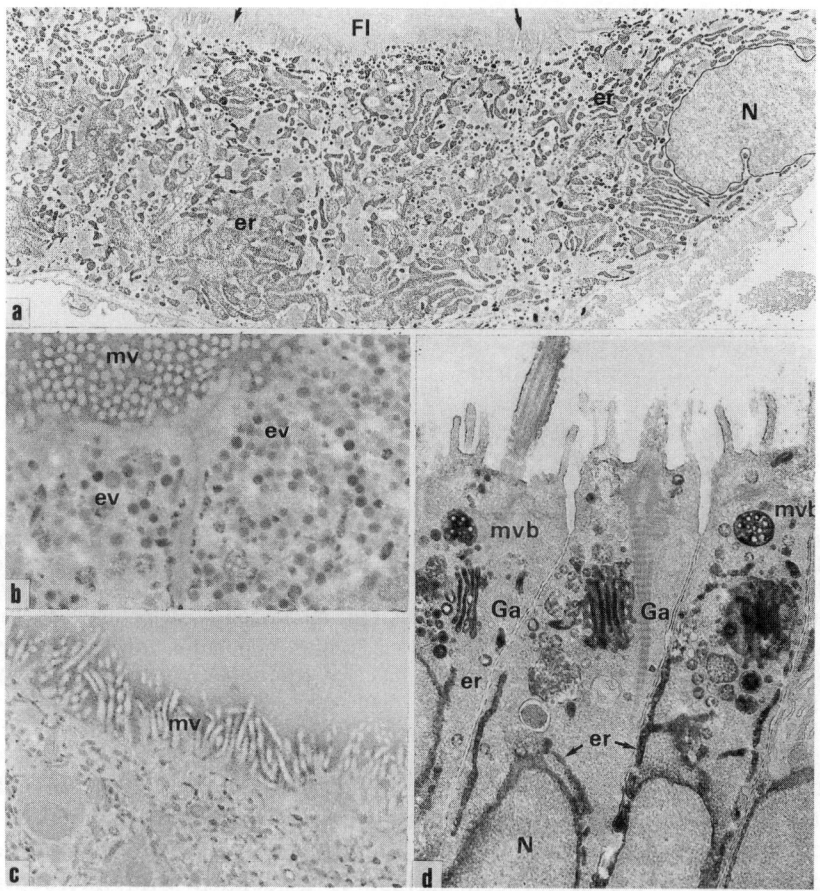

Fig. 1. Electron microscopic peroxidase cytochemistry. - **a.** Part of a rat thyroid follicle. The dense reaction product fills intracellular compartments, including the rough endoplasmic reticulum (er), and is also present along the apical surface (arrows). Fl = Follicle lumen, N = Nucleus. x 4,000. - **b.** Apical part of rat thyroid follicle cell. Dense reaction product surrounds transversely cut microvilli (mv). Exocytotic vesicles (ev) are filled with reaction product. x 16,000. - **c.** Apical part of human follicle cell. The reaction product at the apical surface surrounds microvilli (mv). x 9,000. - **d.** Protothyroid cell in the endostyle of larval amphioxus. Peroxidase activity is present in the endoplasmic reticulum (er), including the nuclear (N) envelope, in Golgi areas (Ga), apical vesicles, multivesicular bodies (mvb) and along the apical surface, furnished with microvilli and cilia. x 20,000.

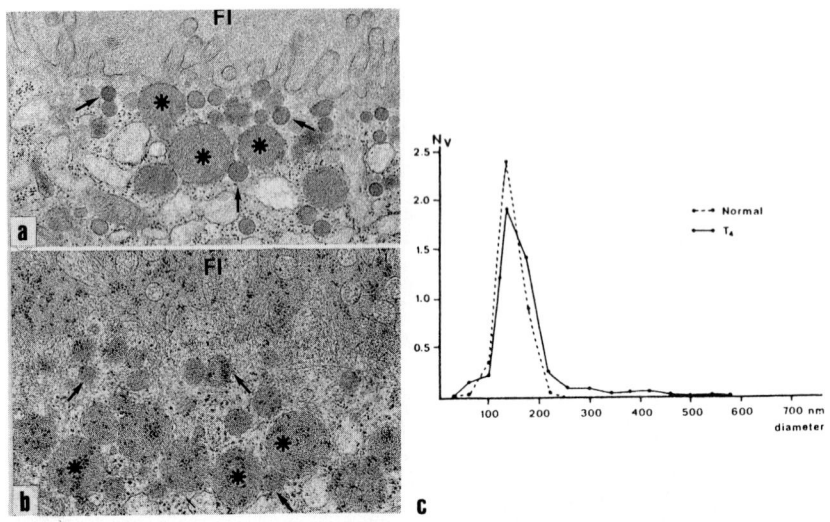

Fig. 2. Exocytotic vesicles in T_4-treated rats. - **a.** Apical cytoplasm contains typical, peroxidase-containing (cf. Fig. 1b) exocytotic vesicles (arrows) as well as large vesicles (*). x 18,000. - **b.** Thyroglobulin immunocytochemistry. Gold particles are located over the follicle lumen (Fl) as well as over typical exocytotic vesicles (arrows) and large vesicles (*) in the apical cytoplasm. x 27,000. **c.** Electron microscopic stereology. N_v = number of vesicles/um^3 follicle cell. In normal rats a single population of peroxidase-containing exocytotic vesicles is present. In T_4-treated rats an additional population of thyroglobulin-containing, peroxidase-negative vesicles with diameters >200 nm are present in the apical cytoplasm.

selective binding of antibodies to the apical surface of the polarized cells can be demonstrated by electron microscopic immunocytochemistry using colloidal gold technique (Nilsson et al., 1987). Quantitative evaluation shows that 90% of the gold particles at the apical cell surface is associated with microvilli and that the concentration of gold particles at the microvillus membrane is, although with great intercellular variation, several times higher than at smooth portions of the apical plasma membrane. This distribution, also demonstrated in Fig. 3a, suggests that TPO is organized in microdomains. The functional importance of this is not clear. A possibility might be that organization in microdomains to the microvillus membrane might provide a mechanism by which the TPO molecules escape internalization by micropinocytosis which occurs at smooth membrane portions between the microvilli. As will be further discussed below neither peroxidase activity (Tice and Wollman, 1974; Öfverholm and Ericson, 1984) nor binding of anti-TPO antibodies can be demonstrated in the membrane of pseudopods formed from the apical plasma membrane.

Effect of TSH on peroxidase activity in the apical plasma membrane
An early effect of TSH, detectable within two minutes, is stimulation of exocytosis. TSH-stimulated exocytosis and endocytosis are functionally related

in that the amount of membrane added by exocytosis to the apical plasma membrane determines the amount of membrane appearing in endocytotic structures (Ericson, 1983). Stimulation of exocytosis results in a release of newly synthesized thyroglobulin into the follicle lumen, a decrease in the number of exocytotic vesicles in the apical cytoplasm and a temporary expansion of the apical plasma membrane surface (Ericson and Engström, 1978). As thyroglobulin-containing exocytotic vesicles show peroxidase activity this implicates that also TPO is added to the apical surface during TSH-stimulated exocytosis. In fact an increased amount of reaction product along the apical plasma membrane has been observed in TSH-injected rats (Öfverholm et al., 1985). Recently Perrild et al. (1988) using a quantitative cytochemical technique noticed an increased peroxidase activity in the apical plasma membrane region upon TSH stimulation. It appears quite possible that this is related to a rapid transfer of intracellular TPO to the the apical plasma membrane by exocytosis. Besides stimulation of exocytosis, TSH also acutely increases the production of hydrogen peroxide, generated by a NADPH-oxidase present in the apical plasma membrane (Ekholm, 1990) and stimulates iodide efflux selectively across the apical plasma membrane (Nilsson et al., 1990). Thus, TSH acutely increases the four components (thyroglobulin, TPO, hydrogen peroxide, iodide) required for the iodination process taking place only at the luminal border of the follicle cell. The synergistic result of these acute TSH effects is an increased rate of iodination (Ekholm, 1990).

Internalization of thyroperoxidase

The apical plasma membrane is internalized by macropinocytosis as well as micropinocytosis. Macropinocytosis, which shares many features with phagocytosis in other cells, includes the formation of pseudopods, protruding into the colloid, and colloid droplets. Macropinocytosis is dependent of the presence of TSH. Micropinocytosis implies the formation of small vesicles by invagination of the apical plasma membrane. This process continues in the absence of TSH, but morphometric observations indicate that micropinocytosis is also stimulated by TSH (Ericson and Engström, 1978).

As mentioned above, TPO is excluded from the pseudopod membrane and also from colloid droplets. The absence of cytochemical peroxidase activity from the colloid droplet is not related to an inactivation of the enzyme, as peroxidase-positive membrane fragments, representing shed apical plasma membrane, retained their peroxidase activity when internalized by colloid droplets (Öfverholm and Ericson, 1984). Thus, available evidence indicates that TPO is not internalized by macropinocytosis and that micropinocytosis is the predominant internalization pathway. However, positive evidence for micropinocytotic uptake of TPO is scarce. Following immunocytochemical labelling of the apical plasma membrane of human thyroid follicle cells with anti-TPO antibodies, gold particles are internalized in vesicles and appear later on in multivesicular bodies and lysosomes (Fig. 3b) (Nilsson et al., 1987). However, it is uncertain to what extent this process reflects an antibody-induced uptake or the normal internalization of TPO.

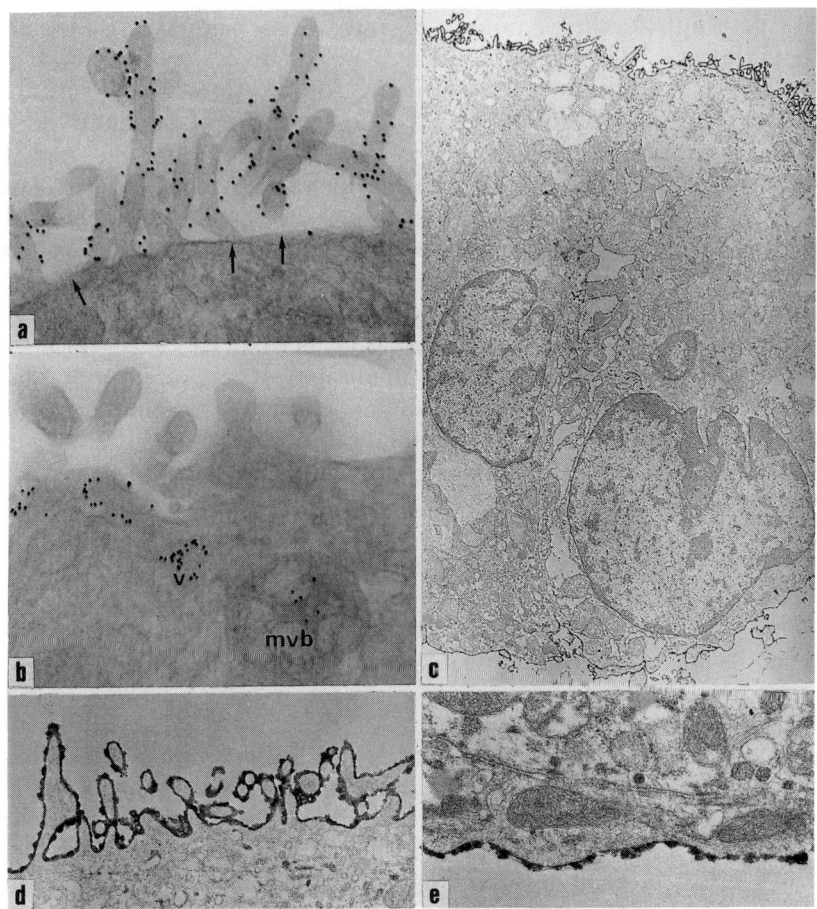

Fig. 3. - a. Open, unfixed human thyroid follicles incubated with anti-TPO antibodies at 4°C. Very thick section (500 nm). The antibodies are detected with a secondary antibody labelled with colloidal gold. Gold particles are preferentially bound to microvilli and only few are associated with smooth portions (arrows) of the apical membrane. x 37,000. - **b.** After incubation with anti-TPO antibodies at 4°C, incubation was continued at 37°C for 30 min. Gold particles are internalized in a micropinocytotic vesicle (v) and also located in a multivesicular body (mvb). x 44,000. - **c.** HLA-DR-immunocytochemistry in open, human follicle from Graves' disease. The monoclonal anti-HLA-DR antibody is detected with a peroxidase-labelled secondary antibody. Immunoreactivity is found at the apical as well as basal cell surfaces. x 4,000. - **d.** Detail showing HLA-DR immunoreactivity along the apical plasma membrane. x 16,000. - **e.** Detail showing HLA-DR immunoreactivity along the basal plasma membrane. x 21,000.

Turnover of thyroperoxidase in the apical plasma membrane
In the follicle cell membrane material is added to the apical plasma membrane by exocytosis and removed by endocytosis. Calculations based on data obtained by electron microscopic autoradiography and stereology indicate that in the normal rat thyroid follicle cell the apical plasma membrane is exchanged in 1-2 h; this turnover rate is decreased in T_4-treated rats and acutely increased by TSH (Johanson et al., 1985). However, no conclusions can be drawn from these data on the turnover rate of a particular membrane component like TPO as this might differ from the average estimated for the whole apical plasma membrane domain. Kotani and Ohtaki (1987) recently demonstrated, using open porcine follicles, that TPO immunoreactivity could be removed by trypsinization. The peroxidase epitope reappeared on the cell surface after 2 h incubation in the control medium but already within 30 min in the presence of TSH. This indicates that TPO has a turnover rate which is in the same range as that estimated for the whole apical plasma membrane and that TSH, probably by stimulation of exocytosis, increases the addition rate of TPO as discussed above.

Internalization by micropinocytosis is in all probability the major pathway by which TPO is removed from the surface. However, there are now observations available indicating that peroxidase-positive membrane material is shed from the apical plasma membrane into the follicle lumen and then internalized by macropinocytosis in colloid droplets. In human thyroids such shed membrane material appears to constitute the structural basis for "colloid vacuoles", a typical morphological feature of the hyperactive gland (Nilsson et al., 1988).

Thyroperoxidase as an autoantigen and its relationship to HLA-molecules at the cell surface
As various aspects of TPO as autoantigen will be covered by other contributions in this volume we will only focus on one particular aspect, i.e. the spatial relationship of TPO and HLA molecules at the cell surface of the polarized follicle cell. It is known that the HLA-DR molecule is aberrantly expressed by the follicle cell in autoimmune thyroid disease suggesting that the follicle cell itself might be involved in presentation of autoantigen (Banga et al., 1989). Recent immunocytochemical experiments in our laboratory, comprising both open follicles as well as cryostat sections of thyroid tissue obtained from patients with Graves´ disease, have revealed that in some follicles HLA-DR immunoreactivity is equally expressed at both apical and basolateral domains of the cell surface (Fig. 3c) whereas in other follicles immunolabelling was completely absent or only found at either of the two surfaces. Similar findings were obtained with immunocytochemical detection of HLA-A,B,C molecules. This means that, at least in some follicles of the diseased thyroid, both classes of HLA molecules and TPO are present in the same (apical) domain of the plasma membrane (the same accounts for another thyroid autoantigen: the TSH receptor present in the basolateral plasma membrane), which might be of significance in a discussion by which mechanism(s) a "hidden" autoantigen such as TPO is recognized by immunocompetent cells. From the cell biological point of view, it is also of interest to note that, unlike all hitherto studied thyroid

plasma membrane proteins, HLA molecules are not strictly polarized in their cell surface expression. Possibly, this is a reflection of the aberrant nature of these components in the thyroid follicle cells.

REFERENCES

Banga, J.B., Barnett, P.S., Mahadevan, D., McGregor, A.M. (1989): Immune recognition of antigens and its relevance to autoimmune disease> recent advances at the molecular level. Eur. J. Clin. Invest. 19: 107-116.

Björkman, U., Ekholm, R., Ericson, L.E., Öfverholm, T. (1976): Transport of thyroglobulin and peroxidase in the thyroid follicle cell. Mol. Cell. Endocrinol. 5: 3-17.

Dunn, A.D. (1980): Properties of an iodinating enzyme in the ascidian endostyle. Gen. Comp. Endocrinol. 40: 484-493.

Ekholm, R. (1990): Biosynthesis of thyroid hormones. Int. Rev. Cytol. 120: 243-288.

Ericson, L.E., Engström, G. (1978): Quantitative electron microscopic studies on exocytosis and endocytosis in the thyroid follicle cell. Endocrinology 103: 883-892.

Ericson, L.E. (1983): Ultrastructural aspects on iodination and hormone secretion in the thyroid gland. J. Endocrinol. Invest. 6: 311-324.

Fredriksson, G., Öfverholm, T., Ericson, L.E. (1985): Electron-microscopic studies of iodine binding and peroxidase activity in the endostyle of the larval amphioxus (Branchiostoma lanceolatum). Cell Tiss. Res. 241: 257-266.

Fredriksson, G., Öfverholm, T., Ericson, L.E. (1988): Iodine binding and peroxidase activity in the endostyle of Salpa fusiformis, Thalia democratica, Doliolctta gegenbauri and Doliolum nationalis (Tunicata, Thaliacea) Cell Tiss. Res. 253: 403-411.

Johanson, V., Öfverholm, T., Ericson, L.E. (1984): Turnover of apical plasma membrane in thyroid follicle cells of normal and thyroxine-treated rats. Eur. J. Cell Biol. 35: 165-170.

Kotani, T., Ohtaki, S. (1987): Characterization of thyroid follicular cell apical plasma membrane peroxidase using monoclonal antibody. Endocrinol. Japon. 34:407-413.

Nilsson, M., Mölne, J., Karlsson, F.A., Ericson, L.E. (1987): Immunoelectron microscopic studies on the cell surface location of the thyroid microsomal antigen. Mol. Cell. Endocrinol. 53: 177-186.

Nilsson, M., Mölne, J., Jörtsö, E., Smeds, S., Ericson, L.E. (1988): Plasma membrane shedding and colloid vacuoles in hyperactive human thyroid tissue. Virchows Archive B Cell. Pathol. 56: 85-94.

Nilsson, M., Björkman, U., Ekholm, R., Ericson, L.E. (1990): Iodide transport in primary cultured thyroid follicle cells: Evidence of a TSH-regulated channel mediating iodide efflux selectively across the apical domain of the plasma membrane. Submitted.

Novikoff, A.B., Novikoff, P.M., Ma, M., Woo-Young, S., Quintana, N. (1974): Cytochemical studies of secretory and other granules associated with the endoplasmic reticulum in rat thyroid epithelial cells. In Advances in Cytopharmacology, Cytopharmacology of secretion, Vol. 2. eds B. Ceccarelli, Z.J. Meldolesi and F. Clementi, pp. 349-368. New York: Raven Press.

Öfverholm, T., Ericson, L.E. (1984): Diffusion artefacts and tissue fixation in thyroperoxidase cytochemistry. Histochemistry 81: 1-8.

Öfverholm, T., Björkman, U., Ericson, L.E. (1985): Effects of TSH on iodination in rat thyroid follicles studied by autoradiography. Mol. Cell. Endocrinol. 40: 1-7.

Perrild, H., Loveridge, N., Reader, S.C.J., Robertsson, W.R. (1988): Acute stimulation of thyroidal NAD^+ kinase, NADPH reoxidation and peroxidase activities by physiological concentration of thyroid stimulating hormone acting in vitro: A quantitative cytochemical study. Endocrinology 123: 2499-2505.

Ring, P., Johanson, V. (1987): Immunoelectron-microscopic demonstration of thyroglobulin and thyroid hormones in the rat thyroid gland. J. Histochem. Cytochem. 35: 1095-1104.

Tice, L.W., Wollman, S.H. (1974): Ultrastructural localisation of peroxidase on pseudopods and other structures of the typical thyroid epithelial cell. Endocrinology 94: 1555-1567.

ABSTRACT

Electron microscopic cytochemistry shows that the major fraction of the peroxidase activity, assumed to represent TPO activity, is located in intracellular compartments and that only a minor fraction is present in the apical plasma membrane at the site of iodination. A similar distribution of peroxidase activity is also found in pharyngeal "protothyroid" cells in those chordates lacking a thyroid.

In the normal rat thyroid TPO is co-transported with thyroglobulin in exocytotic vesicles, about 150 nm in diameter. Such typical exocytotic vesicles are also present in T_4-treated rats but in addition a larger type of vesicles, 200-500 nm in diameter, containing thyroglobulin but not TPO appears, indicating that different sorting mechanisms for membrane and secretory proteins exist.

In the apical plasma membrane TPO is concentrated to microvilli. TPO is excluded from TSH-induced pseudopods and colloid droplets and probably internalized only by micropinocytosis. Little is known about the fate of internalized TPO, although a reutilization by recirculation back to the apical plasma membrane appears possible considering the rapid turnover of this membrane domain.

In follicles isolated from thyroids with Graves´ disease HLA-A,B,C and HLA-DR antigens are expressed at the apical as well as basolateral plasma membrane domain, while TPO is only found in the apical plasma membrane. From an immunological point of view this is of interest in a discussion how TPO is recognized by immunocompetent cells. From a cell biological point of view it is of interest to note that HLA molecules, in contrast to all other proteins hitherto examined, are not strictly polarized in their cell surface expression.

Résumé

La cytochimie par microscopie électronique montre que la plus grande partie de l'activité péroxydase - censée représenter celle de la TPO - est localisée dans des compartiments intra-cellulaires et qu'une minime partie seulement est présente sur la membrane plasmique apicale au niveau du site d'iodation. Une distribution identique de l'activité péroxydase se trouve également dans les cellules "protothyroïdiennes" du pharynx. Dans une thyroïde de rat normal, la TPO est co-transportée avec la thyroglobuline dans des vésicules d'exocytose d'un diamètre approximatif de 150 nm. Ces vésicules typiques d'exocytose sont également présentes chez les rats traités à la T4 mais apparaissent également des vésicules plus grosses d'un diamètre de 200 à 500 nm, contenant de la thyroglobuline, mais pas de TPO, ce qui indique qu'il existe, pour la membrane et pour les protéines secrétées, différents mécanismes d'exocytose. Sur la membrane plasmique apicale, la TPO est concentrée dans des microvillosités. La TPO est absente des pseudopodes induits par la TSH, ainsi que des gouttelettes colloïdales; elle est probablement internalisée seulement par micropinocytose. On sait peu de choses du devenir de la TPO internalisée, quoiqu'une réutilisation par retour à la membrane apicale paraisse possible compte-tenu du turnover rapide de cette région de la membrane. Dans les follicules isolés à partir de thryoïdes de Basedow, l'expression des antigènes HLA-A, B, C et HLA-DR, se situe dans la région de la membrane plasmique apicale. Ceci est intéressant d'un point de vue immunologique pour comprendre comment la TPO est reconnue par les cellules immunocompétentes. D'un point de vue biologique, il est intéressant de noter que les molécules HLA, contrairement à toutes les autres protéines jusqu'ici examinées, ne sont pas strictement polarisées sur la surface cellulaire où elles s'expriment.

Immunolocalization of functional thyroperoxidase and expression of thyroid cell differentiation

B. Rousset, Z. Kostrouch, J. Pommier and Y. Munari-Silem

INSERM U. 197, Faculté de Médecine Alexis Carrel, Lyon and INSERM U.96, Hôpital de Bicêtre-Le Kremlin-Bicêtre, France

ABSTRACT

Thyroperoxidase (TPO) is a membrane-bound enzyme thought to be selectively transported to the apical membrane domain of the polarized epithelial thyroid cells where it catalyzes the formation of thyroid hormone residues within thyroglobulin molecules. Using polyclonal anti-pig TPO antibodies and either immunofluorescence labeling or immunogold labeling on ultrathin cryosections, we have studied the localization of TPO at different stages of the expression of thyroid cell polarized phenotype in vitro. Immunoreactive TPO was found in intracellular compartments and rather evenly distributed all around thyroid cells which were freshly isolated from the intact tissue. Incubation of isolated cells in suspension in the presence of TSH led to the formation of intracellular lumina (ICL) which contained thyroglobulin (Tg); the membrane delimiting the ICL as well as the very numerous microvilli bore TPO. The appearance of immunoreactive TPO in ICL was accompanied by a decrease of the TPO at the plasma membrane. Structures of the ICL-type, positive for Tg and TPO, were also occasionally observed in thyroid cells cultured as monolayers. Isolated cells cultured in the presence of TSH reorganized in follicular structures : the in vitro reconstituted thyroid follicles (RTF) exhibiting a closed intrafollicular lumen (IL). Immunofluorescence and immunogold-labeling showed a) the accumulation of large amounts of Tg molecules in the IL of RTF and b) the presence of TPO on the membrane delimiting the neoformed IL (preferentially near or on microvilli). In RTF, the distribution of plasma membrane TPO was clearly polarized. These data indicate that the TSH-dependent in vitro morphogenesis of ICL or IL is coupled with the vectorial transport of membrane TPO and soluble Tg for the reconstitution of functional hormonogenetic compartments.

Keywords
Thyroxperoxidase, thyroid cell differentiation, intracellular lumen, thyroid follicles, immunogold labeling.

INTRODUCTION

The synthesis of thyroid hormones is dependent on the ability of thyroid cells to generate a well defined compartment in which, Tg, the precursor protein, accumulates and undergoes enzymatic iodination. The requirement of such a differentiated locus is demonstrated by in vitro studies. Thyroid cells cultured as monolayers, polarized or not, are not capable of synthetizing thyroid hormones (Lissitzky et al, 1971) although polarized cells keep the ability to trap iodide and synthetize and secrete Tg (Chambard et al, 1983). Upon the action of TSH, thyroid cells cultured on solid substratum reorganized in follicular structures on the inside of which one can identify lumina comparable to those observed in vivo (Kerkof et al, 1964). The neoformed intrafollicular lumina (IL) represent functional sites of Tg iodination (Fayet et al, 1971) and hormone synthesis (Lissitzky et al, 1971). Thyroid cells maintained in suspension in serum-free medium exhibit the capacity to iodinate Tg and synthetize and secrete thyroid hormones (Rousset et al, 1976, 1977, 1980a, 1981, 1989a). These activities are related to the development of intracellular structures morphologically identical to intrafollicular lumina (Rousset et al, 1985). Electron microscope autoradiographic studies revealed that these intracellular lumina (ICL) are actually the sites of Tg iodination (Remy et al, 1977 ; Ekholm and Björkman, 1984 ; Rousset et al, 1985). In the present work, using mainly immunoelectron microscopy, we have studied the localization of TPO in thyroid cells at different stages of morphological and metabolic differentiation : freshly isolated thyroid cells, isolated cells exhibiting ICL, thyroid cells in monolayer, reconstituted thyroid follicles.

MATERIAL AND METHODS

Cell preparation and culture

Isolated thyroid cells were prepared by the discontinuous trypsinization procedure previously described (Rousset et al, 1976) and either incubated in suspension for short period of time or cultured on tissue-culture Petri dishes for 3 to 4 days. Incubations in suspension were carried out in Earle's medium pH 7.4 with or without TSH (10 mU/ml) for 3 hr at 37°C under constant agitation to generate intracellular lumina (ICL) (Rousset et al, 1985). Cells were cultured in F12 medium + 10 % calf serum without or with TSH (1 mU/ml) (Munari-Silem, 1986, 1990) to obtain monolayers or RTF, respectively.

Western blot analysis

Thyroid cell proteins were fractionated by SDS-PAGE (Rousset and Wolff, 1980b) and electrophoretically transfered onto nitrocellulose sheet. Incubations with anti-TPO antibodies, goat anti-rabbit Ig antibody as amplifier and ^{125}I-labeled protein A were performed as previously described (Durrieu et al, 1987). Immune complexes were revealed by autoradiography.

Antibodies

Anti-TPO immune serum was raised in rabbit using purified pig TPO (J. Kaniewski and J. Pommier, INSERM U. 96, Le Kremlin-Bicêtre). Anti-Tg immune sera were obtained in rabbit using pure pig Tg as immunogen. These antibodies have been previously characterized (Selmi and Rousset, 1988 ; Rousset et al, 1989b).

Immunofluorescence method

Cells cultured on Petri dishes were fixed with 4 % formaldehyde in phosphate buffered saline, permeabilized with 0.05 % Triton and allowed to react with anti-TPO, anti-Tg rabbit immune sera or normal rabbit serum at a 1:100 to 1:1000 dilution. Fluorescence labeling was performed with biotinylated F(ab)2 fragments of donkey anti-rabbit Ig antibody and FITC-streptavidin.

Immunogold labeling

Isolated cells or cultured cells were fixed in 4 % paraformaldehyde and 0.5 % glutaraldehyde in 200 mM Pipes buffer pH 7.2, embedded in fibrin cloth and resubmitted to the same fixation procedure. Samples were mounted on copper stubs to prepare cryosections. Immunolabeling with anti-TPO or anti-Tg antibodies was conducted according to Griffiths et al, 1984. Anti-TPO and anti-Tg were used at 1:300 and 1:1000 dilution respectively. Immune complexes were visualized with Protein A colloidal gold complexes, the diameter of the gold particles being 6 or 9 nm (a kind gift from G. Griffiths, EMBL, Heidelberg, FRG).

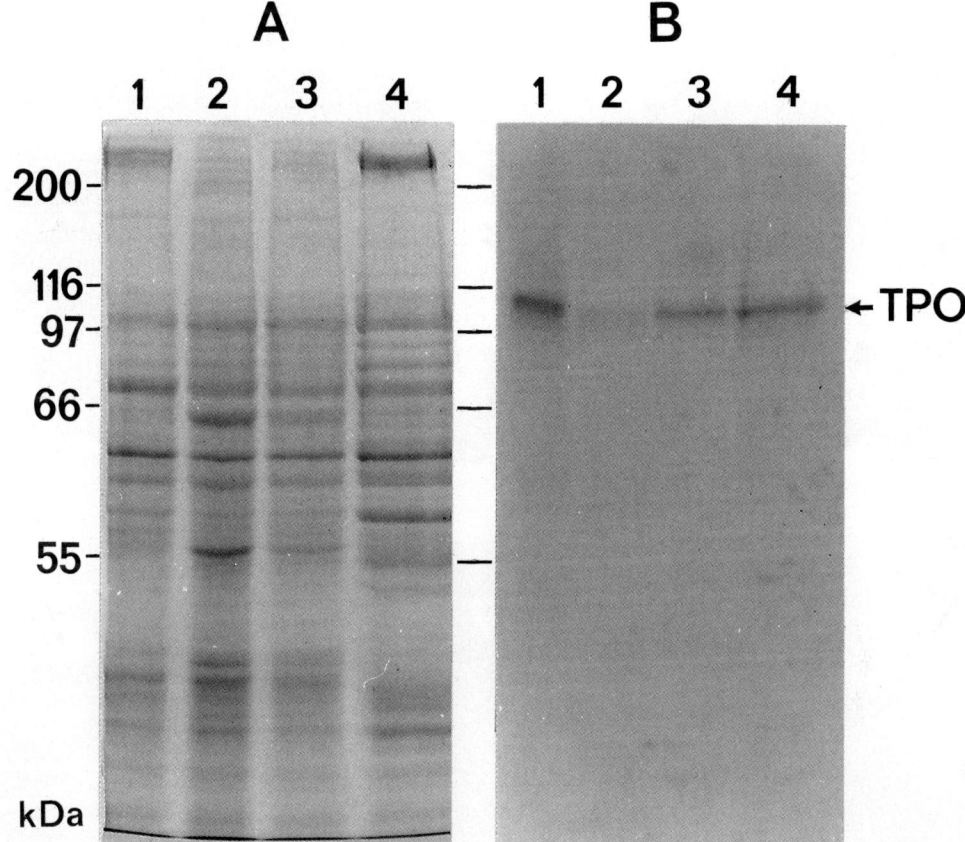

FIGURE 1 : **Western blot analysis of thyroperoxidase (TPO) in pig thyroid cells at different stages of differentiation.** Freshly isolated thyroid cells and cells cultured for 4 days as monolayers (in the absence of TSH) or in the form of reconstituted thyroid follicles (in the presence of TSH) were homogenized in an isoosmotic buffer and the particulate material sedimenting at 100,000 g was analyzed by SDS-PAGE (panel A) and Western Blot (panel B) using rabbit polyclonal anti-pig TPO antibodies (1:400 dilution). Lane 1 : Isolated thyroid cells ; lane 2 : monolayer cells ; lane 3 : reconstituted thyroid follicles ; lane 4 : microsomal fraction prepared from intact pig thyroid tissue by isopycnic centrifugation on Percoll gradient (Rousset et al, 1989). Each lane contains 150 µg protein.

RESULTS AND DISCUSSION

Polyclonal anti-pig TPO antibodies detected a single polypeptide with a molecular mass of 105-110 kD in different particulate cell extracts analyzed by Western blot (fig. 1). Thyroid cells cultured as monolayers in the absence of TSH exhibited a decreased TPO content when compared to either starting isolated cells or cells cultured in the presence of TSH giving rise to reconstituted thyroid follicles (RTF). These data on the expression of TPO at the protein level are in keeping with previous analyses on mRNA (Gerard et al, 1988 ; Damante et al, 1989) showing that TSH regulates TPO expression at transcriptional and post-transcriptional levels.

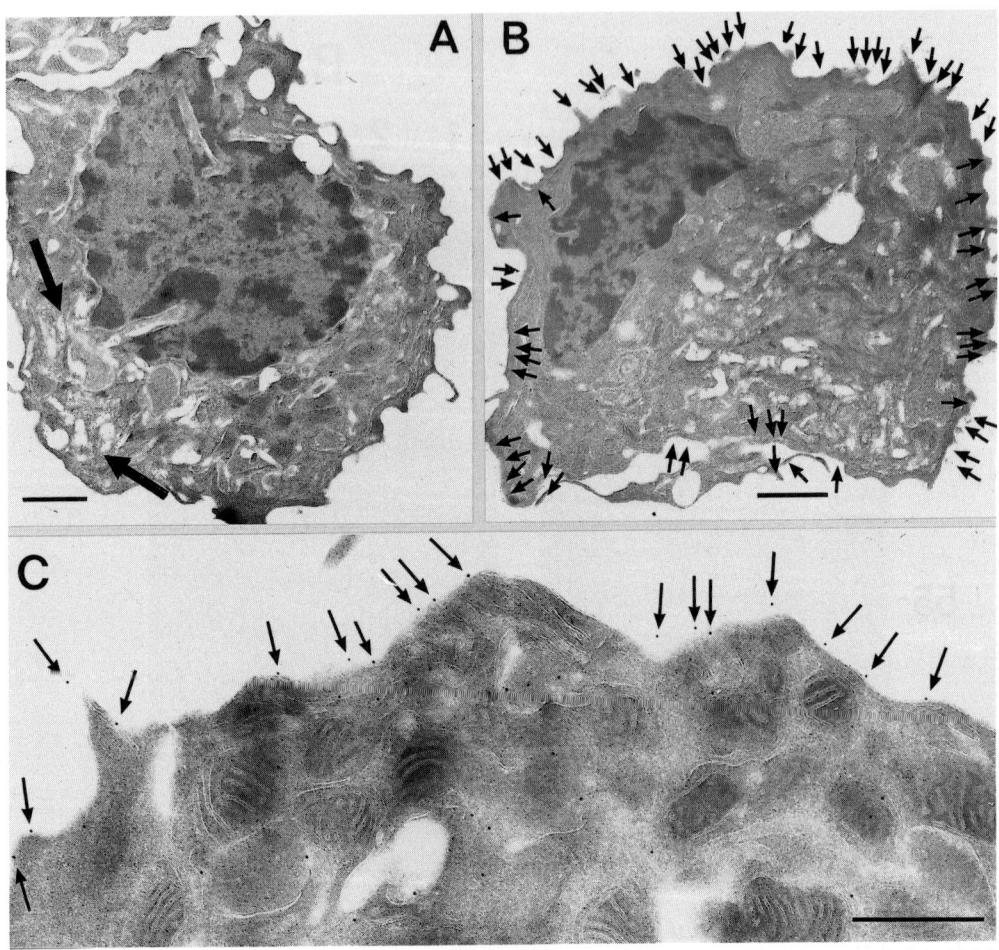

FIGURE 2 : Immunogold labeling of TPO in freshly isolated pig thyroid cells. Comparative localization of Tg and TPO. Cells were labeled with anti-pig Tg antibodies (A) or anti-pig TPO antibodies (B and C). Large arrows in A identify intracellular structures which contained Tg. Arrows in B and C identify individual gold particles located on the plasma membrane bars : 1 µm in A and B and 500 nm in C.

Freshly isolated thyroid cells bore a large number of TPO molecules at their surface as shown in fig. 2B on which gold particles are identified by arrows. For comparison, there was no labeling at the plasma membrane with anti-Tg antibodies whereas many intracellular structures or vesicles were heavily labeled. TPO was evenly distributed on the plasma membrane as the result of the loss of cell polarity. This is in agreement with previous results showing the existence of extracellular sites of iodination in isolated thyroid cells (Rousset et al, 1980a). TPO was also detected inside the cell but the density of labeling of intracellular structures was about 10 times lower than the density of labeling of the plasma membrane. Our finding is in marked contrast with the expected distribution based on earlier cytochemical analysis (Tice and Wollman, 1972). In this study and many others, peroxidase, localized through its oxidized products seemed to be essentially inside the cells. Preliminary morphometric analysis of the gold particle distribution indicate that plasma membrane TPO could account for 30 to 50 % of total cellular TPO.

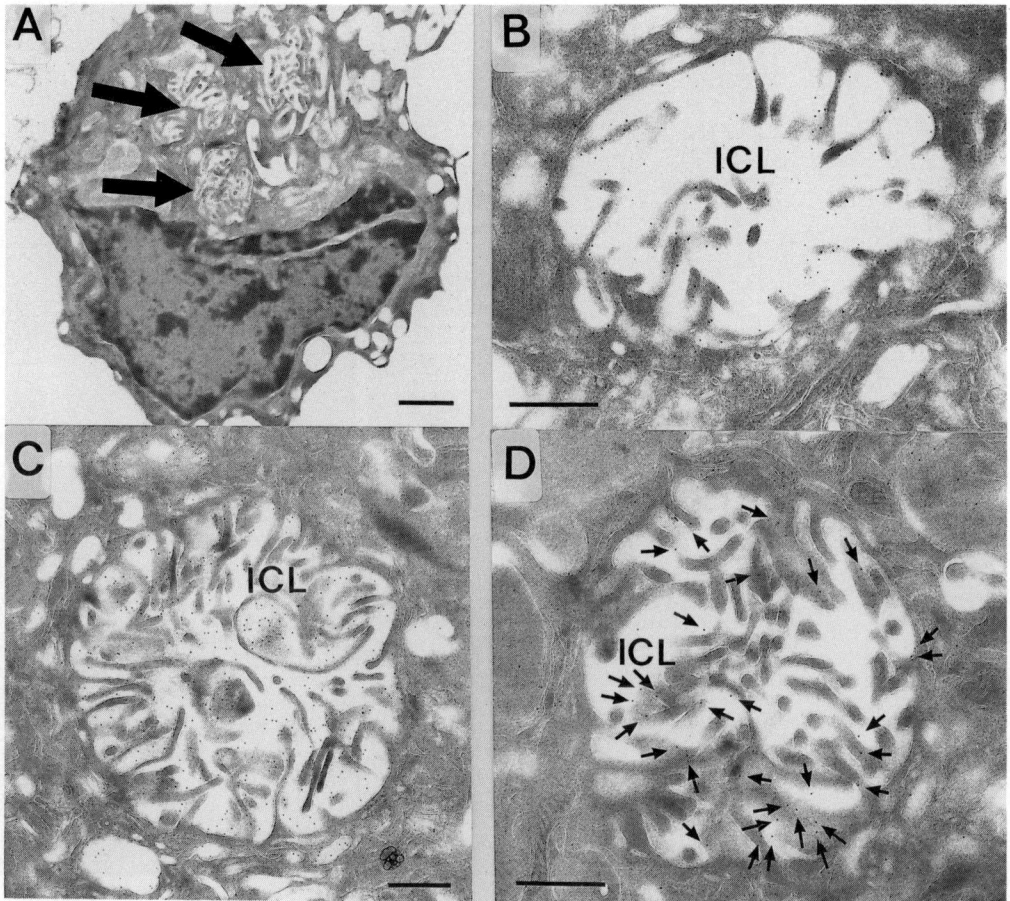

FIGURE 3 : Identification of intracellular lumina (ICL) in isolated thyroid cells acutely stimulated by TSH. Localization of TPO and Tg by immunogold labeling. Freshly isolated cells were incubated in suspension in serum-free medium in the presence of TSH (10 mU/ml) for 3 hr. A and C : labeling with anti-Tg antibodies ; B and D : labeling with anti-TPO antibodies. Large arrows in A identify ICL ; small arrows in D indicate the position of gold particles. Bars : 1 μm in A and 500 nm in B, C and D.

Isolated cells incubated in suspension expressed a peculiar differentiation pattern: the formation of intracellular lumina, a process which is TSH-dependent (Rousset et al, 1985). The structure and the Tg and TPO content of ICL are reported in fig. 3. Neoformed ICL were characterized by a very large number of long microvilli. Several ICL were often present in the same cell. Whereas immunoreactive Tg was homogenously distributed over the IL, gold particles attached to TPO-anti TPO antibody complexes were found on the membranes delimiting the ICL and for a major part along microvilli. The appearance of TPO in ICL was accompanied by a reduction of plasma membrane TPO. Up to 30 % of cellular TPO was found in ICL. As far as the hormone synthesis is concerned, ICL play in the isolated thyroid cell system the role of IL in the intact tissue or RTF (Rousset et al, 1981, 1985).

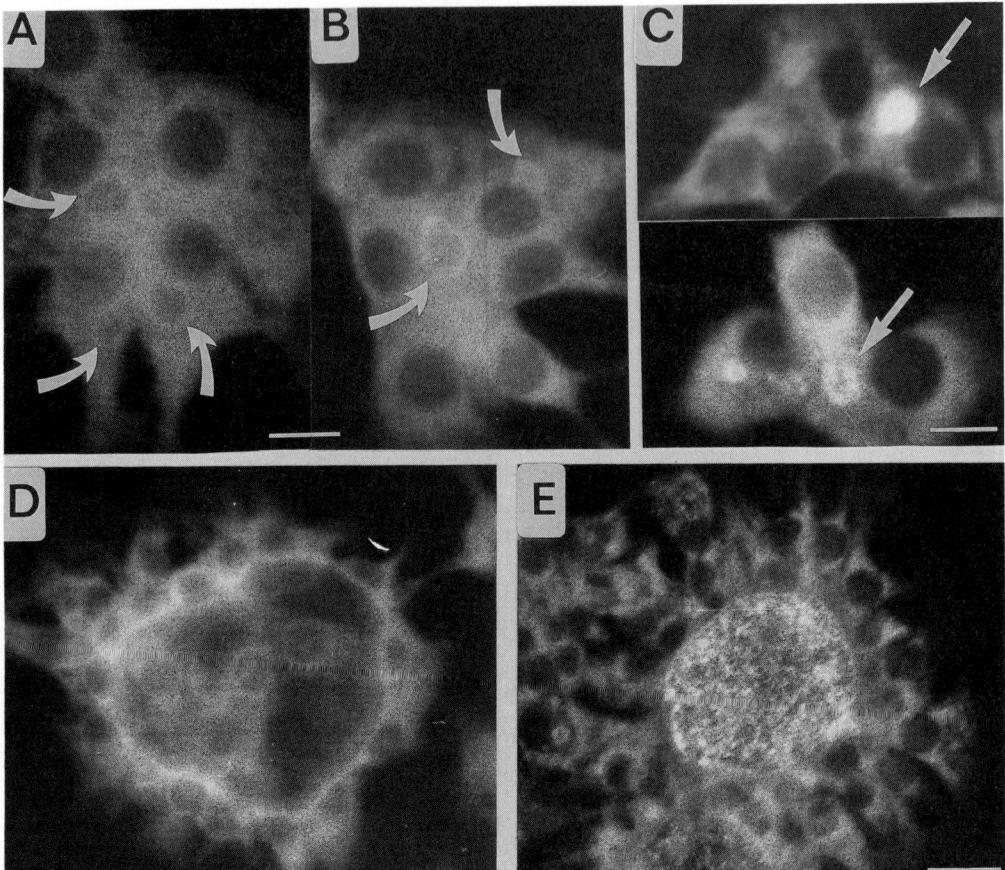

FIGURE 4 : Immunofluorescence staining of thyroid cells in culture with anti-TPO or anti-Tg antibodies. *A, B and C : thyroid cell in monolayer ; D and E : reconstituted thyroid follicles (RTF) exhibiting a well-defined lumen (IL). The antibodies used were : rabbit polyclonal anti-pig TPO antibodies (A, B and D) and rabbit polyclonal anti-pig Tg antibodies (C and E). Arrows identify intracellular vacuoles, probably ICL, the circumference of which is faintly stained by anti-TPO antibodies (bended arrows) in A and B. The same type of structures are heavily labeled with anti-Tg antibodies in C. Bars: 5 µm in A, B and C ; 10 µm in D and E.*

The distribution of TPO and Tg in thyroid cells cultured as monolayers or RTF was studied by indirect immunofluorescence. As shown on fig. 4A, B and C, intracellular vacuoles probably ICL are present in thyroid cell monolayer. Interestingly, the contour of these structures appear slightly TPO positive whereas the interior was Tg-positive. A diffuse fluorescence was also observed over the cells both with anti-Tg and anti-TPO antibodies. Panels D and E of fig. 4 show the TPO and Tg distribution in RTF. Anti-TPO antibodies delineated the contour of IL whereas anti-Tg antibodies labeled the interior of the IL. Since RTF are formed from non-polarized isolated cells exhibiting TPO on their entire surface, it was of interest to determine whether the reconstitution of follicles involving the re-polarization of thyroid cells (fig. 5A) was accompanied by a plasma membrane redistribution of TPO. The immunogold labeling of fig. 5B demonstrates the

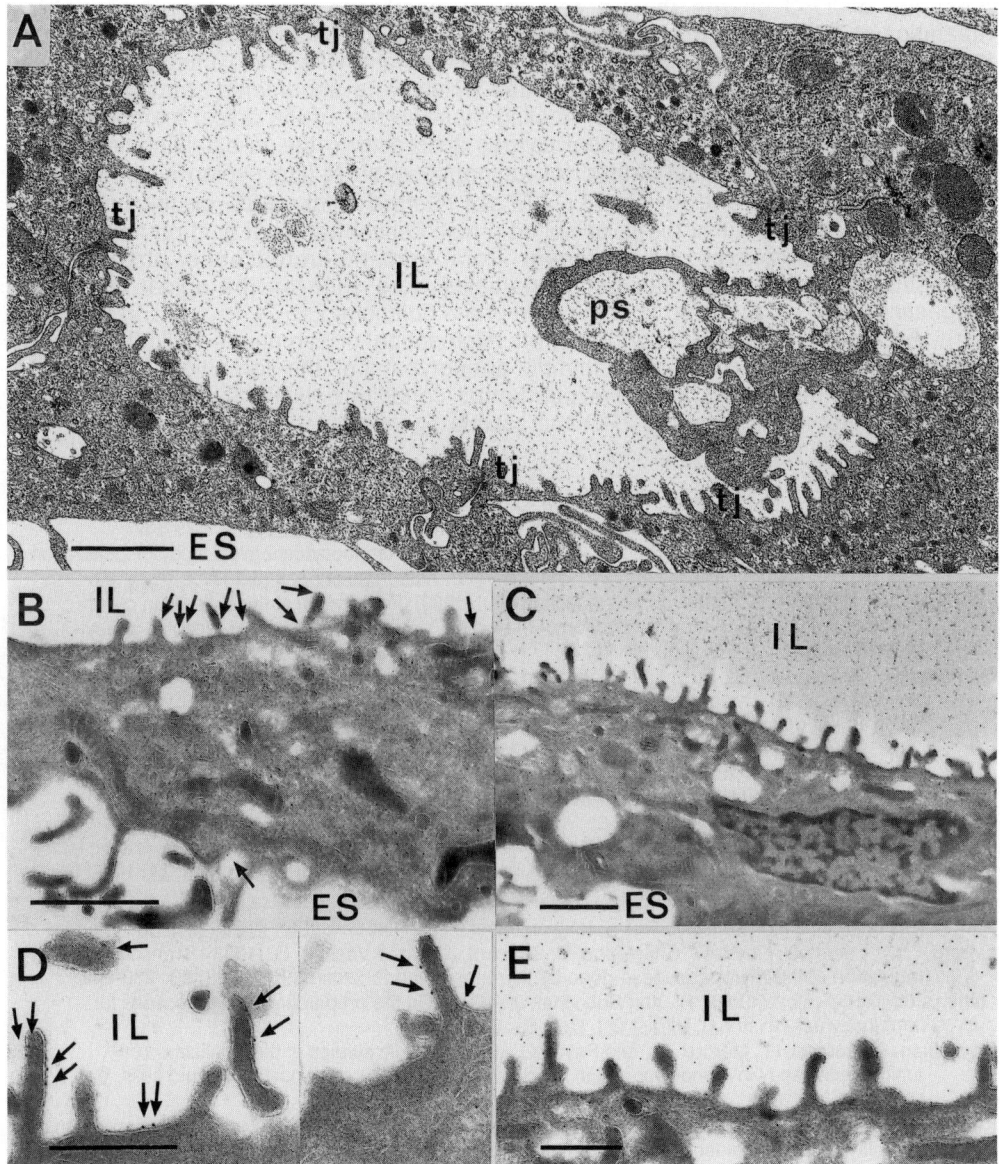

FIGURE 5 : **Electron microscope immunolocalization of TPO and Tg in the lumen (IL) of in vitro reconstituted thyroid follicles.** Overall structure of the IL observed on ultrathin section prepared from Epon embedded sample (A). Note the presence of tight junctions (tj) ; microvilli and a pseudopode (ps). Immunogold labeling on cryosections with anti-TPO antibodies (B and D) or anti-Tg antibodies (C and E). ES : extracellular space. Arrows identify gold particle TPO-anti TPO antibody complexes on the apical plasma membrane. Bars : 1 μm in A, B and C ; 500 nm in D and E.

presence of TPO on the thyroid cell apical membrane and a clear asymmetrical repartition of TPO between basal and apical surface of the polarized cells. It was counted that the density of labeling for TPO on apical membrane was 7 to 10 times higher than that on the basal membrane. Pseudopodes which were uncommun structures in RTF exhibited a substantially lower TPO labeling than the rest of the apical membrane. The re-localization of thyroid membrane enzymes according to the re-establishment of the cell polarity has been demonstrated for aminopeptidase N (Hovsepian et al, 1982) on the apical membrane and for Na^+/K^+ ATPase (Gerard et al, 1985) on the basolateral membranes. The interior of the IL exhibited a high concentration of gold particle Tg-anti-Tg antibody complexes as expected from immunofluorescence observations. Interestingly, a rather high number of particles were seen on the apical membrane suggesting that Tg could bind to some membrane components.

All together these immunoelectron microscope observations indicate that the expression of the morphological thyroid phenotype, i.e. the formation of ICL or IL compartments depending on the experimental conditions, is tightly coupled with the vectorial transport of membrane TPO and soluble Tg towards these compartments.

REFERENCES

Alquier, C., Guenin, P., Munari-Silem, Y., Audebet, C., and Rousset, B. (1985): Isolation of pig thyroid lysosomes. Biochemical and morphological characterization. Biochem. J. 232: 529-537.

Alquier, C., Ruf, J., Athouel-Haon, A.M., and Carayon, P. (1989): Immunocytochemical study of localization and traffic of thyroid peroxidase/microsomal antigen. Autoimmunity 3: 113-123.

Chambard, M., Verrier, B., Gabrion, J., and Mauchamp, J. (1983): Polarization of thyroid cells in culture : Evidence for the basolateral localization of the iodide "pump" and of the TSH receptor-adenyl-cyclase complex. J. Cell Biol. 96: 1172-1177.

Damante, G., Chazenbalk, G., Russo, D., Rappaport, B., Foti, D., and Filotti, S. (1989): TSH regulation of thyroid peroxidase messenger ribonucleic acid levels in cultured rat thyroid cells. Evidence for the involvement of a non transcriptional mechanism. Endocrinology 124: 2889-2894.

Durrieu, C., Bernier-Valentin, F., and Rousset, B. (1987): Binding of glyceraldehyde 3-phosphate dehydrogenase to microtubules. Mol. Cell. Biochem. 74: 55-65.

Ekholm, R., and Björkman, U. (1984): Localization of iodine binding in the thyroid gland in vitro. Endocrinology 115: 1558-1567.

Fayet, G., Michel-Bechet, M., and Lissitzky, S. (1971): TSH-induced aggregation and reorganization into follicles of isolated porcine thyroid cells. II. Ultrastructural studies. Eur. J. Biochem. 24: 100-111.

Gerard, C., Gabrion, J., Verrier, B., Reggio, H., and Mauchamp, J. (1985): Localization of the Na^+/K^+ ATPase and of an amiloride sensitive Na^+ uptake on thyroid epithelial cells. Eur. J. Cell Biol. 38: 134-141.

Gerard, C.M., Lefort, A., Libert, F., Christophe, D., Dumont, J.E., and Vassart, G. (1988): Transcriptional regulation of the thyroperoxidase gene by thyrotropin and forskolin. FEBS Lett. 60: 239-242.

Griffiths, G., McDowall, A., Back, R., and Dubochet, J. (1984): On the preparation of cryosections for immunocytochemistry. J. Ultrastruct. Res. 89: 65-78.

Hovsepian, S., Feracci, H., Maroux, S., and Fayet, G. (1982): Kinetic studies of the localization of aminopeptidase N in monolayer and in follicle-associated cultures of porcine thyroid cells. Cell Tissue Res. 224: 601-611.

Kerkof, P.R., Long, P.J., and Chaikoff, I.L. (1964): In vitro effect of TSH. I. On the pattern of organization of monolayer cultures of isolated sheep thyroid gland cells. Endocrinology 74: 170-179.

Lissitzky, S., Fayet, G., Giroud, A., Verrier, B., and Torresani, J. (1971): Thyrotropin-induced aggregation and reorganization into follicles of isolated bovine thyroid cells. I. Mechanism of action of TSH and metabolic properties. Eur. J. Biochem. 24: 88-99.

Munari-Silem, Y., Champier, J., Riou, J.P., Audebet, C., Rabilloud, R., and Rousset, B. (1986): Cyclic AMP-dependent phosphorylation of high molecular mass proteins in pig thyroid cells. Mol. Cell. Endocrinol. 44: 251-260.

Munari-Silem, Y., Mesnil, M., Bernier-Valentin, F., Rabilloud, R., and Rousset, B. (1990): Cell-cell interactions in the process of differentiation of thyroid epithelial cells into follicles. A study by microinjection and fluorescence microscopy on in vitro reconstituted thyroid follicles (submitted).

Remy, L., Michel-Bechet, M., Cataldo, C., Bottini, J., Hovsepian, S., and Fayet, G. (1977): The role of intracellular lumina in thyroid cells for follicle morphogenesis in vitro. J. Ultrastruct. Res. 61: 243-253.

Rousset, B., Poncet, C., and Mornex, R. (1976): Thyroxine secretion by isolated hog thyroid cells. Biochim. Biophys. Acta 437: 543-561.

Rousset, B., Munari, Y., Rostagnat, A., and Mornex, R. (1977): Thyroxine secretion by isolated hog thyroid cells. A cyclic AMP-independent pathway. Mol. Cell. Endocrinol. 9: 33-43.

Rousset, B., Poncet, C., Dumont, J.E., and Mornex, R. (1980a): Intracellular and extracellular sites of iodination in dispersed hog thyroid cells. Biochem. J. 192: 801-812.

Rousset, B., and Wolff, J. (1980b): Lactoperoxidase-tubulin interaction. J. Biol. Chem. 255: 2514-2523.

Rousset, B., and Mornex, R. (1981): Identification of an intracellular pathway of thyroxine synthesis by dispersed thyroid cells. Biochim. Biophys. Acta 675: 8-18.

Rousset, B., Authelet, M., Munari-Silem, Y., Dumont, J.E., and Neve, P. (1985): Formation of intracellular lumina in dispersed pig thyroid cells. Eur. J. Cell. Biol. 39: 432-442.

Rousset, B., Selmi, S., Alquier, C., Bourgeat, P., Orelle, B., Audebet, C., Rabilloud, R., Bernier-Valentin, F., and Munari-Silem, Y. (1989a): In vitro studies of the thyroglobulin pathway. Biochimie 71: 247-262.

Rousset, B., Selmi, S., Bornet, H., Bourgeat, P., Rabilloud, R., and Munari-Silem, Y. (1989b): Thyroid hormone residues are released from thyroglobulin with only limited alteration of the thyroglobulin structure. J. Biol. Chem. 264: 12620-12626.

Selmi, S., and Rousset, B. (1988): Identification of two subpopulations of thyroid lysosomes. Relation to the thyroglobulin proteolytic pathway. Biochem. J. 253: 523-532.

Tice, L.W., and Wollman, S.H. (1974): Ultrastructural localization of peroxidase on pseudopods and other structures of the typical thyroid epithelial cells. Endocrinology 94: 1555-1567.

Résumé

La thyroperoxydase (TPO) est une enzyme membranaire qui serait transportée sélectivement vers le domaine apical de la membrane plasmique des cellules thyroïdiennes épithéliales, où elle catalyse la formation des hormones thyroïdiennes au sein des molécules de thyroglobuline. En utilisant des anticorps polyclonaux anti-TPO et la technique d'immunofluorescence ou des immunomarquages aux particules d'or sur des coupes ultrafines à congélation, nous avons étudié la localisation de la TPO à différents stades de l'expression in vitro du phénotype polarisé des cellules thyroïdiennes. La TPO immunoréactive a été trouvée dans des compartiments intracellulaires mais aussi assez homogènement distribuée tout autour des cellules fraîchement isolées à partir de tissu thyroïdien. L'incubation de cellules isolées en suspension en présence de TSH conduit à la formation de lumières intracellulaires (ICL) qui contiennent de la thyroglobuline (Tg); la membrane délimitant les ICL, ainsi que les très nombreuses microvillosités portent de la TPO. L'apparition de TPO dans les ICL s'accompagne d'une réduction de la TPO localisée sur la membrane plasmique. Des structures de type ICL, contenant Tg et TPO, sont observées occasionnellement dans les cellules thyroïdiennes cultivées en monocouches. Les cellules thyroïdiennes cultivées en présence de TSH se réorganisent en structures folliculaires : les follicules thyroïdiens reconstitués (RTF) qui présentent une lumière intrafolliculaire (IL) complètement close. Les études en immunofluorescence et immunomarquage à l'or montrent : a) l'accumulation de grandes quantités de Tg dans les IL des RTF et b) la présence de TPO sur la membrane délimitant les IL néoformés (préférentiellement près ou sur les microvillosités). Dans les RTF, la distribution de la TPO membranaire est clairement polarisée. Ces données montrent que la morphogénèse des ICL ou des IL in vitro, qui est contrôlée par TSH, est couplée avec le transport vectoriel de TPO membranaire et de Tg soluble pour la reconstitution d'un compartiment fonctionnel pour la synthèse des hormones thyroïdiennes.

Microscopic imaging of human thyroid hormonosynthesis : digital correlation of ion and optical microscopic images

P. Fragu[(1)], S. Halpern[(1)], J.C. Olivo[(2)] and E. Kahn[(2)]

INSERM U.66, [(1)] Equipe de Microscopie Ionique, [(2)] Equipe de Méthodologie de l'Imagerie Biologique, Institut Gustave-Roussy, 39, rue Camille Desmoulins, 94805 Villejuif Cedex, France

Most of the data on thyroid hormonosynthesis has been obtained from biochemical studies (Taurog 1986). The respective roles of iodine, thyroglobulin (Tg), peroxidase, and TSH have been progressively evidenced with the development of technical approaches more and more sensitive : chemistry, immunology, radioimmunology, molecular biology. In human, qualitative mapping of these different parameters has been also developed : evaluation of exchangeable iodine pool with radioiodine (Studer et al. 1989), and localisation of TSH receptor by autoradiography, (Schmid et al. 1988) detection of Tg and peroxidase by immunohistochemistry (De Micco 1989), and of their mRNA messengers by in situ hybridization (Berge Lefranc et al. 1983).

More recently the analytical ion microscope (AIM) has been used for direct imaging and relative quantification of organified ^{127}I in human thyroid tissue (Fragu et al. 1989). Futhermore the development of an original image processing system in our laboratory (Olivo et al. 1989) allowed to combine different microscopic approaches (ion and optical) of thyroid tissue and to study in situ the capacity of thyroid cell to express Tg gene, to synthetize Tg and to iodinate it.

I - Analytical ion microscopy

Principle : AIM is based on secondary ion mass spectrometry (SIMS) (Fig.1). A primary ion beam is focused onto the surface of a resin embedded biological tissue section (2 - 3 µm thickness). Under ion bombardment the atoms of the most superficial molecular layer (1-5nm) of the specimen are progressively sputtered ; some of them are ionized. These secondary ions, characteristic of the atomic composition of the analyzed area, are focused and energy filtered. The different ion species are separated by a mass spectrometer. An analytical image of the selected element is displayed on a fluorescent screen ; the selected secondary ion beam intensity can also be measured with an electron multiplier. Thus, AIM is a quantitative method of microscopic imaging of thyroid gland.

Elemental Imaging : Direct ion imaging is performed on areas from 25 to 400 µm in diameter. A mass resolution ($M/\Delta M \geq 2000$) is used in order to eliminate interferences between cluster ions and the specific ion studied (Halpern et al. 1988). The main advantage of AIM is its capacity to preserve elemental mapping in relation with histological structure which is defined by the distribution of ^{31}P associated with the cell nuclear DNA and the phosphorylated cytoplasmic molecules (Fig.2). A microcomputer based digital imaging system achieving acquisition at low light level has been developed (Olivo et al. 1989). It includes a high sensitivity video camera connected to a specialized image processor subsystem. Acquired images consists of 512 x 512 pixels with 8 bits accuracy. Real time image processing software has been implemented. Allowing on and off-line superimposition of 2 or 3 ion images (Fig. 2D).

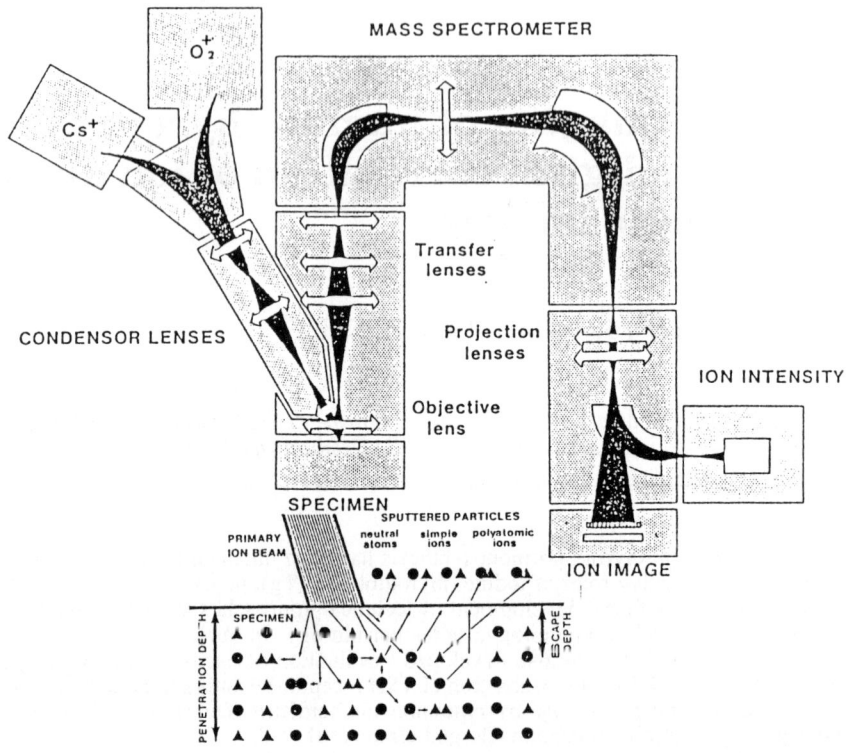

Fig.1. Scheme of the CAMECA IMS 3F. The instrument is fitted with a Cs+ primary ion source which increases the sensitivity and the detection limits of electronegative elements : i.e. hydrogen, phosphorus and halogens. The mass resolution is adjustable from 200 to 10,000 and the lateral resolution is 0.5 µm. The analyzed area varies from 1.5 to 400 µm in diameter.

Elemental quantification : As computerized images do not directly reflect the exact elemental concentration, quantitative evaluation is performed using the electron multiplier which allows the measurement of the secondary ion beam intensity on small areas (1.5 - 8 µm) of histological structure with adapted apertures. In SIMS, there is a direct relationship for a given element A between the secondary ion beam current I_A and the analyzed elemental concentration C_A :

$$I_A = C_A \cdot S \cdot Y_A \cdot I_p$$

S = analyzed surface ; Y_A = useful yield ; Ip = primary ion beam current.

However, when dealing with insulating specimens such as biological samples, electronegative ion extraction ($^{12}C^-$, $^{31}P^-$, $^{127}I^-$, ...) creates a build-up of positive charges repelling the primary electropositive Cs+ ion beam. The real ion beam intensity Ip is unknown and the relation between I_A and C_A is not directly applicable. Nevertheless, a relative quantitative approach is possible by measuring the intensity I_R of an internal reference R, such as carbon, present in a large homogeneous and constant concentration in the specimen. Then $I_A/I_R = K \cdot C_A$. With the use of an iodine standard curve established with an iodized resin (Telenczak et al. 1989) it is possible to express the results of measurements in ^{127}I µg/mg of thyroid within the analyzed area (cell or colloid). The specific detectable minimum (Resin background + 3SD) is $3.12 \cdot 10^{-4}$ µg/mg. Figure 3 shows the results of measurements of ^{127}I concentration in human thyroid follicle (Fragu et al. 1989).

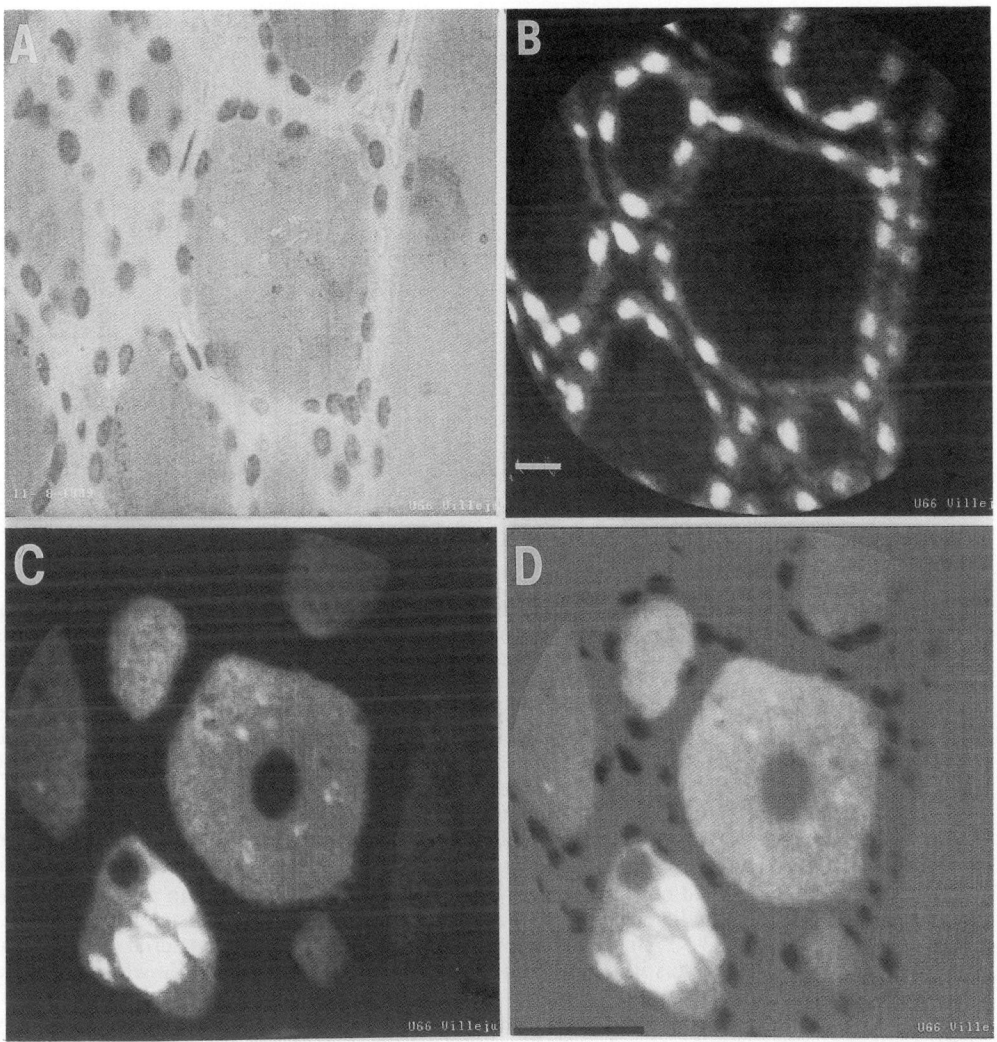

Fig.2. Computerized Ion images of human thyroid tissue. The histological structure (A) is given by phosphorus distribution (B). Iodine (C) is directly visualized on the same area. Computerized images of iodine mapping can be superimposed onto that of ^{31}P (D) and compared on serial section with the Tg mapping revealed by immunohistochemistry (A).

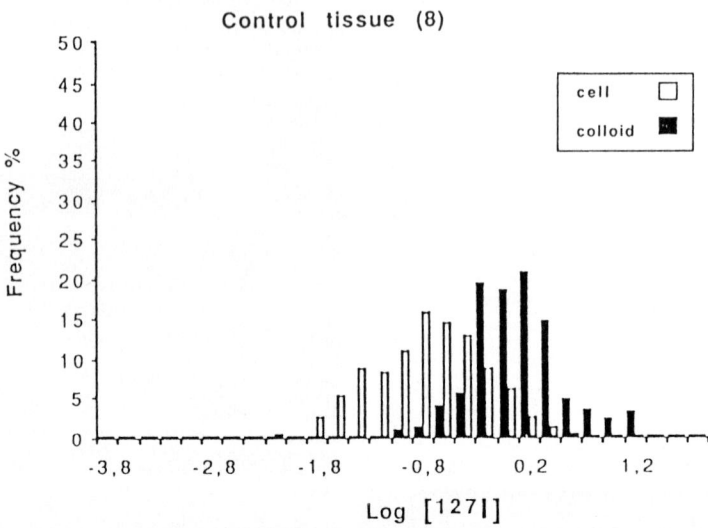

Fig.3. ^{127}I concentration within thyroid follicle in normal tissue. For each tissue, the analyses (mean of 10 measurements of the same area) were performed in 30 follicular lumina and 30 follicules cells selected from phosphorus images with adapted apertures.

Sample preparation : The chemical fixation methods are very suited to preserving localization and local concentration of element bound to macromolecules as for example iodine bound to Tg (Rognoni et Simon 1974). Then the sample must be embedded in metacrylate resin in order to obtain perfectly plan section which are deposited on gold holder for AIM analysis.

For the study of the diffusible elements, the specimen needs to be cryofixed to arrest physiological processes and cryopreparative techniques are necessary to prevent movement of the elements during specimen preparation (Wroblewski et al. 1988). High speed freezing of the tissue (5000 K sec^{-1}-) can be carried out in surgery room by plunging the specimen in a liquid cooland (liquid propane subscooled by liquid nitrogen). Freeze substitution is the second step in which water is replaced by acetone at 183 K. After embedding in lowycril resin at 213 K, material can be cut at room temperature for AIM. Thus it is possible to evaluate by AIM the role of Ca which seems to regulate $H_2 O_2$ generating system in iodination process (Dupuy et al. 1989) as well as the role of unbound iodine in thyroid disease. Furthermore this technique enhances the immunohistochemistry quality in preserveting most of molecule antigens.

II - Digital correlation of ion and optical microscopic images

In order to relate the modifications of chemical distribution to molecule maps, a digital correlation method has been developed which allows to superimpose ion and optical microscopic images. This method has been used to assess the heterogeneous iodination and sulfuration of this protein within human pathological tissue. Two serial sections, (2 µm thick), are obtained from a chemically fixed thyroid sample. One section is analyzed by AIM and produces a serie of images showing different chemical distributions. The second one is treated by immunohistochemistry in order to reveal thyroglobulin. Ion and optical images are correlated by means of a registration algorithm based on cell position. This algorithm combines an affine global transformation and an elastic transformation which are necessary to correct for geometrical distorsions introduced by the ion microscope (Olivo et al. 1990). Preliminary results suggest major modifications of the Tg chemical composition from one follicle to another in human pathological tissue. Futhermore these modifications can be related to the images of thyroperoxidase revealed by immunohistochemistry or mRNA messagers of Tg or thyroperoxidase revealed by in situ hybridization.

In the next future, this unique and original methodology will allow, in the one hand, to combine different microscopic in situ approaches of a thyroid tissue and, in the second hand, to display on the same image, structural and functional information.

REFERENCES

Berge-Lefranc J.L., Cartouzou G., Bignon C., Lissitzky S. (1983) : Quantitative in situ hybridisation of ^{3}H labeled complementary dexoxyribonucleic acid (cDNA) to the messenger ribonucleacid of thyroglobulin in human thyroid tissues. J. Clin. Endocrinol. Metab. 57, 470-476.

De Micco C., (1989) : Immunohistochimie des carcinomes thyroidiens. I carcinomes d'origine vesiculaire et tumeurs indifférenciées. Ann. Pathol. 9, 233-240.

Dupuy C., Kaniewski J., Deme D., Pommier J., Virion A. (1989) : NA DPH-dependant $H_2 O_2$ generation catalyzed by thyroid plasma membranes. Studies with electron scavengers. Europ J. Bruchem, 185, 597-603.

Fragu P., Briançon C., Noel M., Halpern S. (1989) : Imaging and relative quantification of ^{127}I in human thyroid follicle by analytical ion microscope : characterization of benign thyroid epithelial tumors. J. Clin. Endocrinol. Metab.69 : 304-309.

Halpern S., Fragu P., Briançon C., Larras-Regard E. (1988) : Contribution of the high mass resolution in trace elements imaging in biology. In : Secondary ion mass spectrometry (SIMS VI), A Benninghoven, M Huber, HW Werner, pp 897-900, Chichester (England), : John Wiley and sons.

Olivo J.C., Kahn E., Halpern S., Briançon C., Fragu P., Di Paola R. (1989) : Microcomputer system for ion microscopy digital imaging and processing. J. Microscopy, 156 : 105-114.

Olivo J.C., Kahn E., Halpern S., Fragu P., Di Paola R. (1990) : Ion and light microscopic images superimposition and correlation.SPIE Image Processing III, 1989, pp 56-61.

Rognogni J.B., Simon C. (1974) : Critical analysis of the glutaraldehyde fixation of the thyroid gland : a double labelling experiment. J. Microp. 21, 119-128.

Schmid K.W., Jasani B., Morgan J.M., Williams E.D., (1988) : Light microscopic immunocytochemical demonstration of thyroid stimulating hormone (TSH) receptors on normal rat thyroid cells. J. Histochem. cytochem. 36, 977-982.

Studer H, Peter H.J, Gerber H : (1988 : Natural heterogeneity of thyroid cells ; the basis for understanding thyroid function and nodular goiter growth. Endorc. Rev., 10, 125-145.

Taurog A., (1986) : Hormone synthesis ; thyroid iodine metabolism. In : Werner's : the thyroid gland, eds SH Ingbar, IE Braverman, pp 53-97, Philadelphia (USA) : Lippincott.

Telenczak P., Bessode M., Ricard M., Halpern S., Fragu P (1989) : Quantification de l'iode par microscopie ionique analytique (MIA). CR Acad Sci. 308 série D : 479-484.

Wroblewski J, Wroblewski R, Roomans C.M.(1988) : Low temperature techniques for X-ray microanalysis in Pathology : alternative to cryoultramicrotomy. J. Elect. Micr. Techn. 9 : 83-95.

Acknowledgments : we thank Mrs Dupont and Omri for their help in the manuscript preparation.

Résumé

Depuis ces 10 dernières années, le développement des techniques immunohistochimiques en microscopie optique et électronique a donné une nouvelle dimension à l'étude des tissus thyroïdiens normaux et pathologiques. Il est maintenant possible de révéler la distribution tissulaire des principales molécules impliquées dans la synthèse des hormones thyroïdiennes : thyroglobuline (Tg), peroxydase, T3 et T4, grâce à l'utilisation d'anticorps monoclonaux spécifiques dirigés contre leurs sites antigéniques. Par ailleurs, l'hybridation in situ permet l'étude des modifications de l'expression génique au niveau transcriptionnel par l'évaluation quantitative des messagers de Tg de la peroxydase, de calcitonine et dans un avenir très proche du récepteur à la TSH. Bien que le métabolisme thyroïdien soit étroitement lié à celui de l'iode, il n'existait jusqu'à ces dernières années aucune méthode d'évaluation directe de l'iode stable (^{127}I) au niveau tissulaire. Les méthodes autoradiographiques lorsqu'elles sont réalisées après une injection unique d'iode radioactif (^{125}I, ^{131}I), n'évaluent que l'iode renouvelable. Elles sont en pratique peu utilisées dans le diagnostic microscopique des maladies thyroïdiennes. La microscopie ionique analytique (MIA) qui permet d'obtenir une cartographie quantitative des éléments chimiques présents dans un échantillon biologique donne directement la distribution tissulaire d'^{127}I. De plus, le développement d'un système de traitement d'images microscopiques permet de corréler, à partir de coupes sériées, les informations chimiques élémentaires fournies par la MIA aux informations moléculaires données par l'immunohistochimie, ouvrant la voie à des possibilités d'investigation entièrement nouvelles. Il est en effet maintenant possible de corréler les variations de concentration de l'iode, à la capacité de synthèse de son support protéique la Tg, et à sa capacité d'iodation par la peroxydase thyroïdienne.

TPO as marker of malignancy in thyroid tumors : immunohistochemical study

C. de Micco, J. Ruf, M.A. Chrestian, N. Gros, J.F. Henry and P. Carayon

Laboratoire d'Anatomie Pathologique et INSERM U.38, Faculté de Médecine, 27 Bd J. Moulin, 13385 Marseille Cedex 05, France

RESUME

La fixation de deux anticorps monoclonaux spécifiques de la TPO, appelés respectivement mAb30 et mAb47 a été étudiée par immunocytochimie sur des échantillons de 65 carcinomes thyroïdiens, 70 adénomes et 10 cas de maladie de Basedow. Le mAb30 se fixe normalement sur tous les tissus bénins et 75 % des tissus carcinomateux. Avec le mAb47 la détection de TPO est réduite ou négative dans 96,9 % des tumeurs malignes mais normale dans 94,2 % des tumeurs bénignes. Ces résultats montrent que la TPO des tumeurs thyroïdiennes malignes comporte une anomalie immunologique décelable par immunocytochimie. Cette anomalie est présente avec une fréquence suffisante pour servir de marqueur de malignité utilisable en histopathologie diagnostique.

INTRODUCTION

The histopathological diagnosis of malignancy in well differentiated thyroid tumors is unreliable in about 5 to 15 % of the cases (De Micco 1989a). A broad range of thyroid associated antigens can easily be investigated in these tumors by immunohistochemistry (De Micco 1989b) but, to date, none of these antigens is able to discriminate malignant from benignant tumors. A decrease in TPO activity was previously reported in about 50 % of malignant thyroid tumors by biochemical analysis (Valenta et al., 1973, Nagasaka et al., 1975, Fragu et al., 1977, Mizukami et al., 1981, Valenta et al., 1977) and histochemistry (Yamashita et al., 1987). By histochemistry however, the TPO activity can be disclosed only at the ultrastructural level. This prompted us to study possible alterations of TPO in thyroid tumors by immunohistochemistry on histological sections.

METHODS AND RESULTS

In the course of studies on microsomal antigen and TPO (Ruf et al., 1987), monoclonal antibodies (mAb) to TPO were produced and characterized (Ruf et al., 1989). Ten mAb directed against various TPO antigenic sites were applied

on paraffin-embedded sections of various thyroid tissues and their fixation was evidenced by the avidin-biotin-peroxidase complex method as previously reported (De Micco et al., 1987). Two mAb, termed mAb30 and mAb47, were selected for their clear cut fixation on normal thyroid tissue and then characterized on other tissues to assess their specificity. This specificity was restricted to the thyroid for mAb47 whereas mAb30 also produced slight reactions on bone marrow cells, some glandular epithelial cells, muscular and glial cells. First results on tumors showed that mAb47 failed to react with most malignant thyroid tumors and thus could serve as marker of malignancy in these tumors (De Micco et al., 1988). We subsequently performed a systematic study of the fixation of mAb30 and mAb47 on various pathological thyroid tissues to confirm and extend these data. This study concerned specimens of 145 surgically removed pathological thyroid glands (43 papillary carcinoma, 22 follicular carcinoma, 25 colloïd adenoma, 25 foetal adenoma, 10 oncocytoma, 10 toxic adenoma and 10 cases of Graves'disease). Tumors were classified separately by two pathologists according to the W.H.O. (Hedinger, 1988). Adjacent normal thyroid tissue was used as positive control.
The number of cases with normal, reduced or negative fixation of mAb47 are presented in the following table :

HISTOLOGY	mAb47 Fixation		mAb30 Fixation	
	Normal	Reduced or Negative	Normal	Reduced or Negative
CARCINOMA				
Papillary	0	43	18	8
Follicular	2	20	3	7
ADENOMA				
Follicular	25	0	25	0
Foetal	22	3	25	0
Oncocytoma	10	0	10	0
Toxic	9	1	10	0
GRAVES'DISEASE	10	0	10	0

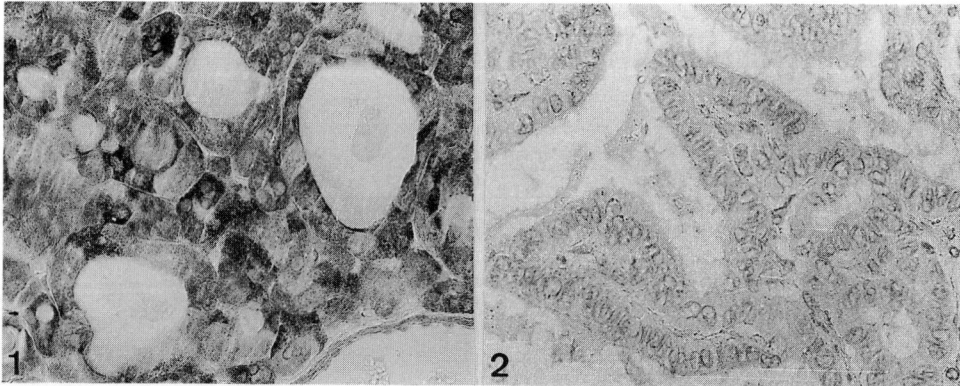

Fig. 1 : Positive detection of TPO with mAb47 in an oncocytic adenoma. Fig. 2 : With the same mAb47, negative reaction in a papillary thyroid carcinoma.

The staining in normal tissue was always diffuse, finely granular, cytoplasmic for mAb47, sometimes concentrated along cytoplasmic or nuclear membranes for mAb30. All hypersecreting tissues (Graves'disease, toxic adenoma), colloïd adenoma and oncocytoma (Fig. 1) exhibited intensely positive reactions with both mAb even in areas showing atypical features on histological examination : papillary formations resulting from degenerative changes always appeared deeply stained. Results in foetal adenoma were more inconstant with mAb47 : one case was negative and two others gave pale reactions. In all papillary carcinoma and 70 % of follicular carcinoma the TPO was found with mAb30. The staining however was lower than normal in 30 % of the papillary and 40 % of the follicular carcinoma. With mAb47 the reaction was negative in 90,7 % of the papillary (Fig. 2) and 68,1 % of the follicular carcinoma and feeble in 4 papillary and 5 follicular carcinoma, so that only 3,1 % of all malignant tumors produced a significantly positive reaction.

DISCUSSION

The presence of TPO in pathological thyroid tissues was studied by immunohistochemistry with two mAb directed against two different antigenic sites of the TPO molecule. These two mAb yielded strikingly different results. With mAb30, the TPO is detected in all benignant tumors just as in normal tissues ; in malignant tissues the reaction is reduced or negative in about 40 % of the cases : these results are consistent with those previously found by histochemistry (Yamashita et al., 1987).
With mAb47, the TPO is also normally found in most benignant tumors but not in 96,9 % of malignant tumors : comparison of the results obtained with both mAb suggests that the TPO is usually present in neoplastic tissues, often at a lowered level, but that it presents antigenic changes and thus cannot be recognized by some mAb as mAb47. Such alterations of TPO in neoplastic tissues have already been suspected by biochemical and enzyme-linked immunosorbent assay analysis (Neary et al. 1978 ; Hamada et al., 1987).
The failure of mAb47 to detect TPO in malignant thyroid tissues is of interest in diagnostic histopathology : it is in accordance with the histological diagnosis of malignancy in 95,6 % of the cases. The discrepancy between a lowered or negative mAb47 test and a histological diagnosis of benignancy in 3 cases of foetal adenoma is not surprising as the biological frontiere between foetal adenoma and encapsulated follicular carcinoma is not clear : in these cases the modification of TPO detected by mAb47 could be related to a progression toward a preinvasive malignant state. In tumors with papillary formations, the distinction "benignant/malignant" was clear-cut : the papillae of benignant conditions reacted always with mAb47 whereas those in carcinoma were negative. The most puzzling are cases of histologically malignant tumors with positive mAb47 test (false negative for the diagnosis of malignancy). As they represent less than 2 % of all the cases one can accept mAb47 as a reasonably good marker of malignancy in thyroid tumors, to be used in conjonction with standard histological examination.

REFERENCES

De Micco, C. (1989a) Immunohistochimie des carcinomes thyroïdiens I. Carcinomes d'origine vésiculaire et tumeurs indifférenciées. Ann Pathol 4:233-248.

De Micco, C. (1989b) Carcinomes thyroïdiens différenciés d'origine folliculaire : faits nouveaux en 1988. Arch Anat Cytol Path 37:21-27.

De Micco, C., Ruf, J., Carayon, P., Chrestian, M.A., Henry, J.F., Toga, M. (1987) Immunohistochemical study of thyroglobulin in thyroid carcinomas with monoclonal antibodies. Cancer 59:471-476.

De Micco, C., Ruf, J., Chrestian, M.A., Gros, N., Henry, J.F., Audiffret, J., Toga, M. (1988) Immunohistochemical study of thyroid peroxidase in thyroid neoplastic disorders. Ann Endocrinol 1988, 3:194 (Abst).

Fragu, P., Nataf, B.M. (1977) Human thyroid peroxidase in benign and malign thyroid disorders. J Clin Endocrinol Metab 45:1089-1096.

Hamada, N., Yamakawa, J., Hinotani, A., Ohno, M., Morii, H., Noh, J., Ito, K., Portmann, L. (1987) Analysis of thyroid microsomal antigen in various thyroid disease (Abstr). Ann Endocrinol 48:145.

Hedinger, C. (1988) Histological typing of thyroid tumours. In : Hedinger C. International histological classification of tumours, vol. 11. World Health Organization. Springer-Verlag Berlin, Heidelberg.

Mizukami, Y., Matsubara, F. (1981) Correlation between thyroid peroxidase activity and histopathological and ultrastructural changes in various thyroid diseases. Endocrinol Jpn 28:381-389.

Nagasaka, A., Hidaka, H., Ishizuki, Y. (1975) Studies on human iodide peroxidase : its activity in various thyroid disorders. Clin Chim Acta 62:1-4.

Neary, J.T., Nakamura, C., Davidson, B., Soodak, M., Vickery, A.L., Maloof, F. (1978) Studies on membrane-associate nature of human thyroid peroxidase : a difference in the solubility of the enzyme from benign and malignant thyroid tissues. J Clin Endocrinol Metab 46:791-798.

Ruf, J., Czarnocka, B., De Micco, C., Dutoit, C., Ferrand, M., Carayon, P. (1987) Thyroid peroxidase is the organ-specific "microsomal" autoantigen involved in thyroid autoimmunity. Acta Endocrinol (Copenh) suppl 281:49-56.

Ruf, J., Toubert, M.E., Czarnocka, N., Durand-Gorde, J.M., Ferrand, M., Carayon, P. (1989) Relationship between immunological structure and biochemical properties of human thyroid peroxidase. Endocrinology 125:1211-1218.

Valenta, L.J., Michel-Bechet, M. (1977) Ultrastructure and biochemistry of thyroid carcinoma. Cancer 40:284-300.

Valenta, L.J., Valenta, V., Wang, C.A., Vickery, A.L., Caulfield, J., Maloof, F. (1973) Subcellular distribution of peroxidase activity in human thyroid tissue. J Clin Endocrinol Metab 37:560-569.

Yamashita, H., Noguchi, S., Murakami, N., Yokoyama, S., Nakayama, I. (1987) Loss of intracellular peroxidase and anaplastic change of differentiated carcinoma of human thyroid gland. Acta Pathol Jpn 37:425-430.

Long term iodination of thyroglobulin by porcine thyroid cells cultured in porous bottom culture chambers. Regulation by thyrotropin

D. Gruffat, S. Gonzalvez and O. Chabaud

INSERM U. 270, Faculté de Médecine Nord, boulevard P. Dramard, 13326 Marseille Cedex 15, France

Thyroid cells cultured as monolayers on the porous bottom of culture chambers have been shown to express some specific thyroid follicle functions (1-4). This system which allows one independent access to apical and basal media, is suitable for the long term study of polarized processes, as the cells maintain their polarized organization. Iodination of thyroglobulin has been investigated under different culture conditions in the presence or absence of thyrotropin. Apical thyroglobulin accumulation, apical iodide concentration and thyroglobulin iodination have been followed simultaneously. Iodide was added (0.5 µM) to basal medium at various stages : only once for four day incubations and at each medium change or daily for longer experiments. Thyrotropin increased the amount of thyroglobulin secreted into the apical medium (5-6 fold), whereas high basal iodide concentrations (>5 µM) inhibited thyroglobulin secretion by thyrotropin stimulated cells. Thyrotropin increased iodide uptake giving an iodide concentration ratio between apical and basal media of about 5. Thyroglobulin was iodinated only in the apical compartment. Secretion and iodination of thyroglobulin were polarized phenomenons but the polarity of iodination was total whereas the polarity of secretion was only partial. This functional assymetry was maintained up to 29 days. Thyroglobulin iodination was thyrotropin-dependent but the maximal incorporation obtained was never higher than 3,5 atoms/mole. Apical iodide concentrations from 1 to 15 µM, depending on culture conditions, did not increase this value. These results suggest that our culture system is able to reproduce several steps of thyroidal iodide metabolism although there may be other unknown factor that could interfere and reduce the efficiency of thyroglublin iodination.

1. Chambard M., Verrier B., Gabrion J. & Mauchamp J. (1983). J. Cell Biol. 96 : 1172-1177.
2. Chambard M., Mauchamp J. & Chabaud O. (1987). J. Cell Physiol. 133 : 37-45.
3. Chabaud O., Chambard M., Gaudry N. & Mauchamp J. (1988). J. Endocr. 116 : 25-33.
4. Chambard M., Depetris D., Gruffat D., Gonzalvez S,. Mauchamp J. & Chabaud O. (1990). J. Mol. Endocr. "in press".

Inherited defects
Anomalies congénitales

Iodine organification defect. Permanent and transient cases diagnosed early in infancy

J. Léger, N. Hoog and P. Czernichow

Département d'Endocrinologie pédiatrique et Diabète, Hôpital Robert Debré, 48 Boulevard Sérurier, 75019 Paris, France

Most of the published cases of iodine organification defects concern children or young adults with long standing hypothyroidism and goiter.
The systematic screening for congenital hypothyroidism (CH) has changed the clinical picture of the disease. CH is a frequent disease occurring once in every 4000 neonates and is due to various causes. Non genetic CH due to absence or ectopic thyroid gland is by far the most common form of the disease. The prevalence of dyshormogenesis among the various causes of CH is believed to be approximately 20 % (Fisher & Klein, 1981).
Among the congenital anomalies producing defects in the biosynthesis of thyroxine, the organification defect is the most common (Maenpaa, 1972).
Thyroid scintigraphy ^{123}I imaging including a perchlorate washout test has been used in the rapid diagnosis of an organification defect in neonates with CH (Takeushi et al., 1970 ; Cone, 1988).
We report 6 cases of CH due to organification defect. 2 patients had a severe form of hypothyroidism with a complete organification defect. Three of the the cases were transient related to immaturity of iodine organification (Delange et al., 1978 ; Nose et al., 1986). One was euthyroid probably with a partial enzyme defect.

PATIENTS AND METHOD

Five infants were identified between 1980 and 1988 through the neonatal screening program using TSH measurement on filter paper spots. At screening, the TSH level was 85 ± 30 µU/ml (mean ± SEM). Patients were assessed at a mean age of 20 ±7 days (m ± SD) through a complete history, physical and radiological examination, thyroid function tests and thyroid scan (table I). The mean age at the beginning of therapy was 23 ± 8 days.
Thyroxine therapy was initiated at a dosage of 5-8.6 µg/kg/day and the dosage was modified thereafter according to clinical evaluation and thyroid hormone levels (Leger & Czernichow, 1986). Therapy was gradually withdrawn at various ages (Davy et al., 1985) and serum TSH carefully monitored every weeks or months during this period. LT_4 therapy could not be withdrawn in patient 1.
Patient 6 was seen for the first time at the age of 27 months. The FP-TSH was normal at screening. She had a moderately well- compensated hypothyroidism and no treatment was administered.

Serum TSH, T4^t or FT4 , T3^t or FT3, antithyroglobulin and antimicrosomal antibodies were measured by radioimmunoassay with the use of commercial kits. Bone maturation was assessed by measurement of the knee epiphyseal surface as reported previously (Léger & Czernichow, 1989).
For the ^{123}I thyroid uptake and perchlorate discharge tests, 20 µCi ^{123}I was admnistered IV. Thyroidal radioactivity was measured and a thyroid scintigram obtained. Then 400 mg perchlorate was given and thyroidal radioactivity was measured.
Normal subjects have less than a 10% discharge of thyroidal radioiodine after perchlorate administration. In the iodine organification defect, iodine is not organified. The administration of perchlorate within 2 hours after administration of radioiodine is followed by a dramatic drop (between 30 to 90 %) in thyroid radioactivity.

RESULTS

The initial clinical data at the time of diagnosis is shown in Table I. The diagnosis of hypothyroidism (patiens 1 - 5) was established on the basis of high TSH levels and undetectable (cases 1 - 2) or low (cases 3 - 5) T4 levels. Patient 4 presented a goiter but the perchlorate washout test was not performed. His 18 year old brother has been treated for hypothyroidism since the age of one year. Initial thyroid scan including a perchlorate washout test indicated an organification defect. Patient 6 was seen at the age of 27 months because of hypothermia. She was clinically euthyroid but the serum TSH was moderately elevated.
For all the patients at the time of diagnosis, the mother was clinically and biologically euthyroid with no detectable antithyroid antibodies. No history of iodine intoxication was found either during pregnancy or at birth, even if the child was born by cesarean section (n = 2). Serum or urinary iodine was normal. All the patients were full term. None of them was admitted to a neonatal intensive care and no disorders, hypothyroid signs excluded, either at birth or during the neonatal period, were noted.
Iodine intoxication was biologically excluded for all the patients but one (case 5) on whom the dosage was not done.
The evolution of the thyroid function is shown in Table II. During treatment serum TSH levels reverted to normal within two weeks (patients 3 - 5) and after and two five months for patients 1 and 2 respectively. In patient 1 LT$_4$ therapy was maintained. After 43 months, treatment was withdrawn in patient 2. This was followed by a quick rise in serum TSH to 60 µU/ml and the treatment was given again. These patients had a severe form of hypothyroidism related to a complete organification block which remained a cause of permanent hypothyroidism. Patients 3, 4, 5 were treated by L thyroxine for 8 to 23 months. They remained euthyroid during the follow up period of 1 to 5 years after withdrawal of therapy which demonstrated that they had presented a transitory form of hypothyroidism. Partial organification block defect was demonstrated during the neonatal period for patients 3 and 5 and was strongly suspected for patient 4. After therapy withdrawal, these three patients had shown normal thyroid glands both clinically and after thyroid scan. At that time a second perchlorate test was performed and found to be normal even in the brother of patient 4 who remained euthyroid after withdrawal of therapy at the age of 18 years. Patient 6 only received no treatment and was euthyroid after 3 4/12 years.

TABLE I : THYROID PARAMETERS. TSH was measured on filter paper blood spots before five days of age and in serum at diagnosis. Normal values in brackets. Total T_4 (TL) in µg/100 ml (normal value 8 - 14)

CASE NUMBER	TSH (µU/ml) Filter paper (< 30)	TSH (µU/ml) serum (n<3.5)	FT_4 pmol/l (11-28)	FT_3 pmol/l (4.2-11.7)	Perchlorate test % discharge radioiodine (< 10)
1	> 200	> 200	1	0.3	80
2	> 90	> 90	T_4^t:0.2	-	85
3	32	44	10	7,5	30
4	60	60	-	-	-
5	42	294	T_4^t:4.8	-	40
6	<30	7	T_4^t:11.9	-	30

TABLE II : TSH VALUES AFTER THERAPY WITHDRAWAL IN 4 PATIENTS

CASE NUMBER	AGE AT DIAGNOSIS (days)	AGE AT THERAPY WITHDRAWAL (months)	THERAPY WITHDRAWAL Duration (months)	THERAPY WITHDRAWAL TSH* (µU/ml)
2	29	43	2	60
3	27	12	3	3.5
			12	2.9
4	10	8	1	1.1
			24	0.7
5	28	23	1.5	5.2
			5 years	1.8

LT_4 therapy could not be interrupted in patient 1.
Patient 6 was never treated.
* TSH measured in patient off therapy for various period of time.

DISCUSSION

These 6 patients had complete or partial iodine organification block. In this study soon after their birth, five of the six infants had clinical and biochemical features typical of primary thyroid insufficiency which required substitutive L thyroxine therapy. Three of these 5 infants presented a severe hypothyroidism during the fetal period as demonstrated by the severe delay in the bone maturation. Three of them were transient. As demonstrated by clinical and biochemical parameters, they were euthyroid after a 1 to 5 years period of LT4 withdrawal.

In patient 6, in whom the defect was partial, thyroid function was moderately altered with a small goiter and elevated TSH, but since the clinical picture and the plasma T4 were normal, no treatment was undertaken. The first patient with an inborn defect in thyroid hormonogenesis was described in 1950 as having an absent or deficient peroxidase enzyme for oxidizing thyroidal iodine to reactive iodine (Stambury & Hedge, 1950). The complete block in the biosynthesis of thyroxine usually occurs in a severe form of congenital goitrous hypothyroidism while partial enzyme defects in euthyroid or mildly hypothyroid patients with goiter and partial perchlorate induce discharge of radioiodine (Furth et al., 1967). Different organification defects have now been characterized. Peroxidase deficiency or absence has been reported. The nature of the peroxidase defect can be caused by an abnormal peroxidase apoenzyme (Hagen et al., 1971 ; Niepomniszcze et al., 1972 ; Niepomniszcze et al.,1975) or by a deficient peroxidase activity (Niepomniszcze et al., 1973 ; Niepomniszcze et al.,1975). The criterion for differentiation of the two abnormalities is restoration of enzyme activity when peroxidase preparations are preincubated with hematin in vitro. Hematin has no effect if peroxidase is absent, but produces a dramatic restoration of enzyme activity in the apoenzyme prosthetic group defect (Pommier et al., 1976).

Congenital goiter and hypothyroidism with impaired iodine organification but with normal or elevated thyroid peroxidase concentrations have also been described (Pommier et al., 1974 ; Medeiros-Neto et al., 1979). The presence of an endogenous inhibitor or a genetically abnormal thyroid peroxidase or a quantitative defect involving an abnormality in the binding of substrate for oxidation have been discussed (Niepomniszcze et al., 1980; Medeiros-Neto et al., 1982). Deficient organification also occurs in Pendred syndrome which associates deafness, goiter and hypothyroidism. The biochemical defect is not clear. Thyroid peroxidase activity is normal. The cause of deafness is not known.

More recently, transient neonatal hypothyroidism probably related to immaturity of thyroidal iodine organification an detected through newborn screening programs, has been discussed (Nose et al., 1986). These patients had no history of exposure to iodine during fetal or early postnatal life. In our study, 2 of the 3 transient hypothyroidism patients had normal urinary iodine and/or serum iodine during the neonate period. None of these full term infants have an history of iodine intoxication likely to lead to severe iodine-induced hypothyroidism which would require L thyroxine treatment (Leger & Czernichow, 1988).

Delayed maturation of thyroidal peroxidase activity is suggested, as demonstrated by normal discharge perchlorate tests later in life.

At present children with neonatal hypothyroidism are diagnosed early in infancy. A dyshormonogenesis disorder is discussed in the presence of clinical and biological signs of hypothyroidism with a thyroid gland in normal position and usually enlarged.

Once iodine intoxication is excluded the diagnosis of dyshormonogenesis should be envisaged. The iodine perchlorate test is the most appropriate in young children to demonstrate the organification defect. When the diagnosis and therapy is established it should be remembered that this case may be transient. These can be ascertained only by progressive therapy withdrawal after a year of LT4 treatment.

REFERENCES

CONE L., OATES E., VASQUEZ R. : Congenital hypothyroidism : diganostic scintigraphic evaluation of an organification defect. Clinical Nuclear Medicine 1988, 13 : 419-20

DAVY T., DANEMAN D., WALFISH .PG. and EHRLICH R.M. : Congenital hypothyroidism. The effect of stopping treatment at 3 years of age. Am J Dis Child 1985, 139 : 1028-30

DELANGE F., DODION J., WOLTER R., BOURDOUX P., DALHEM A., GLINOER D., ERMANS A.M. : Transient hypothyroidism in the newborn infant. J Pediat 1978, 92 : 974-76

FISHER D.A.,KLEIN A.H. : Thyroid development and disorders of thyroid function in the newborn. New Engl J Med 1981, 12 : 702-10

FURTH E.D., GARVALHO M., VIANNA B.: Familial goiter due to an organification defect in euthyroid siblings. J Clin Endocr 1967, 27 : 1137-40

HAGEN G.A., NIEPOMNISZCZE H., HAIBACH H., BIGAZZI M., HATI R., RAPOPORT B., JIMENEZ C., DE GROTT L., FRAWLEY T. : Peroxidase deficiency in familial goiter with iodine organification defect. N Engl J Med 1971, 285 : 1394-98

LEGER J., CZERNICHOW P. : L'hypothyroïdie congénitale pendant les deux premières années de vie. Evolution des paramètres biologiques et recommandations thérapeutiques. Arch Pédiatr 1986, 33 : 291-95

LEGER J., CZERNICHOW P. : Congenital hypothyroidism : decreased growth velocity in the first weeks of life. Biol Neonate 1989, 55 : 218-23

LEGER J., CZERNICHOW P.: Hypertryorotropinémie néonatale transitoire. Arch Fr Pediatr 1988, 45 : 783-6

MAENPAA J. : Congenital hypothyroidism. Aetiological and clinical aspects. Arch Disease Child 1972, 47 : 914-23

MEDEIROS-NETO G.A., NAKASHIMA T., TAUROG A., KNOBEL M., SIONETTI J.P., MATTAR E. : Congenital goitre and hypothyroidism with impaired iodine organificationand high thyroid peroxidase concentration. Clin Endocrinology 1979, 11 : 123-39

MEDEIROS-NETO G.A., OKAMURA K., CAVALIERE H., TAUROG A., KNOBEL M., BISI H., KALLAS WG., MATTAR E. : Familial thyroid peroxidase defect. Clinical Endocrinology 1982, 17 : 1-14

NIEPOMNISZCZE H., DE GROOT J.L., HAGEN G. A. : Abormal thyroid peroxidase causing ioding organification defect. J Clin Endocri Metal 1972, 34 : 607-16

NIEPOMNISZCZE H., CASTELLS S., DE GROOT L., REFETOFF S., LIM O.S., RAPOPORT B., HATI R. : Peroxidase defect in congenital goiter with complete organification block. J Clin Endocr Metab 1973, 36 : 347-57

NIEPOMNISZCZE H., ROSEMBLOOM A.L., DE GROOT L.J., SJIMAOKA K., REFETOFF S., YAMAMOTO K. : Differenciation of two abnormalities in thyroid peroxidase causing organification defect and goitrous hypothyroidism. Metabolism 1975, 24 : 57-67

NIEPOMNISZCZE H., COLEONI A.H., TARGOVNIK H.M., IORGANSKY S., DEGROSSI O.J. : Congenital goitre due to thyroid peroxidase-iodinase defect. Acta Endocrinologica 1980, 93 : 25-31

NOSE O., HARADA T., MIYAI K., HATA N. and al. : Transient neonatal hypothyroidism probably related to immaturity of thyroidal iodine organification. J Pediatr 1986, 108 : 573-6

POMMIER J., TOURNIAIRE J., RAHMOUN B., DEME D., PALLO D., BORNET H., NUNEZ J. : Thyroid iodine organification defects : a cause with lack of thyroglobulin iodination and a cause without any peroxidase activity. J Clin Endocr Metab 1976, 42 : 319-29

POMMIER J., TOURNIAIRE J., DEME D., CHALENDAR D., BORNET H., NUNEZ J. A. : defective thyroid peroxidase solubilized from a familial goiter with iodine organification defect. J Clin Endocr Metab 1974, 39 : 69-80

STANBURY J.B., HEDGE A.N.: A study of a family of goitrous cretins. J Clin Endocrinol Meta 1950, 10 : 1471-84

TAKEUCHI K., SUZUKI N., HORIUCHI Y. and MASHIMO K. : Significance of Iodine-Perchlorate Discharge Test for detection of iodine organification defect of the thyroid. J Clin Endocrinol 1970, 31 : 144-46

VALENTA J.L., BODE H., VICKERY A.L., GAULFIED J.B., MALOOF F. : Lack of thyroid peroxidase activity as the cause of congenital goitrous hypothyroidism. J Clin Endocr Meta 1973, 36 : 830-44

Résumé

ANOMALIES DE L'ORGANIFICATION DE L'IODE : formes permanentes et transitoires diagnostiquées chez de très jeunes enfants.

La plupart des cas des anomalies de l'organification de l'iode ont été observées chez des enfants ou de jeunes adultes. Le dépistage de l'hypothyroïdie congénitale a mis les endocrinologues en situation de diagnostiquer ces malades très tôt dans la vie. Nous rapportons 6 cas qui ont pu être observés chez de très jeunes enfants. Cinq de ces malades ont été identifiés dans le premier mois de vie grâce au dépistage de l'hypothyroïdie congénitale et un cas a été observé à l'âge de 27 mois et le papier filtre qui avait servi à doser la TSH a pu être retrouvé, démontrant que cet enfant n'avait pas d'hypothyroïdie à la naissance. Les 5 cas avaient une hypothyroïdie profonde. Le dernier cas avait une hypothyroïdie extrêmement modérée avec un goître et une TSH à la limite supérieure de la normale.

Le trouble de l'organification a été confirmé chez tous ces enfants par un test au perchlorate démontrant une diminution de la radioactivité au niveau de la glande thyroïde supérieure à 10 % après prise du perchlorate.

Un traitement a été institué chez tous les enfants. Le dernier cas qui avait une hypothyroïdie compensée avec des taux normaux d'hormones thyroïdiennes n'a pas été traité.

Après un temps variable allant de 8 mois à 4 ans, le traitement a été progressivement arrêté, sauf dans le cas n° 1 chez lequel très rapidement la TSH augmentait et la chute de la thyroxine plasmatique a provoqué une reprise du traitement. Dans le cas n° 2 la TSH était à 60 µU/ml après deux mois d'arrêt de traitement démontrant la nécessité d'une poursuite de la thérapeutique. Par contre dans les trois derniers cas, l'arrêt de la thérapeutique n'a pas entraîné d'augmentation de la TSH et la chute de la thyroxine. Un deuxième test au perchlorate s'est révélé normal chez 3 patients.

En conclusion, nous présentons 6 cas d'hypothyroïdie de sévérité variable liée à un trouble d'organification. Deux cas sont permanents et 4 cas sont transitoires.

Le dépistage néonatal de l'hypothyroïdie congénitale permet donc de faire ce diagnostic dans les premières semaines de la vie. Une fois le traitement institué, il faut savoir que des formes transitoires existent. L'arrêt progressif du traitement permet de mieux définir cette situation.

DNA polymorphisms in the TPO gene and hereditary defects in iodide organification

J.J.M. de Vijlder, H. Bikker and T. Vulsma

Department of Experimental Pediatric Endocrinology, Academic Hospital of the University of Amsterdam, Meibergdreef 9, 1105 AZ Amsterdam, The Netherlands

INTRODUCTION

The neonatal thyroid screening reveals that permanent congenital hypothyroidism occurs with an incidence of 1 to 3000 neonates. In the Netherlands ten to fifteen percent of permanent congenital hypothyroidism appears to be hereditary. Most hereditary defects can be classified in two classes; thyroglobulin (Tg) synthesis defects [1,2,3] and defects in the organification of iodide [1,3,4]. The latter defects can be caused by defects in the H_2O_2 generation or by defects in thyroid peroxidase (TPO) [1,4].
Since cDNA and genomic probes from both TPO and Tg are available [5,6,7,8], DNA polymorphism analysis can be performed in families with defects in the synthesis of both proteins. In this paper we describe polymorphism studies in families with TPO defects.

PATIENTS

Patients with a complete absence of iodide organification [9] were investigated in the neonatal period or after a short interruption of the T4 replacement therapy at least three years after birth. Serum T4 levels became below 5 nmol/l and serum Tg was more than 1000 pmol/l (normal range for neonates: 15-375 pmol/l; above one year: 10-60 pmol/l). Radioiodide uptakes were performed with i.v. injected $^{123}I^-$ (1-2 MBq). All thyroid glands showed a high uptake rate with a maximum of about 30% of the dose within 30 min. Sodium perchlorate (100-200 mg) administered i.v., 120 min after $^{123}I^-$, led to a complete discharge of the tracer within 30 min. In most of the younger patients with a complete absence of iodide organification, thyroids were not palpable, however thyroid ultrasound imaging showed in these cases always a normal sized or enlarged gland at the normal location.
Urinary iodine excretion was essentially within the reference range for young Dutch children (120-600 nmol I/day or 15-75 ug I/day) and low molecular weight iodinated material (LOMWIOM) was absent [10]. With an early and conscientious therapy goitre formation and thyroidectomy will be avoided and as a consequence the future possibilities for biochemical analysis of thyroid glands with such defects will be limited.

MATERIALS AND METHODS

In infants detected by neonatal thyroid screening serum T4, T3, Tg, TBG and FT4 were measured by radioimmunoassays and TSH by immunoradiometric assay. Thyroid ultrasound imaging was performed with a 5.0 or 7.5 MHz linear array transducer.
Urinary iodine and LOMWIOM concentrations were measured as described by Gons et al [10].
Available thyroid tissue thyroglobulin was purified [11] and iodination degree was determined [12]. TPO activity was measured spectrophotometrically in the microsomal fraction by I_3^- formation at 420 nm [13]. RNA was isolated from goitrous tissue, homogenized in 6 M urea/3 M lithium chloride at 0°C and centrifuged (90 min, 0°C, 60.000 x g). Samples of 25 ug RNA were electrophoresed in formaldehyde-treated gels [14] blotted on nitrocellulose and hybridized with a 3 kb TPO cDNA probe [15]. Chromosomal DNA for polymorphism studies was isolated from white blood cells out of 5-10 ml blood samples containing sodium EDTA as anticoagulant. DNA was treated with EcoRI, electrophoresed, blotted on nitrocellulose and hybridized with cDNA clones [2]. The cDNA probes used were a 3 kb TPO cDNA [15] or a 0.7 kb TPO cDNA [8].

RESULTS

In recent years we obtained thyroid tissue of two adolescents with a complete absence of iodide organification. Both glands contained a normal amount of Tg (Mw: 660,000; 19S). The iodination degree of Tg was less than 0.1 mol I/mol Tg. Normal Tg contains 6-60 mol I/mol Tg. In both goitres the peroxidase activity measured by I_3^- formation, was absent in the microsomal fraction. Looking for TPO mRNA, we found in one goitre that this messenger was absent (Fig. 1), while in the other normal sized TPO mRNA was present.

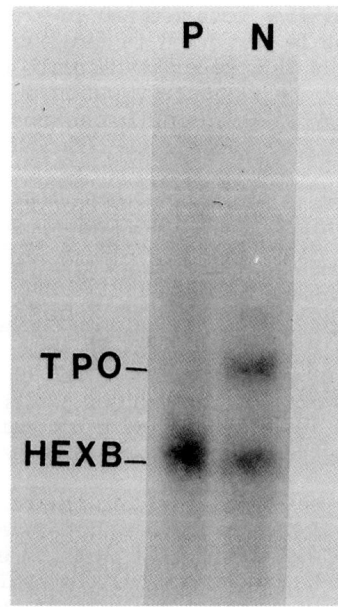

Fig. 1. Northern blot showing the absence of TPO mRNA in one of the patients with an iodide organification defect. HEXB cDNA was used as a control probe.

With the TPO cDNA clones we looked for RFLPs in the TPO gene. The 0.7 kb cDNA fragment identified in chromosomal DNA, treated with EcoRI, a polymorphism based on the occurrence of a VNTR (variable number of tandem repeats) in the genomic DNA. In 50 caucasians at least nine different alleles with a DNA fragment between 3.0 and 4.1 kb hybridized with the TPO cDNA fragment. As can be observed from Fig. 2 codominant segregation of this EcoRI RFLP was found. (Fig. 2).

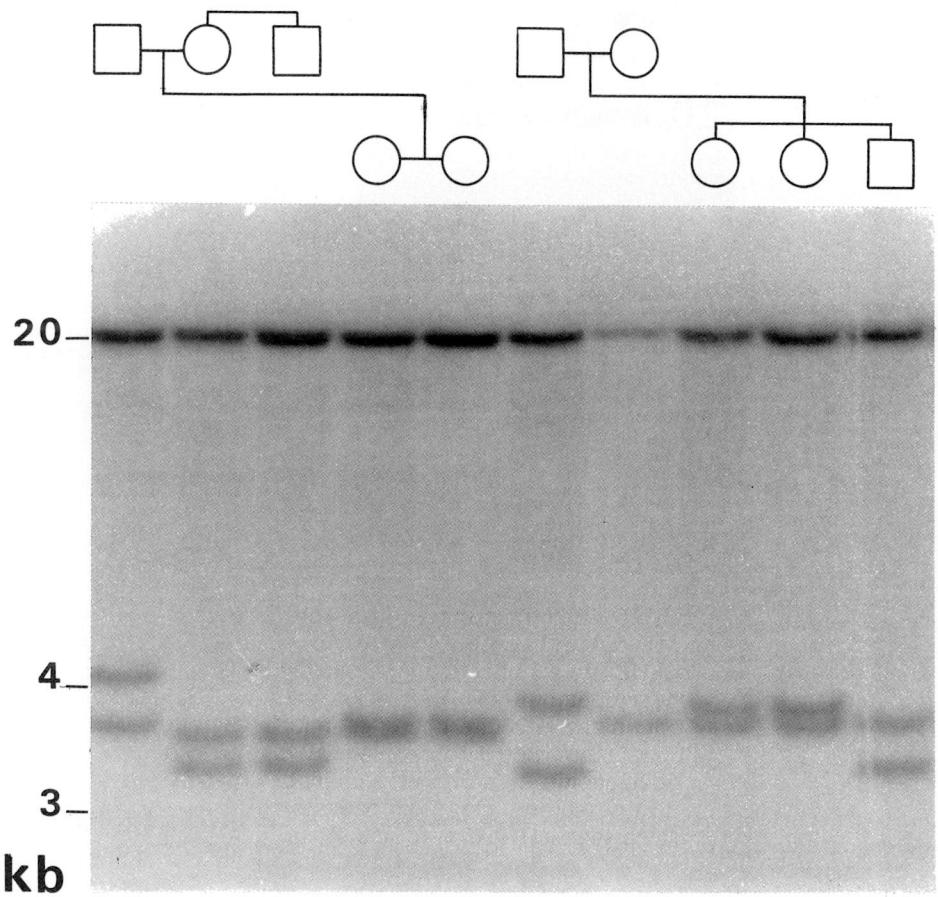

Fig. 2. Southern blot of genomic DNA of two different families. DNA was digested with EcoRI, and hybridized with the 0.7 kb TPO cDNA probe.

The 3.0 kb cDNA probe [15] detected with EcoRI another RFLP with DNA fragments of 10.5 and 11.5 kb. The minor allele (11.5 kb) frequency was 4%.
These EcoRI polymorphisms are used to study families in which defects in the organification of iodide occur (Fig. 3). The phenotypically normal daughter shows 3.3 and 3.4 kb fragments and must be heterozygous for the defect. Since the children with the TPO defect both show a band at 3.3 kb.

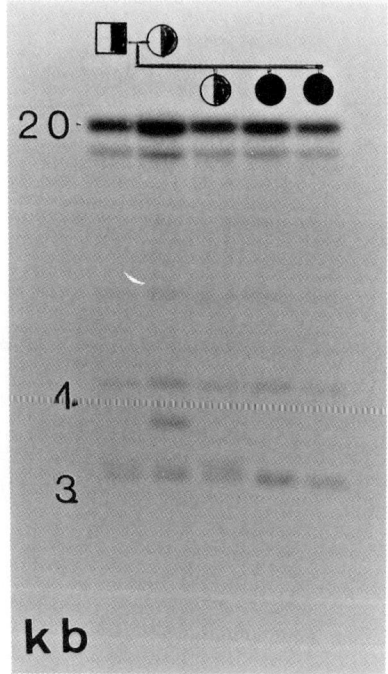

Fig. 3. Southern blot of genomic DNA from a family with two affected daughters. DNA was digested with EcoRI and probed with the 0.7 kb cDNA fragment.

The other EcoRI polymorphism identified with the 3.0 kb TPO cDNA probe was not informative in this family.
In another family the EcoRI-VNTR polymorphism was not informative. In this family the heredity of the aberrant gene was followed with the EcoRI 11.5/10.5 kb RFLP.

DISCUSSION

Via the follow-up studies of patients found in the neonatal thyroid screening, we were able to investigate families in which a complete absence of iodide organification occurs.
In stimulated glands, as in case of Tg synthesis defects, TPO activity was 10-30 times higher than normal (results not shown). In the equally stimulated glands of the two patients with a complete organification defect no TPO activity could be measured and Tg was not iodinated. This means that hypothyroidism was a result of absent peroxidase activity. In one case no TPO mRNA was detected while in the other patient TPO mRNA of normal size was present. This shows that these TPO disorders can have different genetic origins. One of the defects is probably caused by deregulation of the promotor. The other defect may be caused by alterations in the structural gene.
To perform DNA polymorphism studies the TPO gene appears to be more accessible that the Tg gene. The polymorphisms found in the well conserved Tg gene (2) were only informative in two of the seven investigated families with Tg synthesis defects (results not shown). For the TPO gene several RFLPs are known for the restriction enzymes EcoRI (8; this paper), Bgl2 and PstI (G. Vassart; personal communication).
These RFLPs appeared to be useful for studies in families with defects in TPO.

CONCLUSION

From the nation-wide evaluation of all hypothyroid patients, found in the Dutch national screening on congenital hypothyroidism, the most frequent thyroid dyshormonogenesis is the total absence of iodide organification. The incidence is 1:60,000 in a population of 1.7 million newborn children.
In two goitres from patients with a total organification defect it was shown that the peroxidase activity was absent and thyroglobulin was not iodinated.
In one goitre TPO mRNA was absent while in the other normal sized TPO mRNA was found in concentrations comparable with controls. With TPO cDNA probes various RFLPs have been found. A 0.7 kb TPO cDNA probe detected an EcoRI VNTR (variable number of tandem repeats) polymorphism, identifying at least nine alleles with a band between 3.0 and 4.1 kb. Another EcoRI-RFLP was found with the 3.0 kb TPO cDNA probe giving bands of 10.5 and/or 11.5 kb. These RFLPs appeared to be informative markers in families, in which a total absence of iodide organification occur.

ACKNOWLEDGEMENTS

We thank Dr. P. Bolhuis for discussions, Dr. G. Vassart for the TPO cDNA probes. Mrs. S. Majoor for preparing the manuscript and the department of medical photography and illustration for their service. Part of this work was supported by the Netherlands Organization for Scientific Research (NWO) and the Ludgardine Bouwman Stichting.

REFERENCES

1. Dumont JE, Vassart G, Refetoff S (1989): Thyroid disorders In <u>The metabolic basis of inherited disease</u> sixth edition. Scriver CR, Baudet AL, Sly WS, Valle D (eds.). p.p. 1843-1879. New York: McGraw Hill.

2. Baas F, Bikker H, van Ommen GJB, de Vijlder JJM (1984): Unusual scarcity of restriction site polymorphism in the human thyroglobulin gene. A linkage study suggesting autosomal dominance of a defective thyroglobulin allele. <u>Hum. Genet. 67:</u> 301-305.

3. Vulsma T, Gons MH, de Vijlder JJM (1986): The etiology of congenital hypothyroidism in the Netherlands. <u>Ann Endocrinol 47,</u> 79.

4. Vulsma T, Kootstra PR, Leer LM, Bikker H, Gons MH (1988): Absence of thyroid peroxidase activity in patients with a total organification defect. <u>Ann Endocrinol 49,</u> 244.

5. Brocas H, Christophe D, Pohl V, Vassart G (1982): Cloning of human thyroglobulin complementary DNA. <u>FEBS-Lett. 137,</u> 189-192.

6. Baas F, van Ommen GJB, Bikker H, Arnberg AC, de Vijlder JJM (1986): The human thyroglobulin gene is over 300 kb long and contains introns of upto 64 kb. <u>Nucleic Acids Res 14,</u> 5171-5186.

7. Libert F, Ruel J, Ludgate M, Swillens S, Alexander N, Vassart G, Dinsart C (1987): Thyroperoxidase, an auto-antigen with a mosaic structure made of nuclear and mitochondrial gene modules. <u>EMBO J 6,</u> 4193-4196.

8. Bikker H, Bolhuis PA, Vassart G, Libert F, Massaro G, de Vijlder JJM (1989): EcoRI RFLP in human thyroid peroxidase (TPO) gene on chromosome 2. <u>Hum Genet 82,</u> 95.

9. Vulsma T, Gons MH, de Vijlder JJM (1989): Maternal-fetal transfer of thyroxine in congenital hypothyroidism due to total organification defect or thyroid agenesis. <u>N Engl J Med 321,</u> 13-16.

10. Gons MH, Kok JH, Tegelaers WHH, de Vijlder JJM (1983): Concentration of plasma thyroglobulin and urinary excretion of iodinated material in the diagnosis of thyroid disorders in congenital hypothyroidism. <u>Acta Endocrinol 104,</u> 27-34.

11. Van Voorthuizen WF, de Vijlder JJM, van Dijk JE, Tegelaers WHH (1978): Euthyroidism via iodide supplementation in hereditary congenital goitre with thyroglobulin deficiency. <u>Endocrinology 103,</u> 2105-2111.

12. De Vijlder JJM, van Voorthuizen WF, van Dijk JE, Rijnberk A, Tegelaers WHH (1978): Hereditary congenital goitre with thyroglobulin deficiency in a breed of goats. <u>Endocrinology 102,</u> 1214-1222.

13. Taurog A (1986): Hormone synthesis: Thyroid iodine metabolism. In <u>Werner's The Thyroid,</u> Ingbar SH, Braverman LE (eds). pp. 53-97. Philadelphia: JB Lippincott Company.

14. Maniatis T, Fritsch EF, Sambrook J (1982): Molecular cloning, A laboratory manual, pp 188-209. Cold Spring Harbor Laboratory, New York.

15. Libert F, Ruel J, Ludgate M, Swillens S, Alexander N, Vassart G, Dinsart C (1987). Complete nucleotide sequence of the human thyroperoxidase microsomal antigen cDNA. <u>Nucleic Acids Res 15,</u> 6735.

Résumé

L'étude menée sur l'ensemble de la population néerlandaise sur l'hypothyroïdisme congénital, a montré que le dérèglement le plus fréquent de la formation des hormones thyroïdiennes était l'absence totale d'organification de l'iode. L'incidence est de 1/60 000 sur une population de 1.7 millions de nouveaux-nés. On a montré que dans deux goitres de patients présentant une totale déficience d'organification, l'activité péroxydase était absente, et que la thyroglobuline n'était pas iodée. Dans un goitre, l'ARN messager de la TPO était absent, tandis que dans l'autre, de taille normale, l'ARN messager de la TPO présentait des concentrations comparables à celles du groupe contrôle. A l'aide de sondes cADN de la TPO, différents RFLPs ont été trouvés. Une sonde cADN de TPO de 0.7 kb a détecté un EcoRI-VNTR (nombre variable de zones répétitives en tandem) identifiant au moins 9 allèles avec une bande comprise entre 3.0 et 4.1 kb. Un autre EcoRI-RFLP a été découvert, à l'aide d'une sonde du cADN de la TPO de 3.0 kb, donnant des bandes de 10.5 et/ou 11.5 kb. Ces RFLPs se sont avérés être des marqueurs informatifs dans les familles chez lesquelles on note une absence complète d'organification de l'iode.

Defective expression of the thyroid peroxidase gene

G. Medeiros-Neto*, A. Mangklabruks**, N.J. Cox**, D. Rosenthal*, D.P. Carvalho-Guimarães and L.J. DeGroot**

* Thyroid Laboratory, Hospital das Clínicas, The University of São Paulo Medical School, São Paulo and Instituto de Biofísica C. Chagas Filho, Rio de Janeiro, Brazil
** Thyroid Study Unit, Department of Medicine, The University of Chicago, USA

Defective expression of thyroid peroxidase function at the clinical level is caused by a group of defects (Lever et al,1983). The common patho-physiologic denominator is the discharge of a significant percentage of labelled iodide from the thyroid upon administration of perchlorate, indicating a defect in converting accumulated iodide to organically bound iodine. The defect may be partial or complete. The inheritance mode is typically autosomal recessive (Medeiros-Neto,1980). In the thyroid tissue obtained at surgery TPO activity is usually absent, or defective for iodide oxidation or unable to perform iodotyrosine coupling (Niepomniszce et al, 1977; Medeiros-Neto et al, 1979 and 1982), but the possibility of the presence of TPO inhibitor was also raised in the past (Pommier et al, 1977).

Since the cDNA of the human TPO was already reported (Seto et al, 1987; Massaro et al, 1989), we used this cDNA to study the RFLP of human TPO in five unrelated families (A,C,G,P,R) which included nine patients with complete TPO deficiency. Using this probe and six restriction enzymes, we were unable to find any polymorphisms in one family (A). We could obtain blood samples from only two family members who had complete TPO deficiency from family (C), and it is consequently not possible to determine linkage in this family. Samples from affected and unaffected members from families (G),(R) and (P) were used for the linkage analysis.

MATERIALS AND METHODS

Subjects

The affected subjects belong to five unrelated families and demonstrated severe or complete TPO deficiency defined by congenital goiter, varying degree of hypothyroidism, a positive perchlorate discharge test (> 20% of the accumulated iodide is discharged after an oral dose of 2 g of $KClO_4$) and, when tissue studies were performed, absent or diminished TPO activity in the thyroid tissue. In four families the affected subjects came from consanguineous marriages, the parents being first cousins (Table 1). In four families two siblings were affected in the same generation. Judging from these studies and reported cases (Medeiros-Neto,1980; Lever et al, 1983) the inheritance mode was autosomal recessive. The parents are believed to be heterozygous and the affected patients homozygous for the defective gene.

Table 1: Clinical and genetic characteristics of the five families studied.

Family	Affected members	Goiter present in other members*	Consanguinity	RFLPs**	Obs
A	2 siblings	2	yes	no	Presence of TPO inhibitor
C	2 siblings	1	no	Bgl II	---
G	2 siblings	4	yes	Bgl II	2 members became hypothyroid late in life
P	1	2	yes	Bgl II	---
R	2 siblings	2	yes	Bgl II Pst I	Genetic linkage of disease and TPO gene

* Two were previously thyroidectomized.
** DNA was obtained from 25 relatives and the 10 parents of the affected subjects.

In the five families studied, a total of 25 relatives and the ten parents were also tested for thyroid function. Eleven relatives have goiter and euthyroidism; two of these were previously thyroidectomized for goiter. Five relatives had either an abnormally exaggerated TSH response to TRH or an abnormally elevated basal serum Tg level with a subsequent increase after bovine TSH stimulation. Late in life, two siblings from the affected subjects in the (G) family had clinical and laboratory diagnosis of primary hypothyroidism, and normal auto-antibodies (microsomal) tests. It is unknown whether these family members, some of whom may be carriers of the TPO gene, develop goiter from the partial TPO enzyme defect or because of other causes.

Thyroid tests

Serum T_4, T_3, TSH and Tg were assayed using commercial kits (Diagnostic Co., USA). The TRH test was performed using an IV bolus of TRH (200 µg) and blood samples were collected at -15,0,15,30 and 45 min. The bovine TSH stimulation test was performed as previously described (Medeiros-Neto et al,1985) using a single injection of 10 IU of bovine TSH (Ambinon, Organon Pharm. Co., São Paulo).

RFLP Analysis

Genomic DNA was separated from 20-30 ml EDTA blood obtained from patients and family members (Madisen et al,1987).10 µg of genomic DNA was digested by restriction enzymes TaqI, PstI, BglI, and BglII in the conditions suggested by the manufacturers (Bethesda Research Laboratories, Bethesda, MD and New England Biolabs, Beverly, MA), and electrophoresed in 1% agarose gels along with HindIII digested lambda DNA and HaeIII digested phi-X DNA which served as molecular size markers. The DNA was transferred to nylon membranes (Zetabind, AMF, Cuno, Inc.,)hybridized to ^{32}p-oligo labelled probe, washed under high stringency (0.1 x SSC, 0.1%SDS at 65º C for one hour),and autoradiographed using Kodak XAR-5 film for 3-7 days with an intensifying screen.

DNA probe

The DNA probe used in these studies was pM5, an 0.8 kb cDNA clone encoding 30% of the cDNA of thyroid peroxidase gene downstream from bp 730 (Seto et al, 1987).

Linkage Analysis

Data obtained from the RFLP studies in families were analysed for possible linkage disequilibrium using two methods for analysis , one with an inbreeding factor and the other without.

RESULTS

Thyroid tests

The perchlorate discharge test was positive in all nine patients, ranging from 36 to 77% discharge of the accumulated iodide in the thyroid gland. All patients had an exaggerated TSH response to TRH, including the two patients with a normal basal serum TSH level. Serum T_4 and serum T_3 were within normal limits in five patients; the remaining four subjects were hypothyroid. One patient had a normal serum Tg level; the others had serum Tg above 30 µg/L. After injection of bTSH, all patients exhibited an abnormally elevated serum Tg peak.

Thyroid tissue studies

Thyroid tissue was obtained from four patients with varying degrees of hypothyroidism and a positive perchlorate discharge test. Two siblings were from family (A) and two siblings from family(R). No intrinsic TPO iodide-oxidation activity was found in the solubilized particulate fraction from thyroid tissues from the (A) family. The tissue Tg was weakly labeled and yielded only DIT and MIT after diggestion and thin-layer chromatography. The TPO preparations from (A) family siblings were added to a very active TPO obtained from Graves' disease tissue and produced a 60% reduction of the enzyme activity on iodide organification and on incorporation of iodine to protein. The inhibitory activity had an UV absorption maximum around 250-260 nm. was not modified after treatment at 100ºC for 30 min but was clearly diminished after 18h dialysis.

RFLP Analysis

No polymorphisms were observed in family (A). In this (A) family a TPO inhibitor was found in thyroid tissue studies. DNA from families (C), (P) and (G), showed polymorphisms when digested with BglII using pM5 probe. The polymorphisms observed at 8.7 and 8.5 kb are biallelic polymorphisms. No other polymorphism was found when using other enzymes in these family members. The RFLPs found in (R) family differ from other previously reported polymorphisms (Massaro et al,1989). There were two allelic polymorphisms at the 9.0 and 8.5 kb. The 9.0 kb bands were definitely larger than the 8.7 kb bands found in the other subjects. Also, there was an absence of the 4.0 - 3.9 kb band. This band is also a biallelic polymorphism which occurs in normal individuals. The absence of this band may represent a partial gene deletion responsible for the deficiency of TPO in this family.

With PstI restricted DNA, no polymorphisms were observed in any families except a possible deletion of a 5.5 kb band in affected siblings from the (R) family. These are the same subjects in whom we found possible deletions using BglII enzyme. The TaqI enzyme revealed a two allelic pattern at 3.0 and 2.6 kb, which shows segregation in these families. Using BglI enzymes, the (R) family also shows the same allelic polymorphism at 7.8 and 6.6 kb.

Genetic linkage

Lod scores were obtained from linkage analysis of the gene with TPO deficiency. Because of the consanguineous marriage in these families, we included an inbreeding factor in the analysis. The Lod score analyzed from the (R) family with inbreeding factor was highly compatible with linkage of disease and TPO gene (Lod=2.078). When this method was used with the (G) and (P) families, the Lod score was inconsistent with linkage between disease and TPO genes. [Lod= -2.54 in the (G) family and -3.14 in the (P) family]. When the linkage analysis was done without inbreeding factor, the (R) family showed a Lod score of 1.476, and in the (G) and (P) families with Lod scores of 0.425 and -0.176, respectively, which are inconclusive because of small family size.

DISCUSSION

The TPO defect is probably the most prevalent of the inherited defects in thyroid metabolism. In our experience it may account for nearly 40% of all cases studied at the Hospital das Clinicas in the past 25 years (Medeiros-Neto,1980). About half of these patients have congenital goiter. Thyroid hyperplasia compensates to some degree for the lack of adequate iodide organification, and some patients may remain borderline euthyroid/hypothyroid until midlife. Others present with clinical and laboratory signs of hypothyroidism early in childhood, with all consequences of lack of an adequate supply of thyroid hormones.

Consanguinity of the parents is common, and more than one sibling may be affected in one generation. Some presumably heterozygous relatives have manifestations of disturbed thyroid function such as goiter, abnormal TRH or bTSH stimulation tests, and progressive thyroid failure. The reasons for this late-in-life hypothyroidism are not known, but there is no evidence for associated autoimmune thyroid disease. The possibility of a dialysable TPO inhibitor was raised on tissue studies performed "in vitro" on thyroid specimens from siblings of family (A). The inhibitor could be removed by extensive dialysis. The chemical nature of this inhibitor remains unknown but it seems to be similar to a TPO inhibitor described by Pommier et al (1977).

To characterize the defect of incomplete TPO deficiency at the gene level, we investigated the disease related RFLPs from nine affected individuals. Apart from two possible deletions in the (R) family, no disease specific polymorphisms were observed among other affected individuals. We found by linkage analysis that the TPO gene defect may be the cause of TPO deficiency in the (R) family. The results are inconclusive in the other two families investigated. Also, when we used the linkage analysis method with inbreeding factor, the analysis was incompatible with linkage in the (G) and (P) families. These data suggested that the cause of TPO deficiency in these families is heterogeneous. In some families such as the (R) family, the affected gene is the TPO gene itself. In other families, the affected gene may be another gene that controls the expression of the TPO gene.

The RFLP pattern of BglII restricted DNA in the (R) family strongly suggests a partial TPO gene deletion has occurred in this family. To investigate the deletion further, a smaller fragment of the probe (bp 733-1100) was used to examine the restricted DNA. Both the deleted fragment at 4.0 kb and the polymorphic fragment at 9.0 and 8.5 kb were observed. This suggests that these fragments of TPO cDNA contain the sequences that indicate polymorphism and possibly deletion. The nature of these deletions and their effect on the TPO molecule is still under investigation.

REFERENCES

Lever, E.G., Medeiros-Neto, G.A. and DeGroot, L. (1983): Inherited disorders of thyroid metabolism. Endocr. Rev. 4: 213-239.
Madisen, L., Hoar, D.I., Holroyd, C.D., et al. (1987):DNA banking the effects of storage of blood and isolated DNA or the integrity of DNA. Am. J. Med. Gen. 27: 379-390.
Massaro, G., Libert, F., Vassart, G., et al. (1989): RFLPs detected at 2 pter-p 12 with a thyroid peroxidase cDNA probe, TPO_3 (McKusick no. 27450). Nucl. Acids Res. 17: 2155.
Medeiros-Neto, G.A., Knobel, M., Yamamoto, K., et al. (1979): Deficient thyroid peroxidase causing organification defect and goitrous hypothyroidism. J. Endocrinol. Invest. 2: 353-357.
Medeiros-Neto, G.A. (1980): Inherited disorders of intrathyroidal metabolism. In Thyroid Research VIII, ed. J.R. Stockigt & S.Nagataki, pp. 101-108, Canberra, Australian Academy of Science.

Medeiros-Neto, G.A., Okamura, K., Cavaliere, H., et al. (1982):Familial thyroid peroxidase defect. Clin. Endocrinol. 17: 1-14.
Medeiros-Neto, G.A., Marcondes, J.A., Cavaliere, H., et al.(1985): Serum thyroglobulin (Tg) stimulation with bovine TSH: a useful test for diagnosis of congenital hypothyroid due to defective Tg synthesis. Acta Endocrinol. (Kbh) 110: 644-650.
Niepomniszcze, H., Medeiros-Neto, G.A., Refetoff, S., et al.(1977): Familial goitre with partial iodine organification defect, lack of thyroglobulin and highlevels of thyroid peroxidase. Clin. En docrinol. 6: 27-39.
Pommier, J., Dominici, R., Bougneres, P., et al. (1977): A dialysable inhibitor bound to thyroglobulin from four simple goiters and from two goiters with iodine organification defect. J. Mol. Med. 2: 169-177.
Seto, P., Hirayu, H., Magnusson, R.P., et al (1987): Isolation of a complementary DNA clone for thyroid microsomal antigen. Homology with the gene for thyroid peroxidase. J. Clin. Invest. 80: 1205-1208.

ABSTRACT

We have conducted biochemical and genetic studies in five unrelated families which included 9 goitrous subjects (five borderline euthyroid; four hypothyroid) with a complete or partial TPO deficiency. In one family (A) a thermostable, dialysable TPO inhibitor was detected in the thyroid tissue. No iodide-organification or iodide incorporation into protein was present in this family. Using four restriction enzymes (Taq I, Pst I, Bgl I e Bgl II) we were unable to find any polymorphisms in this family (A), with a 0.8 kb cDNA clone (pM5) encoding 30% of the cDNA of human TPO gene downstream from bp 730. In another family (C) blood samples were obtained from only 2 family members and consequently it was not possible to determine linkage. DNA from families (G), (P) and (C) showed biallelic polymorphisms when digested with Bgl II, at 8.7 and 8.5 kb. In family (R) we detected 2 biallelic polymorphisms at the 9.0 and 8.5 kb, and the 9.0 kb bands were larger than the 8.7 kb bands found in the other subjects. Also there was an absence of 4.0 - 3.9 kb band that may represent a partial gene deletion. Again with Pst I restricted DNA a possible deletion of 5.5 kb band was present in affected siblings of family (R). These are the same subjects in whom we found possible deletions using Bgl II enzyme. The Lod score analysed from the (R) family with inbreeding factor was highly compatible with linkage of disease and TPO gene (Lod = 2.078). When this method was used with (G) and (P) families the Lod score was inconsistent with linkage between disease and TPO gene. These data suggest that the cause of TPO deficiency in these families is heterogeneous. However the RFLP pattern of Bgl II restricted DNA in the (R) family strongly suggest that a partial TPO gene deletion has occurred in this family.

Résumé

Nous avons réalisé une étude biochimique et génétique de quatre familles différentes présentant un déficit partiel en TPO. Dans la première famille (A), un inhibiteur thermostable et dialysable de la TPO a été détecté dans le tissu thyroïdien et tenu pour responsable d'un défaut complet de l'organification de l'iodure. L'étude génétique de cette famille n'a pas mis en évidence de polymorphisme spécifique. Dans d'autres familles (C, G et P), l'étude de l'ADN à l'aide d'une sonde (pM5) représentant 30% du gène de la TPO, a montré après digestion par Bgl II, un polymorphisme biallélique à 8.7 et 8.5 kb. Dans la famille R, il a été détecté 2 polymorphismes bialléliques à 9.0 et 8.5 kb, la bande de 9.0 kb étant plus importante que la bande de 8.7 kb trouvée chez les autres sujets. De plus, il y avait une disparition de la bande de 3.9 - 4.0 kb suggérant une délétion partielle du gène. En utilisant Pst I, il a été trouvé une délétion de la bande de 5.5 kb chez les sujets atteints de la famille R, qui s'ajoutait à la délétion montrée par Bgl II. Le Lod score calculé dans la famille R était de 2.078 et montrait une liaison entre polymorphisme et anomalie de la TPO. Un tel résultat n'a pas été retrouvé dans les familles G et P. L'ensemble des données suggère que l'anomalie de la TPO retrouvée dans ces familles pouvait avoir des causes variables. cependant, le polymorphisme mis en évidence par Bgl II est en faveur d'une délétion du gène de la TPO dans une des familles étudiées.

Loosely anchored peroxidase. A possible explanation for an iodide organification defect in a hypothyroid cat

M.T. den Hartog[1], B.E. Sjollema[2], A. Rijnberk[2], J.E. van Dijk[3] and J.J.M. de Vijlder[1]

[1] Department of Experimental Pediatric Endocrinology, Academic Hospital, University of Amsterdam, The Netherlands.
[2] Department of Clinical Sciences of Companion Animals and [3] Department of Veterinary Pathology, Faculty of Veterinary Medicine, University of Utrecht, The Netherlands

Abstract

Several congenital disorders in thyroid hormone synthesis have been described. Identification of the molecular nature of the defects has been greatly facilitated for those defects for which an animal as a model has been available. So far the descriptions of these animal models have been limited to defects in the synthesis of thyroglobulin.
Organification defects have been described in animals by in vivo uptake studies of radioactive iodide and competition studies with perchlorate. In two hypothyroid cats we demonstrated that the disorder in thyroid metabolism was caused by this type of defect. From one of the animals thyroid tissue became available. At the moment of hemithyroidectomy the animal was almost euthyroid and the histological examination did not disclose features of functional hyperactivity; the colloidal lumen contained high amounts of protein. Apparently the high iodine content of the food allowed the animal to compensate for the partial defect. In the membrane fraction no peroxidase activity could be demonstrated, however completely unexpected, in the 100,000xg supernatant activity was found. This we have never found in cats or other species. The thyroglobulin (M_r 660,000) in the colloidal fraction was iodinated (0.19%) and contained T4, in amounts comparable to normal (cat) thyroglobulin.
From these experiments we conclude that the described partial organification defect in one of the cats may been caused by loosely anchored thyroid peroxidase that in contrast to normal will be easily released. This might happen already in vivo or on isolation.

Circulating TPO

La TPO circulante

Approaches to the measurement of TPO in serum

T.J. Wilkin and J.L. Diaz

Endocrine Section, Medicine II, Southampton General Hospital, Southampton, UK

Antimicrosomal (anti-TPO, anti-M) antibodies are important clinical markers for autoimmune thyroid disease (Doniach, 1975). Studies by Czarnocka and colleagues (1985) purified human thyroid peroxidase, a haemoprotein enzyme firmly associated with the intracellular membrane and specially with the endoplasmic reticulum of thyroid microsomes, and identified it as the target antigen for antimicrosomal antibodies. The 100,000 molecular weight molecule was subsequently sequenced (Libert *et al.*, 1987) and currently provides a focus of interest as a major immunogen in autoimmune thyroid disease.

Continuing discussions have produced two differing theories to explain the pathogenesis of autoimmunity: one interprets the antigen/antibody interaction primarily as the result of disturbances to the immune system (immune dysregulation theory) (Volpe, 1988); the other explains it as an appropriate response to increased or "pathologically" presented antigen (primary lesion theory) (Wilkin, 1989). It seems reasonable to assume that the immune system does not ordinarily have access to intracellular antigens. An autoantibody response to such antigens might therefore arise in any of three ways: by molecular mimicry (Allison, 1971); by expression of "intracellular" antigens on the outer surface of the cell membrane (demonstrated, for example, by the La(SS-B) nuclear antigen in Sjogren's syndrome) (Baboonian *et al.*, 1989); or by leakage of antigens into the circulation from cells with membrane damage (Wilkin, 1989). We have pursued this last possibility.

Thyroglobulin autoantibodies are common in "non-autoimmune" conditions where circulating thyroglobulin concentrations are nevertheless elevated, such as thyroid cancer (Rochman *et al.*, 1975). This is consistent with the notion that autoantigen release in the context of a primary lesion may result in an autoimmune response. Studies performed by Jansson and colleagues (1985) demonstrated a rise and fall in antimicrosomal antibody titres in response to changes in the concentration of TSH to which the thyroid was exposed, suggesting that the microsomal antibody response (whether from intrathyroidal or circulating lymphocytes) was possibly a function of antigen release. These observations, in addition to a bias towards the primary lesion theory of autoimmunity, led us to question whether the microsomal autoantibodies commonly seen in thyroid diseases were also associated with an increase in circulating TPO antigen. Accordingly, we developed an assay for circulating TPO and measured its concentration in the sera of control subjects and patients with various forms of thyroid disease.

Initially, we attempted to design an enzymatic assay based on the guaiacol assay described by Hosoya et al. (1985) taking advantage of the peroxidase activity of TPO. However, owing to the labile nature of TPO in vitro, the lyophilised samples of purified human TPO available for use as standards exhibited no enzymic activity despite attempts to optimise the conditions.

A radioimmunoassay was subsequently developed with which to determine the concentration of TPO in serum samples. Purified human TPO (courtesy of Dr. P. Carayon) was radiolabelled with 125-iodine, using the iodogen method, to a specific activity of 10 µCi/µg. Radio-labelled TPO (25,000 cpm) was incubated for 24h at 4°C with anti-human TPO polyclonal serum raised in rabbits ($1/10^4$ final dilution) and normal rabbit serum (to act as carrier, $1/10^3$ final dilution) and made up to 250 µl total volume in diluent buffer (phosphate buffered saline, 10 mM EDTA, 0.5% (w/v) BSA, 0.05% (v/v) Tween). The TPO-antibody complexes were precipitated by addition of donkey anti-rabbit globulin (100 µl of a 1/24 working dilution), incubated for 18h at 4°C and pelleted and washed by centrifugation (15 min., 10,000 g). Under these conditions, 50% of the total counts added were consistently precipitated.

The TPO content of sera was assessed by measuring the amount of displacement achieved by adding a 25 µl sample of the test sera in the reaction mixture. Results were interpreted through a standard curve created by displacing the reaction with known amounts of unlabelled TPO (range 0.05 ng - 1 µg). Displacement curves were virtually superimposable irrespective of whether they had been constructed in buffer or in normal human serum, suggesting that displacement was TPO specific and not affected by other factors in human serum.

Forty sera were tested in the assay: 10 normal controls, 16 patients with autonomous (thyrotoxic) nodules, five with untreated hypothyroidism due to autoimmune thyroiditis, five with untreated Graves' disease and four with differentiated thyroid cancer. The scatter of TPO concentration among the 10 control sera was small (mean 5.6 ng/ml, standard deviation 4.4 ng/ml). The TPO concentration corresponding to the mean plus three standard deviations (mean + 3 SD) for the control sera was 18.8 ng/ml. The serum TPO concentrations for all five thyroiditis (mean 3,600 ng/ml, range 1,700-5,0000 ng/ml) and Graves' sera (mean 3,900 ng/ml, range 1,700-8,300 ng/ml) lay above this value. Raised TPO levels were also found in five of 16 sera from autonomous nodule patients (range 600-1,400 ng/ml) and one of four of the thyroid cancer sera (3,800 ng/ml).

Endogenous antimicrosomal antibodies present in patients' sera might be expected to interfere with the assay by competing for labelled TPO, thus giving artificially high apparent concentration of TPO or false positives. However, we found no correlation between antimicrosomal antibody titres and measured TPO concentrations. To assess the influence of these antibodies on the assay, levels of antimicrosomal antibodies in the samples were tested using a M-Serodia AMC kit (Fujirebio) gel particle agglutination assay. The control sera, sera from autonomous nodules and thyroid cancer patients were all found to be antimicrosomal antibody negative. Antimicrosomal antibodies, however, were present in sera from all five thyroiditis (range of titres 1/100 - 1/409,600) and all five Graves' patients (range of titres 1/100 - 1/102,400). Antimicrosomal antibodies were removed from these sera by affinity chromatography using polyclonal anti-human IgG immunoglobulin covalently linked to cyanogen bromide activated sepharose 4B beads. On subsequent re-testing, TPO concentrations in sera from thyroiditis and Graves' patients remained above the mean + 3 SD of the controls. In one thyroiditis patient and in one Graves' patient removal of antimicrosomal antibodies reduced apparent TPO concentration (from 4,400 ng/ml to 76 ng/ml and from 3,900 ng/ml to 400 ng/ml respectively) though both remained positive. In the other sera the drop in the measured TPO concentration after removal of the antimicrosomal antibodies, where observed, was small (0-18%).

These data are preliminary, and the numbers tested small. Nevertheless, they suggest significant TPO concentrations in the systemic circulation of certain patients, discriminating between patients with thyroid pathology from those without, in particular those with diffuse as opposed to localised lesions. These data are consistent with the primary lesion hypothesis which proposes that autoimmune phenomena represent a regulated, physiological and appropriate response to self antigens released or caught up in a conventional immune response to alloantigens such as viral particles expressed on the target cell surface.

Acknowledgements: We are grateful for the gifts of human TPO and anti-TPO antiserum from P. Carayon and to Mrs Wendy Couper for preparing the manuscript.

REFERENCES

Allison A.C. (1971): Unresponsiveness to self antigens. Lancet 2, 1401.
Baboonian C., Venables P.J.W. Booth J., Williams D.G., Roffe L.M., and Maini R.N. (1989): Virus infection induces redistribution and membrane localisation of the nuclear antigen La (SS-B): a possible mechanism for autoimmunity. Clin. Exp. Immunol. 78, 454.
Czarnocka B., Ruf J. et al. (1985): Purification of human thyroid peroxidase and its identification as the microsomal antigen in autoimmune thyroid diseases. FEBS lett. 190, 147.
Doniach D. (1975): Humoral and genetic aspects of thyroid autoimmunity. Clin. Endocrinol. Metab. 4, 267.
Hosoya T., Sato I., Hiyama Y., Yoshimura H., Niimi H., and Tarutani O. (1985): An improved assay method for thyroid peroxidase applicable for a few milligrams of abnormal human thyroid tissues. J. Biochem. 98, 637.
Janssen R., Karlsson A. et al. (1985): Thyroxine, metimazole and thyroid microsomal antibody titres in hypothyroid Hashimoto's thyroiditis. Brit Med J. 290, 11.
Libert F., Ruel J. et al. (1987): Complete nucleotide sequence of the human thyroperoxidase-microsomal antigen cDNA. Nucleic Acids Res. 15, 6735.
Rochman H.L., De Groot C.H.L. et al. (1975): Carcinoembryonic antigen and humoral antibody response in patients with thyroid carcinoma. Cancer Res. 35, 2692.
Volpe R. (1988): The immunoregulatory disturbance in autoimmune thyroid disease. Autoimmunity 2, 55.
Wilkin T.J. (1989): Autoimmunity: attack or defence? Autoimmunity 3, 57.

Résumé

Un dosage radio-immunologique utilisant de la TPO humaine purifiée, marquée à l'iode 125 a été développé pour mesurer la concentration de TPO dans des échantillons de sérum. Le dosage a été utilisé pour déterminer la concentration de TPO dans le sérum de 30 patients atteints de différentes formes de maladies thyroïdiennes et dans celui de 10 sujets contrôles. Des taux élevés de TPO ont été trouvés chez 5 des 16 patients présentant des nodules autonomes, chez un des quatre patients atteints de cancer thyroïdien, chez tous les sujets basedowiens, et chez les 5 patients testés atteints de thyroïdite autoimmune. Un nouveau dosage du sérum effectué après suppression par chromatographie d'affinité, des anticorps anti-microsomiaux, a démontré que les concentration élevées de TPO n'étaient pas un artefact dû à la présence de ces auto-anticorps. La signification de ces données révélant des concentrations de TPO dans le système circulatoire de certains patients atteints de pathologie thyroïdienne, est discutée dans le contexte de l'hypothèse d'une lésion primaire.

Acute release of thyroid peroxidase during subtotal thyroidectomy

U. Feldt-Rasmussen, M. Hoier-Madsen, J. Date and M. Blichert-Toft

Department of Medicine F, Herlev University Hospital, Autoimmune Laboratory, State Serum Institute, Departments of Clinical Chemistry and Surgery, Odense University Hospital, Denmark

An immediate reduction of thyroglobulin autoantibodies (TgAb) during subtotal thyroidectomy of TgAb positive patients has previously been shown to indicate an acute release of thyroglobulin (Tg) into the circulation peroperatively (Feldt-Rasmussen et al. Clin Endocrinol 12:29;1980). The aim of the present study was to investigate if thyroid peroxidase (TPO) was also released by measuring anti-thyroid peroxidase antibodies (anti-TPO) by a quantitative and antigen specific method both per- and postoperatively in patients positive for anti-TPO.

Twelve anti-TPO positive patients (11 females, 1 male) referred for surgery of toxic goitre were studied. Median age was 43 years (range 24-64) and median goitre size 86 g (25-165). All patients had been pretreated with antithyroid drugs and were euthyroid at the time of operation. Anti-TPO was measured before operation, 1-8 hours, 10 days, 1-3 months and 12 months postoperatively by a commercial method (DYNO-test^R, Henning, Berlin).

The median anti-TPO level was before operation 1050 U/ml (range 68-10,520 U/ml) and fell during operation to a fraction of 0.68 (range 0.47-1.30) ($P<0.01$) of initial concentration without further decrease during the next 1-8 hours. The comparative decrease in TgAb was 0.50 (0.27-0.91). The anti-TPO level was increasing after ten days but did not reach initial level until between 3 and 12 months. However in 3 of 10 patients anti-TPO had disappeared after 12 months, all of whom had low levels before operation, whereas anti-TPO was 2-4 times higher than preoperatively in other 3 patients.

The present study thus shows evidence for an acute release of thyroid peroxidase into the circulation during thyroid surgery able to decrease measurable anti-TPO activity to almost the same degree as the Tg induced decrease in TgAb. The binding pattern of one of the monoclonal antibodies utilized in the method indicated that the epitope towards which it is directed was conformational rather than sequential (Ruf et al. Endocrinol, 1989). However, the more precise molecular form of the released TPO requires other methods of determination.

Characterization of TPO autoantibodies

Caractérisation des auto-anticorps anti-TPO

Heterogeneity of human autoantibodies to TPO

L.J. DeGroot

Thyroid Study Unit-Box 138, The University of Chicago, 5841 South Maryland Avenue, Chicago, 60637 IL USA

Antibodies to the "microsomal antigen", recognized by Deborah Doniach and Ian Roitt during the 1950's, were subsequently the subject of extensive investigations which however failed to identify the antigen. Recognition of "microsomal antigen" as a pair of 107 - 101 kb proteins by Hamada et al. (1985), recognition that "anti-microsomal" antibodies reacted with human thyroid peroxidase by Portmann et al. (1985), and Czarnocka et al. (1985), and subsequent cloning of the cDNA for TPO in three laboratories, has conclusively shown that microsomal antigen effectively equals thyroid peroxidase. The antigen exists on the cell surface, and forms part but probably not all of the cell surface antigen recognized by autoantibodies. It is probably the antigen recognized in thyroid antibody dependent complement-mediated cytotoxicity (Khoury et al., 1981). It is probably not one antigen, at least in the sense that at least two molecular forms made by splicing of mRNA are present (Kimura et al., 1987), variable levels of glycosylation may exist, and alleles at the level of nucleotide and amino acid differences also probably exist. How this antigen, normally a part of internal cell membranes and apical cell surface, is recognized by lymphocytes remains uncertain. Surely it is released at cell death. Possibly reverse cell polarity, or enterolimpesis, may allow lymphocytes to recognize it, and there is evidence that the antigen does exist in blood.

Site of antibody production

It is uncertain whether normal autoantibody production is initiated by intrathyroidal or extrathyroidal T and B cells. In time, during the course of AITD, anti-TPO antibody production occurs both in the thyroidal and extrathyroidal compartments. Rarely antibody is produced by cells within the thyroid but does not appear in circulation. Activated B cells are present in a large number in the thyroid and in the peripheral blood in patients with active autoimmune disease, and peripheral blood lymphocytes have clearly been shown to be capable of secreting antimicrosomal antibody by several groups including McLachlan et al. (1983) and Benveniste et al. (1984). These PBLs may come from nodes or thyroid, and probably represent recirculation of educated T and B cells.

Incidence

The occurrence of autoantibodies to TPO must be considered a paranormal phenomenon. Their incidence has been documented in many "normal" individuals in various surveys, including 8% of children and up to 34% of adult women using a highly sensitive assay. In Graves' disease, about 65% of sera are positive, and in

Hashimoto's thyroiditis up to 90%. Whether the antibodies present in individuals who have no evidence of clinical thyroid disease are related to, or are a separate phenomenon from, the presumed "pathogenic" antibodies present in individuals with clinical disease, remains uncertain. "Naturally" occurring antibodies, sometimes of IgM class, which have low affinity for TG, have been reported. Somatic mutation could allow these clones to function as precursors of the "pathogenic" antibodies. Alternatively, antigen driven somatic mutations of unrelated IgG genes could lead to the development of pathogenic autoantibodies, or they may arise from de novo antigen exposure to non-deleted potentially self-reactive T and B cells. Factors which increase the titers of antibodies from the usual low levels found in "normal" individuals to the typically higher levels seen in patients with disease are not fully established, but may include inheritance of specific HLA, immunoglobulin, or TCR genes, exposure to viruses or environmental pathogens with cross-reacting epitopes, stress, defects in suppressor cell function, or exposure to elevated levels of circulating IL-2 or interferon coincident with infection (DeGroot & Quintans, 1989).

Types of antibody

Immunoglobulins in patients with clinically evident autoimmune thyroid disease (Graves' disease, Hashimoto's thyroiditis or primary myxedema) can exist as IgM, or IgA, but are predominantly IgG. IgG classes 1 and 2 predominate among the antibodies, class 3 is unrepresented, and IgG class 4 is increased (Kotani et al., 1986; Weetman et al., 1989). Since IgG 1 and 2 can fix complement, these antibodies could be capable of lysing thyroid follicular cells. Antibodies are clearly polyclonal, as shown by numerous investigators. Epitopes on the antigen recognized by the antibodies are probably both conformational and linear. Ruf et al. (1989) and others have used cross reaction of polyclonal autoantibodies with monoclonal antibodies to map TPO epitopes. Human TPO was found to have seven epitopes clustered in four domains, of which three are conserved between species. Several of these are present at the site of the catalytic domain of the TPO. Autoantibodies recognized primarily two domains. This topology is very similar to that recognized earlier for thyroglobulin, in which case many domains are recognized by heteroantibodies but only a limited number by autoantibodies. Up to two-thirds of TPO autoantibodies react with an 85 amino acid linear (though possibly structured) recombinant peptide representing the carboxy terminal portion of TPO (Ludgate et al., 1989). The molecule appears to share an epitope with thyroglobulin, since cross reaction of antibodies has been clearly demonstrated (Kohno et al., 1988). There is also, not surprisingly, cross reaction with myeloperoxidase epitopes.

We analyzed reaction of autoantibodies and monoclonal antibodies with enzyme digested TPO (Portmann et al., 1988). Staph aureus V8 protease digested TPO into fragments of approximately 80, 55, and 50 kD. All of these were recognized by a monoclonal anti-TPO antibody, suggesting that these fragments represented progressive degradation of one epitope to smaller and smaller subunits. No fragments were recognized by polyclonal antibodies, indicating that the polyclonal antibodies probably reacted primarily with conformational epitopes. Limited trypsin digestion caused the 107 and 101 kD proteins to be reduced to a pair of 88 and 84 kD proteins. This is not surprising, since it had previously been shown that limited trypsin digestion could solubilize thyroid peroxidase without destroying its catalytic subunit function. The 88 and 84 kD peptides strongly reacted with our anti-TPO monoclonal antibodies but reacted weakly and rarely with polyvalent autoantibodies, suggesting that the 20 kD piece of the molecule removed by trypsin carried important epitopes.

In our early studies attempting to characterize thyroid peroxidase, we investigated the distribution of the antigen in Western blots of thyroid proteins run in non-reducing conditions ("native"), after denaturation in the presence of urea and SDS ("denatured"), or with denaturation and reduction by addition of mercaptoethanol ("reduced"). Most sera reacted with a nondescript band when thyroid proteins were electrophoresed in the native state, and with more restricted but still broad bands of protein when the material was denatured. After reduction, most autoantibodies failed to react with proteins on these Western blots. Antibodies from one patient reacted with and characterized the 107 and 101 kD TPO molecules. Our interpretation of this was that some antibodies recognized only native antigen, and others recognized antibody which had been denatured. In these cases the antigen probably exists as large molecular weight complexes held together by sulfhydryl bonds. After reduction, and presumably linearization of the molecule, most of the conformational epitopes were lost, and most sera failed to react. One remained reactive to a (presumed) linear epitope (Hamada et al., 1987b).

We undertook to investigate the characteristics of these different antibodies and their distribution. We developed an Elisa for measuring antibodies to denatured antigen coated on plates after treatment with 3 M sodium thiocyanate. For measurement of antibodies to denatured and reduced antigen, we used a quantitative Western blot procedure. Absorption studies demonstrate that native peroxidase could absorb the antibodies reacting to the denatured or reduced antigen, indicating that these epitopes actually existed in the "non-denatured" peroxidase. This term is used advisedly, since quite possibly some of the "native" molecules are in fact denatured. Assays on about 200 patients' sera showed that there is a high correlation in distribution of all three antibodies, although some patients have high titers of antibodies recognized by microsomal hemagglutination assay or by microsomal Elisa assay, and low titers of antibodies to denatured or denatured and reduced antigen, and vice versa (Hamada et al., 1987a).

Antibodies to the denatured antigen appeared in 22% of Graves' disease patients and 29% of those with thyroiditis, and to the reduced antigen in 11% of Graves' disease patients and 14% of patients with thyroiditis. The denatured and reduced antibodies were increased in Graves' disease patients who had previously been treated by surgery, were hypothyroid after I^{131} therapy, or who had a longer period of illness. They were also increased in patients with thyroiditis who had large goiters or untreated hypothyroidism. Our interpretation was that destruction of the thyroid, or prolonged illness, could lead to liberation of antigen which was damaged and thus denatured, so that antibodies developed to these previously unrecognized epitopes. It also seemed possible that antibodies to denatured antigen might be related to some of the associated autoimmune phenomena in Graves' disease. In preliminary studies, antibodies which recognized the denatured antigen failed to interact, for example, with eye muscle or retrobulbar fat antigens in Elisa assays.

More recently, we have studied reaction of autoantibodies with linear peptides of thyroid peroxidase and have identified specific linear peptides which are recognized by many autoantibodies. These are distributed throughout the molecule and do not overlap the "C2 fragment" recognized as an important antigen by Ludgate et al. (1989).

The function of autoantibodies

The autoantibodies are obviously useful markers of disease. It is possible that the low levels of antibodies found in "normal" subjects serve to scavenge antigens released by the death of thyroid cells, and could help prevent progressive development of immunity. Whether induction of anti-TPO antibodies can in fact lead to development of histologic thyroiditis remains uncertain. It is possible, in experimental animals, to induce antibodies without development of thyroiditis. However, the antibodies are capable of antibody dependent complement-mediated cytotoxicity, and perhaps are involved in T cell-mediated cytotoxicity. They can function to block thyroid peroxidase activity in vitro (Okamoto et al., 1989), although probably do not do this in vivo. There is some evidence that transplacental migration of these antibodies can produce neonatal hypothyroidism (Bogner et al., 1989).

Correlations with disease

Anti-TPO antibody levels tend to be decreased with antithyroid drug therapy of Graves' disease, and increase following RAI therapy. Their presence correlates with the development of post-operative hypothyroidism or post-RAI hypothyroidism in Graves' disease. Possibly propylthiouracil and methimazole have a direct antagonistic effect on lymphocytes to reduce antibody production, although it is more likely that the immunosuppressive effect of these antithyroid drugs is exerted elsewhere than in a direct effect upon B or T cells. In general antibody levels tend to be stable for years but gradually decrease in patients with primary thyroid failure. The presence of TPO antibodies in patients who are pregnant is a marker for the occurrence of postpartum transient thyrotoxicosis or hypothyroidism, and they also correlate with the development of hypothyroidism after "silent" thyroiditis (Yamamoto et al., 1987). The lack of antibodies in patients with Graves' disease correlates with a higher probability of relapse after antithyroid drug withdrawal (Takaichi et al., 1989).

Therapeutic implications

Among the possible modalities that may be considered for control of autoimmune disease are the development of anti-idiotype antibodies, T cells which have immunosuppressive effects on autologous T cells, T cells which can "vaccinate" against development of autoimmunity, and peptides which could compete with autologous pathogenic epitopes for presentation by APCs to T cells. Evidence for the polyclonal nature of the antibody response, and the presence of multiple epitopes recognized in the studies described above, indicates that therapy by these mechanisms will be complicated, since multiple clones of T and B cells with multiple specific cognate epitopes presumably are involved in the immune response. However, a dominant epitope could be the primary or initial pathogen, and other epitopes might be developed during the course of the immune process. If so, then the anti-immune treatments might be more feasible.

REFERENCES

Benveniste, P., Wenzel, B.E., Khalil, A., Row, V. & Volpe R. (1984): Spontaneous secretion of thyroid autoantibodies by cultured peripheral blood lymphocytes from patients with Hashimoto's thyroiditis detected by micro-Elisa techniques. Clin. Exp. Immunol. 58, 273-282.

Bogner, U., Gruters, A., Sigle, B., Helge, H. & Schleusener, H. (1989): Cytotoxic antibodies in congenital hypothyroidism. J. Clin. Endocrinol. Metab. 68, 671.

Czarnocka, B., Ruf, J., Ferrand, M., Carayon, P. & Lissitzky, S. (1985): Purification of the human thyroid peroxidase and its identification as the microsomal antigen involved in autoimmune thyroid diseases. Febs Letters. 190, 147-152.

DeGroot, L.J. & Quintans, J. (1989): The causes of autoimmune thyroid disease. Endocrine Rev. 10, 537-562.

Hamada, N., Grimm, C., Mori, H. & DeGroot, L.J. (1985): Identification of a thyroid microsomal antigen by Western blot and immunoprecipitation. J. Clin. Endocrinol. Metab. 61, 120-128.

Hamada, N., Jaeduck, N., Portmann, L., Ito, K. & DeGroot, L.J. (1987a): Antibodies against denatured and reduced thyroid microsomal antigen in autoimmune thyroid disease. J. Clin. Endocrinol. Metab. 64, 230-238.

Hamada, N., Portmann, L. & DeGroot, L.J. (1987b):Characterization and isolation of thyroid microsomal antigen. J. Clin. Invest. 79, 819-825.

Khoury, E.L., Hammond, L., Bottazzo, G.F. & Doniach, D. (1981): Presence of the organ-specific 'microsomal' autoantigen on the surface of human thyroid cells in culture: its involvement in complement-mediated cytotoxicity. Clin. Exp. Immunol. 45, 316-328.

Kimura, S., Kotani, T., McBride, O.W., Umeki, K., Hirai, K., Nakayama, T. & Ohtaki, S. (1987): Human thyroid peroxidase: Complete cDNA and protein sequence, chromosome mapping, and identification of two alternately spliced mRNAs. Proc. Natl. Acad. Sci. USA. 84, 5555-5559.

Kohno, Y., Naito, N., Hiyama, Y., Shimojo, N., Suzuki, N., Tarutani, O., Niimi, H., Nakajima, H. & Hosoya, T. (1988): Thyroglobulin and thyroid peroxidase share common epitopes recognized by autoantibodies in patients with chronic autoimmune thyroiditis. J. Clin. Endocrinol. Metab. 67, 899-907.

Kotani, T., Kato, E., Hirai, K., Kuma, K. & Ohtaki, S. (1986): Immunoglobulin G subclasses of antithyroid peroxidase autoantibodies in human autoimmune thyroid diseases. Endocrinol. Japon. 33, 505-510.

Ludgate, M., Mariotti, S., Libert, F., Dinsart, C., Piccolo, P., Santini, F., Ruf, J., Pinchera, A. & Vassart, G. (1989): Antibodies to human thyroid peroxidase in autoimmune thyroid disease: Studies with a cloned recombinant complementary deoxyribonucleic acid epitope. J. Clin. Endocrinol. Metab. 68, 1091-1096.

McLachlan, S.M., Dickinson, A.M., Malcolm, A., Farndon, J.R., Young, E., Proctor, S.J. & Rees Smith, B. (1983): Thyroid autoantibody synthesis by cultures of thyroid and peripheral blood lymphocytes. I. Lymphocyte markers and response to pokeweed mitogen. Clin. Exp. Immunol. 52, 45.

Okamoto, Y., Hamada, N., Saito, H., Ohno, M., Noh, J., Ito, K. & Morii, H. (1989): Thyroid peroxidase activity-inhibiting immunoglobulins in patients with autoimmune thyroid disease. J. Clin. Endocrinol. Metab. 68, 730-734.

Portmann, L., Hamada, N., Heinrich, G. & DeGroot, L.J. (1985): Antithyroid peroxidase antibody in patients with autoimmune thyroid disease: possible identity with anti-microsomal antibody. J. Clin. Endocrinol. Metab. 61, 1001-1003.

Portmann, L, Fitch, F.W., Havran, W., Hamada, N., Franklin, W.A. & DeGroot, L.J. (1988): Characterization of the thyroid microsomal antigen, and its relationship to thyroid peroxidase, using monoclonal antibodies. J. Clin. Invest. 81, 1217-1224.

Ruf, J., Toubert, M-E., Czarnocka, B., Durand-Gorde, J.M., Ferrand, M. & Carayon, P. (1989): Relationship between immunological structure and biochemical properties of human thyroid peroxidase. Endocrinology. 125, 1211-1218.

Takaichi, Y., Tamai, H., Honda, K., Nagai, K., Kuma, K. & Nakagawa, T. (1989): The significance of antithyroglobulin and antithyroidal microsomal antibodies in patients with hyperthyroidism due to Graves' disease treated with antithyroid drugs. J. Clin. Endocrinol. Metab. 68, 1097.

Weetman, A.P., Black, C.M., Cohen, S.B., Tomlinson, R., Banga, J.P. & Reimer, C.B. (1989): Affinity purification of IgG subclasses and the distribution of thyroid auto-antibody reactivity in Hashimoto's thyroiditis. Scand. J. Immunol. 30, 73-82.

Yamamoto, M., Sakurada, T., Yoshida, K., Kaise, K., Kaise, N., Fukazawa, H., Suzuki, M., Nomura, T., Itagaki, Y., Saito, S. & Yoshinaga, K. (1987): Thyroid function and anti-microsomal antibody during the course of silent thyroiditis. Endocrinol. Japon. 34, 357-363.

Résumé

Les auto-anticorps dirigés contre la TPO humaine peuvent être hétérogènes si l'on considère leur origine, l'antigène cible spécifique, leur distribution dans différents groupes et différentes maladies, leur site de production, le type d'IgG produite et leur fonction. Il a été suggéré que les anticorps présents chez les individus normaux pouvaient être différents des anticorps pathogéniques de haute affinité rencontrés chez les patients atteints de maladies thyroïdiennes autoimmunes, la TPO pouvant différer par sa structure, sa taille, sa glycolysation et sa structure tertiaire. La réponse immune produit des Igs de tous types, quoique les IgG soient prédominants, et de toutes classes, quoique les classes 1,2 et 4 soient elles aussi prédominantes. Les auto-anticorps reconnaissent de 2 à 7 domaines antigéniques de la TPO et plusieurs épitopes linéaires localisés sur différentes fractions de la molécule. Les auto-anticorps humains reconnaissent l'antigène dénaturé par SM KSCN (D-Ag) et l'antigène réduit et dénaturé par SDS et MSH (RD-ag). Les anticorps reconnaissant ces types d'antigènes ont des taux du même ordre que ceux des anticorps reconnaissant l'antigène natif. Ils sont présents chez 11 à 14% des patients atteints de maladies thyroïdiennes autoimmunes, et apparaissent corréler avec la persistance de la maladie. Le rôle spécifique de ces anticorps n'a pas été défini. Que le rôle premier de ces anticorps anti-TPO soit celui de marqueurs, "d'éboueurs" ou d'agents cytotoxiques, cela demeure obscur, quoique dans les thyroïdites expérimentales chez l'animal ils apparaissent moins thyroïditogéniques que les anticorps anti-Tg.

Cross-reactivity between antibodies to thyroglobulin and thyroperoxidase

J. Ruf, M. Ferrand and P. Carayon

INSERM U. 38, Biochimie Médicale, Faculté de Médecine, Marseille, France

Thyroperoxidase (TPO) is an enzyme implicated in iodination of thyroglobulin (Tg) and subsequent coupling of iodotyrosyl residues to form thyroid hormones T3 and T4 (1,2). It has been recently disclosed that TPO is identical to the thyroid "microsomal antigen" and thus a major autoantigen of the thyroid gland (3-5). Autoantibodies (aAb) to Tg and TPO are found simultaneously in most of the sera from patients with Hashimoto's thyroiditis (6). This led to the striking observation that both enzyme and substrate of the thyroid hormone synthesis pathway are involved in aAb formation. The occurence and role of these aAb in the pathogenesis of the autoimmune thyroid disease is still a matter of debate despite three decades of study. While Tg autoimmunisation process can be explain by presentation to the immune system of Tg which escape intrathyroidal proteolysis (7), TPO autoimmunisation remains unclear as this enzyme is confined to cytoplasm and apical border of the thyroid cell and cannot establish a direct contact to immunocompetent cells (8,9). On the other hand, anti-TPO aAb have been proven to cause tissue damage (10-12) while anti-Tg aAb appear to have no harmful effect even though they are frequently present in high concentrations in the serum of patients with autoimmune thyroid diseases. This is particularly intriguing if one consider that experimental chronic thyroiditis could be induced in various animals by Tg immunization (13-15). Because TPO and not Tg is believed to be the pathogenic autoantigen in destructive thyroid disease, we explored the possibility that cross-reactive anti-TPO aAb could arise from Tg immunization and that patient's sera contain anti-Tg aAb that cross-react with TPO.

MATERIALS AND METHODS

Preparation of human antigens.

From human thyroid tissue obtained by surgery, we prepared Tg according to the procedure of Marriq et al. (16) and we purified TPO according to the procedure of Czarnocka et al. (3). After running in SDS-PAGE under reducing conditions,Tg gave evidence for one major band at 330 KDa and only few minor bands of smaller size. For TPO, we observed a doublet in the 100 KDa region with the upper band more pronounced than the lower one. No band was observed at the Tg position and none below the 100 KDa region.

Production of monoclonal antibodies (mAb).

Production and characterization of anti-Tg (17) and anti-TPO mAb (18) have been previously reported. Anti-Tg and anti-TPO mAb scarcely cross-reacted. Only 1 to 10 anti-Tg mAb (mAb 11) slightly bound to TPO (19.2% of its Tg binding) and only 1 to 10 anti-TPO mAb (mAb 30) slightly bound to Tg (11% of its TPO binding).

Production of anti-Tg antiserum.

Four rabbits were immunized subcutaneously with 50 µg of Tg emulsified in complete Freund's adjuvant. An intramuscular injection of 50 µg Tg, emulsified in incomplete Freund's adjuvant, was given at day 60. Blood was sampled from rabbits by cardiac punction at days 31, 37, 44 and 50 before they were boosted and at days 79, 85, 93, 100, 107 and 114 after boosting. All these samples were tested in ELISA and were shown to contain high titers of both anti-Tg and anti-TPO antibodies. Accordingly, they were pooled and served as polyclonal rabbit antiserum (pAb) source.

Serum samples.

Human sera were obtained from 25 unselected adult patients thought to have Hashimoto's thyroiditis according to their high anti-Tg and anti-TPO titers as assessed by ELISA. They were pooled and served as human autoantibodies (aAb) source.

Antibody purification.

Serum samples (50 ml) of aAb and pAb were precipitated by neutralized ammonium sulfate at 40% saturation, centrifuged and extensively dialyzed against phosphate-buffered saline (PBS) pH:7.3 to give the total IgG fractions. From these IgG fractions, we obtained antigen-specific antibodies (Ab) by affinity-chromatography using Tg- and TPO-coupled gels. Tg (200mg) was coupled to 31 ml CNBr-activated Sepharose 4B (Pharmacia) and TPO (9 mg) to 25 ml Affi-Gel 15 (Bio-Rad) according to the instructions of the respective manufacturers. For each run, the amount of Ab mixed to the coupled gel was inferior to the binding capacity of the gel and incubation was performed under gently shaking overnight at 4°C. Filtrate was then recovered and, after washing, the Ab bound to the gel eluted with 0.1M glycine-HCl buffer pH=2.8 containing 0.5M NaCl. Eluate was immediately neutralized by 1M Tris-HCl buffer pH=8.5 and extensively dialyzed against PBS. Filtrate and eluate were concentrated by dialysis against a 30% polyethylene glycol solution (PEG, mol wt=35000) and then extensively dialyzed again against PBS. The protein concentration of each fraction was determined by the MicroBCA assay (Pierce) with bovine gamma globulin as the standard.

Enzyme-linked immunosorbent assay (ELISA).

This method was used to detect aAb, pAb and mAb binding to Tg and TPO. Wells of polystyrene microtiter plates were filled with 100 µl PBS containing either 10 µg/ml Tg and 3 µg/ml TPO and incubated overnight at 4°C. After antigen coating, the wells were washed, overcoated with bovine serum albumin, washed again and filled with various dilutions of Ab samples. After 90 min. incubation at 37°C, unbound material was removed by extensive washing. Ab bound to coated antigen were detected using successively either affinity-purified anti-human, anti-rabbit and anti-mouse Ab conjugated with alkaline phosphatase and p-nitrophenyl phosphate as a substrate. Quantification was made by OD reading at 405 nm using a Multiskan Spectrophotometer. For aAb and pAb binding inhibition test by soluble Tg and TPO, the amount of Ab giving an OD signal of 0.5 was coincubated overnight at 4°C with serial dilutions of competing antigens before transfer to coated wells. For mAb binding inhibition test by aAb, the amount of mAb giving an OD signal of 0.5 was added after the coated wells were previously incubated overnight at 4°C with serial dilutions of aAb. For aAb and pAb binding to chemicaly altered antigens, we used modified antigens for coating. Denaturation with or without reduction were performed by incubating antigens with 2.5% SDS and 2.25M urea with or without 5% β2-mercaptoethanol for 15 min. at 65°C in PBS. Antigens were oxidized by Chloramine-T (1/1 ratio in PBS) during 1 min. at room temperature. In all cases, the reaction was stopped by 100-fold dilution with PBS and the treated antigens immediately coated for ELISA purpose.

RESULTS

Rabbit immunization.

After immunization with Tg, rabbits produced high levels of antibodies (pAb) reacting with Tg and TPO and these antigenic reactivities followed the same temporal pattern (Fig.1). Anti-Tg and anti-TPO titers were expressed in dilution of rabbit sera giving an OD signal of 0.5 in our ELISA. Maximal Tg and TPO titers occured after the rabbits were boosted and corresponded to a dilution of 1:200,000 and 1:900 respectively. For comparison, rabbits immunized with TPO exhibited maximal anti-TPO titers only 10-fold higher than those found in rabbits immunized with Tg whereas anti-Tg aAb titers were at least 1000-fold lower (data not shown). Preimmune sera as well as sera from bleeds of control rabbits gave anti-Tg and anti-TPO aAb titers consistently < 1:10.

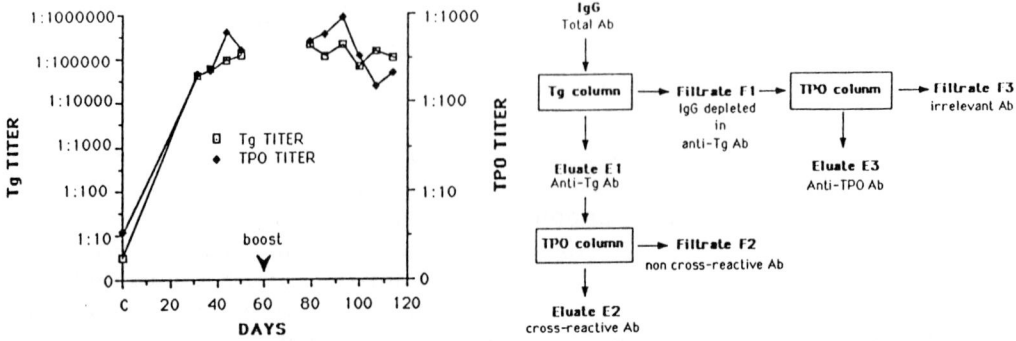

Fig.1. Temporal pattern of anti-Tg and anti-TPO pAb production in rabbits immunized with Tg.

Fig.2. Schematic representation of the affinity purification procedure used to separate specific Ab.

Affinity-purification of aAb and pAb.

Figure 2 shows the strategy we employed to separate the various populations of antibodies specific for Tg, TPO and putatively for both Tg and TPO. The total IgG fractions were put onto a Tg-column which allowed us to separate the anti-Tg reactive fraction in the eluate E1 from the others antibodies. From this eluate E1, we attempted to separate the anti-Tg Ab which cross-reacted with TPO from those which do not by further chromatography onto a TPO-column. These Ab were recovered in eluate E2 and filtrate F2 respectively. Specific anti-TPO Ab were further purified from filtrate F1 by chromatography onto a TPO-column and recovered in eluate E3. All the other irrelevant IgG were in filtrate F3. We tested these various fractions in ELISA for their ability to bind Tg and TPO. Results computed from full titration curves were first expressed in Ab titer (amount of Ab giving an OD signal of 0.5 in the ELISA) and then converted for comparison as percent of maximal titer. The upper panel of Fig.3 shows the results obtained from patients' sera. On a qualitative point of view, maximal anti-Tg and anti-TPO aAb titers were, as expected, present in fractions E1 and E3 respectively. From fraction E1, containing all the anti-Tg reactivity, we obtained anti-Tg aAb which cross-reacted with TPO in eluate E2 whereas fraction F2 contained only Tg specific aAb. From fraction F1 containing all the non Tg-related aAb we purified the anti-TPO aAb which eluted in fraction E3. As a control, the starting material (IgG fraction) was shown to contain both anti-Tg and anti-TPO aAb but, at this stage, their respective titers were lower than in the purified fractions. Conversely, the final material (filtrate F3) was totally depleted in anti-Tg and anti-TPO aAb. The lower panel shows results obtained from rabbit antisera. Maximal anti-Tg titer was, as for human material, in eluate E1 but the maximal anti-TPO pAb titer was in eluate E2 and not E3 as for the aAb. The existence of cross-reactive pAb was ascertained by Tg and TPO binding activities presented by eluate E2. Fraction F2 contained only Tg specific pAb. In contrast, no significant amount of non cross-reactive anti-TPO pAb was shown in fraction E3.

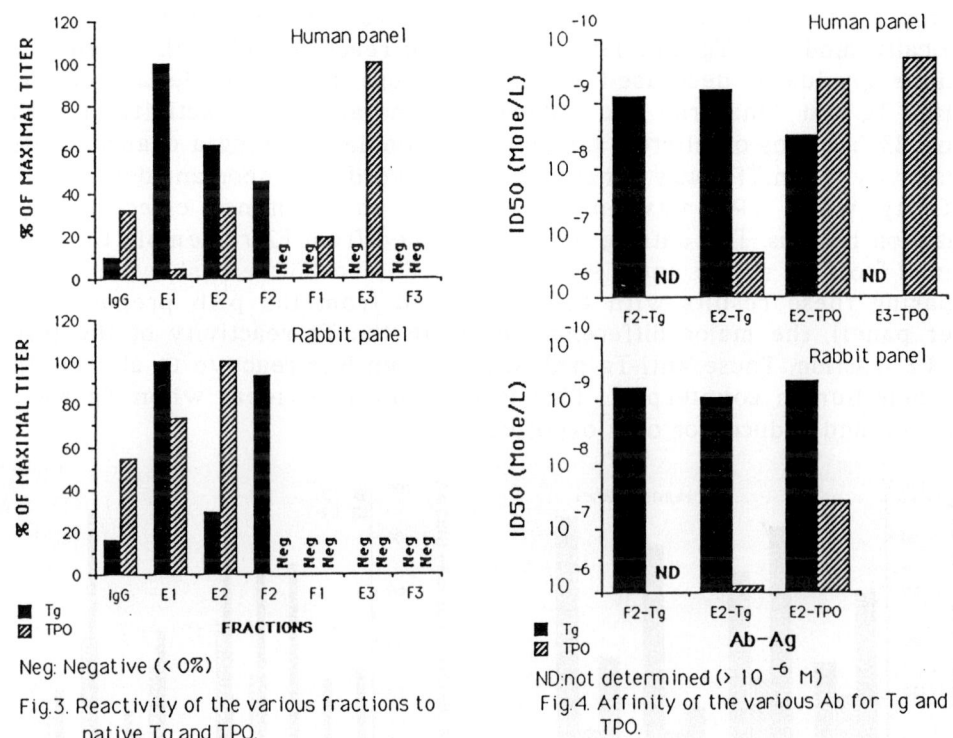

Fig.3. Reactivity of the various fractions to native Tg and TPO.

Fig.4. Affinity of the various Ab for Tg and TPO.

Binding characteristics of the affinity-purified aAb and pAb.

Tg binding of fraction F2, TPO binding of fraction E3 and both Tg and TPO binding of fraction E2 were tested in the presence of increasing amount of Tg and TPO. Results were expressed as the inhibition dose giving 50% binding inhibition (ID50) and were calculated in term of sub-unit molarity taking into account a mol wt of 330 KDa and 100 KDa for Tg and TPO, respectively. As shown in Fig.4 (upper panel), the anti-Tg aAb activity from fraction F2 to Tg and the anti-TPO aAb activity from fraction E3 to TPO were only inhibited by their respective antigens. In contrast, cross-reactive aAb binding from fraction E2 to Tg and TPO were inhibited by both Tg and TPO. TPO was about 350-fold less effective than Tg to inhibit the Tg binding of aAb from fraction E2 and Tg was only 7-fold less effective than TPO to inhibit the TPO binding of aAb from fraction E2. For rabbit pAb (lower panel), TPO was consistently less effective than Tg to inhibit Tg and TPO binding activities in E2 and did not affect Tg binding of the F2 pAb. This latter could be inhibited by Tg as effectively as Tg binding of F2 aAb. In another set of experiments, we compared the antigenic binding of F2, E2 and E3 Ab to antigens chemically altered. Results are reported in Fig.5 and were expressed in percent binding to native, unmodified antigen, the Ab concentration in the test being adjusted to give an OD signal of 1.0 when tested to native antigen in ELISA. The upper panel shows the reactivity of the various aAb preparations to chemically modified Tg and TPO. The anti-Tg reactivity of both F2 and E2 fractions gradually decreased when aAb were tested to denatured Tg, oxidized Tg and denatured and reduced Tg. The anti-TPO reactivity of both E2 and E3 fractions on altered antigens were similar showing a dramatic loss of reactivity when TPO was denatured and reduced, an important decrease of reactivity when TPO was only denatured and a minor effect of the oxidization process. The anti-Tg pattern obtained from E2 ressemble to those obtained from F2 as the anti-TPO pattern of E2 and E3 were shown similar. Comparing these results with those obtained from the pAb preparations (lower panel), the major difference reside in the Tg reactivity of the pAb from F2 fraction. These anti-Tg pAb were shown less reactive to altered Tg than their human counterpart. This is particularly evident when Tg were denatured and reduced or only oxydized.

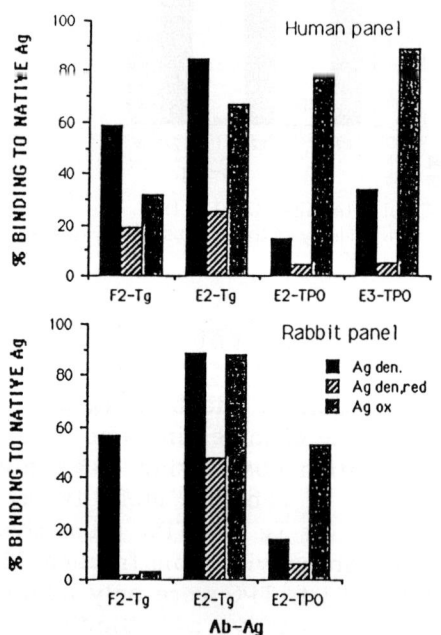
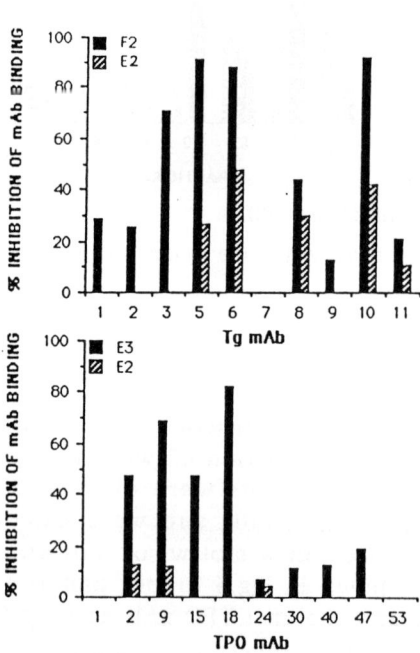

Fig.5. Reactivity of the various fractions to chemically altered Ag.

Fig.6. Fine specificity of anti-TG, anti-TPO and anti-TGPO aAb.

Fine specificities of the various populations of aAb.

We compared the fine specificities of cross-reactive aAb (E2) with those displayed by Tg-specific (F2) and TPO-specific aAb (E3). For this purpose, we use two panel of 10 mAb specific to Tg and TPO respectively. Tg and TPO binding of mAb were tested in ELISA after preincubation of coated antigens with various dilutions of aAb. Results were expressed as percent of mAb binding inhibition. For comparison, we reported in Fig. 6 the results obtained using 3 µg of competing aAb. At this dose, maximal disparities occured between the inhibition pattern displayed by the various aAb for mAb to mAb. The upper panel shows comparison between the Tg pattern of aAb from fractions F2 and E2. F2 aAb cross-reacted strongly (inhibition > 50%) with 4 mAb, weakly (inhibition < 50%) with 5 mAb and does not cross-react with mAb 7. E2 aAb exhibited a more restricted pattern as they weakly cross-reacted only with 5 out of 10 mAb. In all the cases, they were shown to be less potent inhibitors than aAb from F2. The lower panel shows comparison between TPO pattern of aAb from fractions E3 and E2. Similar but more pronounced observations than reported above could be made concerning the comparative extend of inhibition obtained. aAb from E2 very weakly cross-reacted (inhibition < 20%) with only 3 to 10 anti-TPO mAb whereas E3 cross-reacted to various extend with 8 mAb.

DISCUSSION

The results presented here demonstrate that IgG from patients presenting with autoimmune thyroid disorders contain specific aAb directed to Tg and TPO and also an additional aAb population that recognize both Tg and TPO molecules. We termed this aAb anti-TGPO aAb and found that such Ab could be induced in rabbits by Tg immunization. Anti-TGPO Ab could be extracted from affinity-purified anti-Tg aAb and pAb by an additional affinity-purification on TPO coupled gel and represented about 1/4 of the entire anti-Tg reactive Ab population. The dual binding of anti-TGPO Ab to Tg and TPO did not account for minor cross-contamination of the antigenic preparations as specific anti-Tg aAb and pAb from fractions F2 did not bind to TPO and specific anti-TPO aAb from fraction E3 did not bind to Tg. On the other hand, anti-TGPO derived from Tg coupled gel and Tg with respect to its high mol wt and its abundance in thyroid tissue could not be suspected to contain TPO. Moreover, TPO which would be the most likely antigen expected to be contaminated by Tg was obtained by affinity-chromatography using an anti-TPO mAb which was unable to recognize Tg. The dual specificity of the anti-TGPO aAb was further demonstrated by the cross-reactivities they displayed with some anti-Tg and anti-TPO mAb.

Anti-TGPO Ab from E2 fractions are part of the entire anti-Tg Ab population and consequently they displayed a higher affinity for Tg than for TPO. This was particularly evident for E2 pAb binding to Tg and TPO considering ID50 obtained with homologous and heterologous antigens. This was proved for E2 aAb binding to Tg and TPO considering ID50 obtained with heterologous antigens, ID50 obtained with homologous antigens being similar. At the molecular level, such cross-reactivity may be explain by epitopes shared by Tg and TPO; or by the presence of dissimilar epitopic structures (rather conformational) on TPO molecule which accomodate the binding site of some anti-Tg aAb resulting in a low affinity binding to TPO (19). Kohno et al. have previously reported that Tg and TPO share common epitopes recognized by aAb from patients with chronic autoimmune thyroiditis (20). However, the TPO preparation they used was not entirely pure and they do not attempt to isolate these cross-reactive aAb. Our data confirm and extend their finding because we clearly show the existence of the anti-TGPO aAb in patients and the induction of anti-TGPO pAb in rabbit. We also agree with Kohno et al. (20) about the restricted nature of the so-called "thyroiditogenic epitopes" because the mAb-assisted mapping of the anti-TGPO epitopes, albeit conducted with a few mAb revealed only 5 to 10 potential Tg epitopes (compared to 9 for F2 aAb) and 3 to 10 potential TPO epitopes (compared to 8 for E3 aAb). When compared to F2 and E3 aAb, anti-TGPO aAb appeared weakly cross-reactive with mAb suggesting that the epitopes they recognized on Tg and TPO molecules were located at distance from those recognized by F2 and E3 aAb respectively.

Anti-TGPO Ab appeared to be more reactive to denatured Tg than to denatured TPO. In the human panel, both E2 and E3 aAb weakly bound denatured TPO suggesting the conformational nature of TPO epitopes. The dramatic loss of reactivity observed with denatured and reduced TPO emphasized the major role of disulfides bridges in the TPO molecule for aAb recognition as previously reported by other investigators (21,22). Considering the rabbit panel, marked disparities occured between reactivities to altered Tg of pAb from F2 and E2. Such discrepancies were also observed, albeit in a lesser extend, in the human panel confirming that anti-Tg aAb bound weakly to reduced Tg (23). These results suggest that anti-TGPO Ab recognized Tg epitopes more resistant to denaturing process than those recognized by the specific anti-Tg Ab.

The analysis of the temporal pattern of evolution of both anti-Tg and anti-TPO Ab titers in the sera of rabbits immunized with Tg showed a striking correlation in time as well as in titer. This could be interpreted as the appearence of only anti-Tg pAb with a part of this population also reactive with TPO and suggested that similar event could be occur in patient. Thus, anti-TGPO aAb could arise from Tg autoimmunization process directed to some sequential Tg epitopes. No role was attributed to anti-Tg aAb in the development of autoimmune thyroid diseases. Thus, the pathogenic importance of anti-Tg aAb can reside in cross-reactivity that some of them display with other autoimmune thyroid diseases related antigens. For example, anti-Tg aAb (and mAb) were shown to cross-react with an orbital connective tissue membrane antigen. This cross-reactivity was proposed for the association of ophtalmopathy with autoimmune thyroid diseases (24). So, we can hypothesize that such cross-reactivity also occur between anti-Tg and anti-TPO aAb and that these cross-reactive aAb are responsable, at least in part, directly or indirectly, of the tissue damages observed in Hashimoto's thyroiditis which are mediated by humoral events and commonly attributed to anti-TPO aAb.

CONCLUSION

aAb which bind both Tg and TPO are present in sera from patients thought to have autoimmune thyroiditis. These cross-reactive aAb (anti-TGPO aAb) display a higher affinity for Tg than for TPO and recognize Tg and TPO epitopes different of those recognized by Tg and TPO specific aAb. Anti-TGPO aAb bind denatured Tg epitopes more effectively than denatured TPO epitopes. Anti-TGPO Ab can be induced in rabbit by Tg immunization. These results suggest that pathologic anti-TPO aAb can arise from Tg autoimmunization process via related, rather than identical, epitopes on both Tg and TPO molecules. Study of such aAb and the molecular characterization of the corresponding autoepitopes in the antigens should provide information concerning the role of cross-reactivy in autoimmune thyroid diseases.

REFERENCES

1. Taurog A. (1979) : Hormone synthesis. In Endocrinology, eds LJ DeGroot, Jr GF Cahill, WD Odell, L Martini, Jr JT Potts, DH Nelson, E. Steinberger, AI Winegrad, vol 1 : 331, New-York, Grune and Stratton
2. Nunez J (1980) : Iodination and thyroid hormone synthesis. In The Thyroid Gland, eds M De Visscher, p 39, New-York, Raven Press
3. Czarnocka B, Ruf J, Ferrand M, Carayon P, Lissitzky S (1985) : Purification of the human thyroid peroxidase and its identification as the microsomal antigen involved in autoimmune thyroid diseases. FEBS Lett 190 : 147
4. Portmann L, Hamada N, Heinrich G, De Groot LJ (1985) : Anti-thyroid peroxidase antibody in patients with autoimmune thyroid disease : possible identiy with anti-microsomal antibody. J Clin Endocrinol Metab 61 : 1001
5. Kotani T, Umeki K, Matsunaga S, Kato E, Ohtaki S (1986) : Detection of autoantibodies to thyroid peroxidase in autoimmune thyroid diseases by microenzyme-linked immunosorbent assay and immunoblotting. J. Clin Endocrinol Metab 62 : 928
6. Doniach D, Roitt IM (1959) : Autoimmunity in Hashimoto's disease. Proc Roy Soc Med 52 : 178
7. Pinchera A, Mariotti S, Vitti P, Marcocci C, Chiovato L, Fenzi G, Santini F (1989) : Thyroid autoantigens and their relevance in the pathogenesis of thyroid autoimmunity. Biochimie 71 : 237
8. Nilsson M, Molne J, Karlsson F, Ericson L (1987) : Immunoelectron microscopic studies on the cell surface location of the thyroid microsomal antigen. Molec Cell Endocrinol 53 : 177
9. Alquier C, Ruf J, Athouel-Haon AM, Carayon P (1989) : Immunocyto chemical study of localization and traffic of thyroid peroxidase/ microsomal antigen. Autoimmunity 3 : 113

10. Khoury EL, Hammond L, Bottazzo GF, Doniach D (1981) : Presence of the organ-specific "microsomal" autoantigen on the surface of human thyroid cells in culture : its involvement in complement-mediated cytotoxicity.Clin Exp Immunol 45 : 316
11. Bogner U, Schleusener H, Wall JR (1984) : Antibody-dependent cell mediated cytotoxicity against human thyroid cells in Hashimoto's thyroiditis but not Graves'disease. J. Clin Endocrinol Metab 59 : 734
12. Wadeleux P, Winand-Devigne J, Ruf J, Carayon P, Winand R (1989) : Cytotoxic assay of circulating thyroid peroxidase antibodies Autoimmunity 4 : 247
13. Weigle WO (1980) : Analysis of autoimmunity through experimental models of thyroiditis and allergic encephalomyelitis. Adv. Immunol 30 : 159
14. Weetman AP, MC Gregor AM (1984) : Autoimmune thyroid disease : Developments in our understanding. Endocr Rev 5 : 309
15. Volpé R (1985) : Autoimmune thyroid disease. In Autoimmunity and Endocrine Disease, ed R. Volpé, p 109, New-York, Marcel Dekker.
16. Marriq C, Rolland M, Lissitzky S (1977) : Polypeptide chains of 19-S thyroglobulin from several mammalian species and of porcine 27-S iodoprotein. Eur J Biochem 79 : 143
17. Ruf J, Carayon P, Sarles-Philip N, Kourilsky F, Lissitzky S (1983) : Specificity of monoclonal antibodies against human thyroglobulin ; comparison with autoimmune antibodies EMBO J 2 : 1821
18. Ruf J, Toubert M.E., Czarnocka B, Durand-Gorde JM, Ferrand M, Carayon P (1989) : Relationship between immunological structure and biochemical properties of human thyroid peroxidase. Endocrinology 125 : 1211
19. Lane D, Koprowski H (1982) : Molecular recognition and the future of monoclonal antibodies Nature 296 : 200
20. Kohno Y, Naito N, Hiyama Y, Shimojo N, Suzuki N, Tarutani O, Niimi H, Nakajima H, Hosoya T (1988) : Thyroglobulin and thyroid peroxidase share common epitopes recognized by autoantibodies in patients with chronic autoimmune thyroiditis J Clin Endocrinol Metab 67 : 899
21. Nakajima Y, Howells, RD, Pegg C, Davies Jones E, Rees Smith B (1987) : Structure-activity analysis of microsomal antigen/thyroid peroxidase Mol Cell Endocrinol 53 : 15
22. Gardas A, Domek H, Czarnocka B (1990) : The effect of dithiotreitol on thyroid peroxidase and microsomal antigen eptiopes recognized by auto and monoclonal antibodies. Autoimmunity (in press).
23. Shimojo N, Saito K, Kohno Y, Sasaki N, Tarutani O, Nakajima H (1988) : Antigenic determinants on thyroglobulin : comparison of the reactivities of different thyroglobulin preparations with serum antibodies and T cells of patients with chronic thyroiditis. J Clin Endocrinol Metab 66 : 689
24. Kuroki T, Ruf J, Whelan L, Miller A, Wall JR (1985) : Antithyroglobulin monoclonal and autoantibodies cross-react with an orbital connective

tissue membrane antigen. A possible mechanism for the association of ophtalmopathy with autoimmune thyroid disorders <u>Clin Exp Immunol</u> 62 : 361

Résumé

L'identification récente de l'antigène microsomal thyroidien à la thyroperoxydase (TPO) souligne le lien immunologique pouvant exister entre cette enzyme et son substrat, la thyroglobuline (Tg).

Dans cette étude, nous avons exploré la possibilité que des réacitivités croisées entre anticorps anti-Tg et anti-TPO puissent être à la base de la présence simultanée de ces deux types d'anticorps chez des patients atteints de thyroidite autoimmune.

Nous avons montré que le sérum de patients contenant des taux élevés d'anticorps anti-Tg et anti-TPO contient aussi des anticorps dirigés contre, à la fois la Tg et la TPO. Ce type d'anticorps (que nous avons appelé anticorps anti-TGPO) est aussi retrouvé dans le sérum de lapins immunisés avec la Tg.

Ces anticorps anti-TGPO représentent une sous-population des anticorps anti-Tg. Ils ont une affinité plus grande pour la Tg que pour la TPO. Ils se distinguent des anticorps anti-Tg par une meilleure reconnaissance de la Tg dénaturée.

L'analyse de leur spécificité fine à l'aide d'anticorps monoclonaux anti-Tg et anti-TPO indique une hétérogénéité apparemment plus restreinte et une reconnaissance épitopique différente par rapport aux anticorps spécificiques soit de la Tg soit de la TPO.

Ces résultats amènent à penser que l'apparition d'anticorps anti-TPO puissent être, à la base, le fait d'une autoimmunisation contre la Tg. Ceci implique, au niveau moléculaire, que la Tg et la TPO partagent des épitopes sinon identiques du moins apparentés.

Cette hypothèse pourrait expliquer la discordance qu'il y a entre le fait qu'une thyroidite expérimentale puisse être induite par immunisation avec la Tg alors que se sont les anticorps anti-TPO qui semblent être responsables des atteintes cellulaires dans la thyroïdie.

B and T cell epitopes on thyroid peroxidase

N. Fukuma, D. Sarsero, J. Furmaniak, C.A.S. Pegg, S.M. McLachlan and B. Rees Smith

Endocrine Immunology Unit, Department of Medicine, University of Wales College of Medicine, Heath Park, Cardiff, and Department of Surgery, University of Nottingham, UK

The epitopes recognised by T and B lymphocytes in the autoimmune response to thyroid peroxidase (TPO) or thyroglobulin (Tg) have not yet been identified. The difficulty in the case of the autoantibodies (i.e. B cell receptors) is associated with the large size and complexity of the autoantigens and often the loss of antibody binding activity following denaturation and/or reduction of the antigen, which suggests that the epitopes are conformational. With respect to T cell recognition, the T cell proliferative response to Tg has proved to be weak and/or variable (McLachlan and Rees Smith 1983, Canonica et al 1984), even with T cell lines and clones (MacKenzie et al 1987, Weetman et al 1986). Responses to TPO have not been reported perhaps because of the difficulty in isolating large amounts of purified human TPO.

However, other approaches to defining autoantigenic epitopes are available and we now report the results of our investigations with respect to TPO.

T cell epitopes on TPO

Recent observations concerning T cell recognition of exogenous antigens in mice and man suggested an approach which could overcome the problem of limited availability of purified TPO. T cells appear to recognise fragments of processed protein antigens in the form of short linear peptides which bind to a cleft in the major histocompatibility (MHC) antigen on the surface of the antigen presenting cell (Bjorkman et al 1987). Further, studies of the nature of T cell epitopes indicate that peptides likely to be T cell epitopes may be predicted from the amino acid sequence of the protein (De Lisi and Berzofsky, 1985, Rothbard and Taylor 1988). In addition, the use of simple peptides could conceivably overcome potential problems associated with limiting numbers of appropriate antigen processing or presenting cells in lymphoid suspensions in culture.

Thirteen synthetic peptides (Table 1), predicted to be T cell epitopes on TPO, were investigated for their ability to stimulate proliferation. Lymphoid suspensions prepared from peripheral blood (n=12), thyroid tissue (n=3) and lymph nodes draining the thyroid (n=7) of 12 Hashimoto and 8 Graves' patients were incubated in 96-well plates in the presence or absence of 2.5 or 25ug/ml of the 13 TPO peptides and 9 control peptides. After 3-6 days, ^{3}H-thymidine was added and the extent of proliferation assessed in terms of ^{3}H-thymidine incorporated.

Table 1. Sequences of thirteen synthetic peptides (single letter amino acid code) predicted to contain T cell epitopes on the extracellular portion of TPO using the algorithms of De Lisi and Berzofsky (1985) and Rothbard and Taylor (1988). A potential epitope shared by TPO and Tg is indicated by asterisks; the sequences of nine control peptides used in the study are included. The peptide sequences were predicted and synthesised by Dr. Basil Rapoport, University of California, San Francisco, who generously made them available to us.

Peptide sequence	Amino Acid residues on TPO
L K K R G I L S P A Q L L S	62-75
S G V I A R A A E I M E T S I Q	84-99
T D A *L S E D L L S I* I A N S	116-131
P P V R E V T R H V I Q V S	203-216
P R Q Q M N G L T S F L D A S	313-327
L T A L H T L W L R E H N R L	403-417
H N R L A A A L K A L N A H W	414-428
A R K V V G A L H Q I I T L	437-450
L P G L W L H Q A F F V S P W T L	514-529
M N E E L T E R L F V L S N S S T	556-572
L D L A S I N L Q R G	572-583
R S V A D K I L D L Y K H P D N	616-631
I D V W L G G L A E N F L P	632-645

Control Peptides

C L P Y M L P P K C	133-142
E A R P A A G T A C	277-286
C A P E P G N P G E T R G P	375-388
E A F Q Q Y V G P Y E G Y D S T A	461-477
Y D S T A N P T V S N V	473-484
R G G G L D P L I R G L	531-542
Y N E W R E F C G L P R L E T P A	591-607
G K F P E D F E S C D S I T G M	712-727
C A D P Y E L G D D G R T C	825-838

Small proliferative responses were observed to some TPO peptides but the stimulatory peptides were different in different individuals, were not always shown by lymphocytes from the same patient on different occasions and did not differ significantly from responses detected in lymphocyte suspensions from control donors with undetectable levels of TPO antibodies (Fukuma et al 1990 and manuscript in preparation). Further, it was not possible to specifically enhance low levels of proliferation by removal of suppressor/cytotoxic (CD8+) cells.

Consequently, using primary lymphoid cultures from a variety of organs, including the thyroid gland which might be expected to be enriched in precursor T cells specific for thyroid antigens (Atherton et al 1985), we were unable to identify TPO epitopes using this selection of peptides. Amongst the peptides from the amino-terminal end of TPO was one of particular interest, as its sequence has a high degree of homology to a sequence in the carboxyl terminus of Tg and it was possible that this potential "shared TPO-Tg epitope" could explain the simultaneous occurrence of autoantibodies to both TPO and Tg in many Hashimoto and some Graves' patients (McLachlan and Rapoport 1989).

Although this approach was unsuccessful in identifying T cell epitopes on TPO, other peptide sequences may prove to be stimulatory. In addition, the number of precursor T cells may be limiting, even in populations of thyroid lymphocytes. Consequently the use of T cell clones, developed from thyroid tissue using autologous thyroid cells and IL-2, together with different peptides, may permit the identification of T cell epitopes on TPO.

B cell epitopes on TPO

Most, if not all, epitopes recognised by autoantibodies on TPO are conformational (Nakajima et al 1987) although Hamada et al (1989) reported the existence of apparently non-conformational autoantibody reactive determinants on TPO. In the case of Tg, the epitopes recognised by autoantibodies are also probably conformational (Male et al 1985; Shimojo et al 1988). The number of epitopes recognised on Tg appears to be relatively restricted, between 4-6 (Nye et al 1980) and there is evidence that the number of epitopes on TPO is also limited (Yokoyama et al 1989, Ruf et al 1989).

We have observed that the IgG subclasses of autoantibodies to TPO and Tg are usually IgG1 or IgG1 and IgG4, with smaller contributions from IgG2 and IgG3 in some patients (Parkes et al 1984). In addition, these IgG subclass patterns form stable, characteristic "fingerprints" for individual patients and we postulated that these restricted IgG subclass patterns might represent the ability of an individual to respond to different epitopes on the autoantigen (McLachlan et al 1987). Some evidence in support of this hypothesis was obtained when we demonstrated that monoclonal human Tg autoantibodies of subclasses IgG2 and IgG4 recognised different epitopes on Tg (Fukuma et al 1989).

We have recently developed a human monoclonal autoantibody to TPO by fusing thyroid lymphocytes from a Hashimoto patient to a mouse myeloma line (X63-Ag8.653) using polyethylene glycol (PEG 4000, Merck, Darmstadt, Germany) and subsequent selection with HAT medium (Goding, 1980). Cell lines secreting autoantibodies to Tg and TPO were detected using ELISA plates coated with Tg or thyroid microsomal antigen respectively (McLachlan et al 1982; Schardt et al 1982). Further analysis showed that cell line 2D10 secreted TPO (mic) antibody of subclass IgG3 and kappa light chain type; serum TPO antibodies in the donor patient were IgG1 $\gg$ IgG4 $>$ IgG3 $>$ IgG2. Although the line was not cloned, the only subclass secreted in amounts readily detectable by an ELISA for human IgG subclasses (The Binding Site, Birmingham UK) was IgG3 and the restriction to one light chain type indicated that the line secreted monoclonal TPO antibody. This monoclonal TPO antibody was used to investigate whether TPO antibodies of different IgG subclasses bind to different epitopes on TPO by ELISA. Replicate wells on two ELISA plates coated with thyroid microsomal antigen were exposed for 1 hour to culture supernatant from 2D10 or to buffer. After washing, duplicate wells on both plates were exposed to a range of dilutions of serum from:-

(a) Hashimoto patient EB, whose TPO (mic) antibodies were known to be predominantly of subclass IgG1, with very low levels of IgG4 TPO antibody and IgG3 Tg antibody undetectable in serum diluted 1:300.

(b) Hashimoto patient MT who had TPO (mic) antibodies predominantly of subclass IgG4 with a smaller contribution from IgG1 and TPO antibodies of subclass IgG3 undetectable in serum diluted 1:100.

After incubation for 1 hour and washing, one plate was exposed to monoclonal murine anti-human IgG1 and one plate to anti-human IgG4 (clones NL16 and RJ4 respectively, Oxoid Ltd., Basingstoke, U.K.). Thirty minutes later, the plates were washed, incubated for a further 30 minutes with anti-mouse IgG peroxidase conjugate (Sigma Chemical Co. Ltd., Poole, U.K.), washed and developed with substrate (o-phenylene diamine + H_2O_2 in citrate buffer pH 5.0) for 10 mins, and the plates read at 492nm after addition of 2M H_2SO_4. The level of IgG3 TPO (mic) antibody present in supernatant from 2D10 was measured using anti-human IgG3 (clone ZG4, Oxoid Ltd.).

As shown in Fig 1A, the optical density values obtained for IgG1 TPO (mic) antibodies for patient EB were essentially similar when measured in wells which had or had not been previously exposed to monoclonal antibody 2D10 and similar results were obtained for the low levels of IgG1 TPO antibody in serum from patient MT (Fig. 1C). TPO antibodies of subclass IgG4 were undetectable in serum from patient EB over the concentration range studied (Fig. 1B), but IgG4 TPO antibody levels in patient MT were virtually identical whether measured in wells exposed initially to 2D10 or not (Fig. 1D).

Fig. 1. TPO antibodies of subclass IgG1 (A and C) and IgG4 (B and D) measured by ELISA on thyroid microsomal antigen coated plates initially exposed to culture supernatant from cell line 2D10 (●-----●) or buffer (o———o) and subsequently to increasing concentrations of serum from patient EB (A and B) or MT (C and D). The level of TPO antibody in 2D10 (subclass IgG3) is indicated by a bar on each graph.

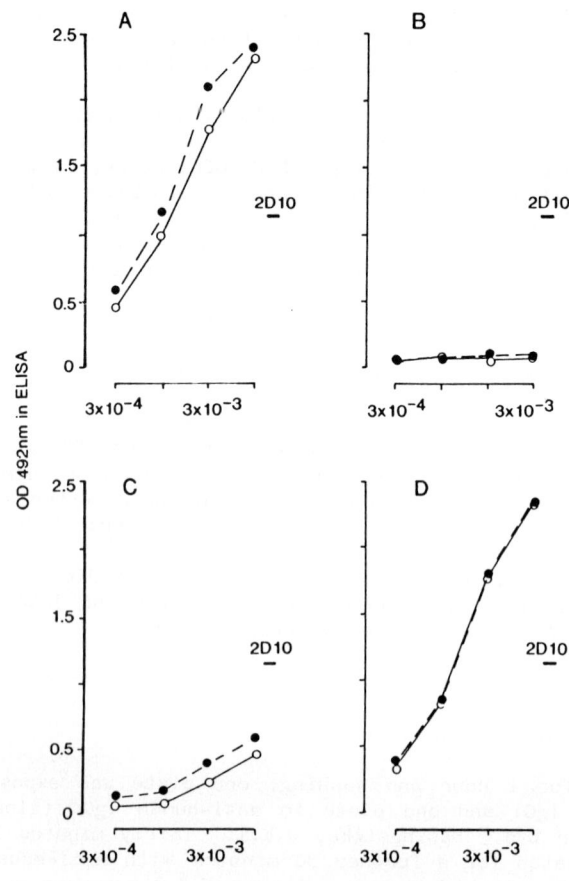

Our investigations indicate that the site to which the monoclonal TPO antibody of subclass IgG3 binds is different from that with which TPO antibodies of subclasses IgG1 and IgG4 interact. These results are consistent with our previous observations for Tg antibodies of subclasses IgG2 and IgG4 (Fukuma et al 1989), and with more recent data we have obtained using two human monoclonal antibodies of subclass IgG1 and two other IgG2 Tg antibodies (manuscript in preparation).

A variety of approaches has been used in attempts to characterise TPO epitopes. Libert et al (1987) isolated clones representing different short segments of recombinant TPO in an expression cDNA library λ gt11 and analysed the interaction of the recombinant proteins with Hashimoto and normal sera. They reported that the amino acid sequence between residues 590 and 675 appears to be an epitope which interacts with autoantibodies to TPO. In addition, Banga et al (1989) reported that TPO autoantibodies interacted with 6 different fragments of TPO expressed in E. coli as a fusion protein with glutathione s-transferase. A similar approach was not successful in the case of studying the interaction of Tg autoantibodies with fragments of Tg expressed in a λ gt11 library (Dong et al 1989) which supports the concept that the secondary structure of Tg is important in forming its antigen binding sites. As TPO requires an intact disulphide bridge to form the TPO antibody binding site (at least in the case of most sera), a study of the effects of reducing agents on different preparations containing TPO fragments seems appropriate.

Acknowledgements

The work was supported in part by the Wellcome Foundation. We acknowledge the skilled assistance of Mrs. Kathy Earlam in preparing the manuscript. We would also like to thank Professor Reginald Hall for assisting us in obtaining Hashimoto thyroid tissue.

References

Atherton, M.C., McLachlan, S.M., Pegg, C.A.S., Dickinson A., Baylis, P., Young, E.T., Proctor, S.J., and Rees Smith, B. (1985) Thyroid autoantibody synthesis by lymphocytes from different lymphoid organs: fractionation of B cells on density gradients. Immunology 55:271-279.

Banga, J.P., Barnett, P.S., Ewins, D.L., Page, M. and McGregor A.M. (1989). Autoantigenic epitopes on thyroid microsome/thyroid peroxidase antigen recognised by autoantibodies reside in the amino acid region, the carboxyl region and the central core of the molecule. Autoimmunity 5:142-144.

Bjorkman, P.J., Saper, M.A., Samraoui, B., Bennett, W.S., Strominger, J.L. and Wiley, D.C. (1987). The foreign antigen binding site and T cell recognition regions of Class I histocompatibility antigens. Nature 329:512-518.

Canonica, G.W., Cosulich, M.E., Croci, R., Ferrini, S., Bagnasco, M., Dirienzo, W., Ferrini O., Bargellesi, A., and Gordiano G. (1984). Thyroglobulin-induced T-cell in-vitro proliferation in Hashimoto's thyroiditis: identification of the responsive subset and effect of monoclonal antibodies directed to Ia antigens. Clin. Immunol. Immunopathol. 32:132-141.

De Lisi, C., and Berzofsky, J.A. (1985). T cell antigenic sites tend to be amphipathic structures. Proc. Natl. Acad. Sci. USA 82:7048-7052.

Dong, Q., Ludgate M., and Vassart, G. (1989). Towards an antigenic map of human thyroglobulin: identification of ten epitope-bearing sequences within the primary structure of thyroglobulin. J. Endocrinology 122:169-176.

Fukuma, N., McLachlan, S.M., Petersen, V.B., Kau, P., Bradbury, P., Devey, M., Bleasdale, K., Grabowski, P. and Rees Smith, B. (1989). Human thyroglobulin antibodies of subclasses IgG2 and IgG4 bind to different epitopes on thyroglobulin. Clin. exp. Immunol. 67:129-131.

Fukuma N., McLachlan, S.M., Phillips, D.I.W., Pegg, C.A.S., Rapoport B., and Rees Smith, B. (1990). T cell epitopes and thyroid peroxidase. Proceedings of a workshop on "Autoimmune Thyroiditis" held in Homburg, West Germany, October, 1989. In press.

Goding, J.W. (1980). Antibody production by hybridomas. J. Immunol. Methods 39:285-308.

Hamada, N., Jaeduck, N., Portmann, L., Ito K., and De Groot, L. (1987). Antibodies against denatured and reduced thyroid microsomal antigen in autoimmune thyroid disease. J. Clin. Endocrinol. Metab. 64:230-238.

Libert, F., Ruel, J., Ludgate, M., Swillens, S., Alexander, N., Vassart, G. and Dinsart F. (1987). Thyroid peroxidase, an autoantigen with a mosaic structure made of nuclear and mitochondrial gene modules. EMBO J. 6:4193-4196.

Male, D.K., Champion, B.R., Matthews, H., and Shepherd P. (1985). Antigenic determinants of human thyroglobulin differentiated using antigen fragments. Immunology 54:419-427.

MacKenzie, W.A., Schwartz, A.E., Friedman, E.W., and Davies, T.F. (1987) Intrathyroidal T cell clones from patients with autoimmune thyroid disease. J. Clin. Endocrinol. Metab. 64:818-824.

McLachlan, S. and Rees Smith, B. (1983) Immune function in autoimmune thyroid disease. In Autoimmune Endocrine Disease, ed. T. F. Davies, pages 139-166. New York, John Wiley and Sons.

McLachlan, S.M., Clark, S., Stimson, W.H., Clark, F., and Rees Smith, B. (1982). Studies of thyroglobulin autoantibody synthesis using a micro-ELISA assay. Immunol Lett. 4:27-33.

McLachlan, S.M., Feldt-Rasmussen, U., Young, E.T., Middleton, S.L., Blichert-Toft, M., Siersboek-Nielsen, K., Date, J., Carr, D., Clark F., and Rees Smith, B. (1987). IgG subclass distribution of thyroid autoantibodies: a "fingerprint" of an individual's response to thyroglobulin and thyroid microsomal antigen. Clin. Endocrinol. 26:335-346.

McLachlan, S.M. and Rapoport, B. (1989). Evidence for a potential common T-cell epitope between human thyroid peroxidase and human thyroglobulin with implications for the pathogenesis of autoimmune thyroid disease. Autoimmunity 5:101-106.

Nakajima, Y., Howells, R.D., Pegg, C., Davies Jones, E. and Rees Smith, B. (1987). Structure activity analysis of microsomal antigen/thyroid peroxidase. Mol. Cell. Endocrinol. 53:15-23.

Nye, L., Pontes de Carvalho, I. and Roitt, I.M. (1980). Restrictions in the response to autologous thyroglobulin in the human. Clin. exp. Immunol. 41:252-

Parkes, A.B., McLachlan, S.M., Bird, P. and Rees Smith, B. (1984). The distribution of microsomal and thyroglobulin antibody activity among the IgG subclasses. Clin. exp. Immunol. 57:239-243.

Rothbard, J.B. and Taylor, N.R. (1988). A sequence pattern common to T cell epitopes. EMBO J. 1:93-100.

Ruf, J., Toubert, M.E., Czarnocka, B., Durand-Gorde, J.M., Ferrand, M. and Carayon, P. (1989). Relationship between immunological structure and biochemical properties of human thyroid peroxidase. Endocrinology 125:1211-1218.

Schardt, C.W., McLachlan, S.M., Matheson, J. and Rees Smith, B. (1982). An enzyme-linked immunoassay for thyroid microsomal antibodies. J. Immunol. Methods 55:155-168.

Shimojo N., Saito, K., Kohno, Y., Sasaki, N., Tarutani, O. and Nakajima Y. (1988). Autoantigenic determinants on thyroglobuliln: comparison of the reactivities of different thyroglobulin preparations with serum antibodies and T cells of patients with chronic thyroiditis. J. Clin. Endocrinol. Metab. 66:689-695.

Weetman, A.P., Volkman, D.J., Burman, K.D., Margolick, J.B., Petrick, P., Weintraub, B.D., and Fauci, A.S. (1986). The production and characterisation of thyroid-derived T-cell lines in Graves' disease and Hashimoto's thyroiditis. Clin. Immunol. Immunopathol. 39:139-150.

Yokoyama, N., Taurog, A. and Klee, G.G. (1989). Thyroid peroxidase and thyroid microsomal autoantibodies. J. Clin. Endocrinol. Metab. 68:766-773.

Résumé

Nous avons testé la capacité de 12 peptides synthétiques -supposés être des épitopes de cellules T sur la TPO- à stimuler la prolifération des cellules T dans des cultures primaires de lymphocytes provenant de sang, de tissu thyroïdien et de nodules lymphocytaires de patients atteints de thyroïdites d'Hashimoto et de Basedow. Aucune prolifération significative n'a été observée. Il est cependant possible que d'autres séquences de peptides soient stimulantes, et il faut peut-être utiliser des clones de cellules T dérivées de thyroïdes de Basedow ou d'Hashimoto, qui sont supposées contenir un nombre important de cellules T spécifiques de la TPO. La plupart des épitopes reconnus par les auto-anticorps humains sur la TPO sont conformationnels, et par conséquent difficiles à identifier. Nous avons récemment développé un autoanticorps anti-TPO monoclonal humain de sous-classe IgG 3 (2 D 10) en fusionnant des lymphocytes de thyroïde d'Hashimoto avec un myélome murin. L'anticorps anti-TPO monoclonal IgG 3 n'interférait pas avec la fixation sur la TPO (antigène microsomal) des anticorps anti-TPO sériques de sous-classe IgG I et IgG 4, en ELISA. Ces observations corroborent notre hypothèse selon laquelle les auto-anticorps de sous-classe IgG différentes reconnaissent des épitopes différents sur la TPO.

Molecular characterization of thyroid peroxidase epitopes

R. Elisei, S. Swillens, G. Vassart and M. Ludgate

Institute of Interdisciplinary Research (IRIBHN), University of Brussels, Campus Erasme, B-1070 Brussels, Belgium

INTRODUCTION

In a previous report (1) we characterized antibodies to a major epitope of thyroid peroxidase (TPO), C2, an 85 amino acid fragment of TPO from 590-675 which was isolated using serum from a patient with Hashimoto's thyroiditis (HT) and which is recognised by two thirds of patients with autoimmune thyroid disease (AITD) who also have antibodies to the intact TPO molecule as measured in a radioimunoassay (RIA). The present work investigates two questions ensuing from that study : 1) Do antibodies which bind to C2 also bind to native TPO ? There is some doubt as to whether or not antibodies which bind to fragments of a protein also bind to the native form (2). 2) Does TPO share an epitope with the $H^+K^+ATPase$ (3) enzyme which has recently been shown to be a major component of the gastric parietal cell antigen (PCA). In our previous report we found 6 out of 9 sera which were positive for PCA antibodies from patients with non-thyroid autoimmune diseases (NTAID) were also positive for C2 antibodies. We have measured C2Ab in a larger series of patients with PCA antibodies (PCA Ab). We have also measured antibodies in these patients to a second fragment of TPO, C21, a 100 amino acid peptide from residues 655 to 755 which was isolated using serum from an HT patient and which overlaps C2 by 20 amino acids. Finally we have investigated whether the alternatively spliced form of TPO demonstrated in Graves' thyroids, in which residues 531 to 589 are spliced out, also exists in normal thyroid.

MATERIAL AND METHODS

Preparation of affinity purified antibodies

Lysis plaques from approximatively 30,000 identical phages (either C2 or an unrelated control) were transferred to nitrocellulose filters soaked in IPTG. The filters, saturated either with C2 or control recombinant proteins, were incubated in PBS containing 1%

BSA to block unoccupied sites and then incubated in sera, diluted to 1:40 in PBS containing 0.25% gelatin and 0.1% NP40 (wash buffer), (plus 50 µl E.coli extract to reduce background staining) at 4°C overnight with agitation. A small piece of each filter was removed for staining by standard procedures (6) to determine whether the serum had bound to the fusion protein or not. The remainder of the filters was washed three times in wash buffer and once in PBS. Bound antibody was eluted by applying 200mM glycine HCl pH 2.5 containing 0.1% gelatin for 3-5 min, the eluates were immediately neutralised by the addition of 100 µl 2M Tris.

Eluates were dialysed against 100 volumes of PBS and tested for binding to C2 in an ELISA and for antibodies to intact TPO in an RIA, as described previously (1). Sera from 10 patients with AITD, as diagnosed by established clinical and laboratory criteria were treated in this way.

Enzyme linked immunosorbent assay

C2 (TPO 590-675) and C21 (TPO 655-755) fragments were used as β-galactosidase fusion proteins to coat microtitre plates at 5 µg/ml as previously described (1). To permit comparison of values obtained in different experiments, results are expressed as a percentage of a standard reference serum. In a typical experiment in which C2 was the antigen, the mean OD_{405} of assays of serum from 20 normal individuals was 0.175 ± 0.045, corresponding to 21 ± 6% of the standard reference serum. Values greater than OD_{405} 0.280 or > 33% of the reference serum were considered positive, i.e. exceeding by 2SD the mean of the normal subjects. When C21 was the antigen, the mean OD_{405} of assays of serum from 17 normal individuals was 0.340 ± 0.096, corresponding to 28 ± 8% of the standard reference serum. Values greater than OD_{405} 0.530 or > 44% were considered positive for C21.

Polymerase chain reaction and hybridisation

The forward and reverse primers were both 18 mer oligo nucleotides of identical GC content located approximatively, 100 nucleotides upstream and downstream respectively from the spliced out fragment. 1 µl aliquots of the lambda gt II normal human thyroid library (containing 10^8 pfu) were subjected to 35 cycles of a standard polymerase chain reaction using the primers described above and Taq polymerase in a temperature cycler (7).

PCR products were separated by electrophoresis in 2% agarose, visualised by ethydium bromide staining and their sizes calculated by comparison with molecular weight markers by standard procedures (8). The amplified DNAs were blotted onto a nylon membrane, by the method of Southern (9) and hybridised overnight at 42°C with a 20 mer corresponding to the TPO junction site, end labelled with P^{32} ATP. After stringent washings, the membrane was exposed to autoradiographic film overnight at -70°C with an intensifying screen.

RESULTS

C2 affinity purification

When eluates were tested for binding to C2 in an ELISA or TPO in an RIA, only C2 eluates from sera containing antibodies both to C2 and TPO were positive in the two assays.

ELISA for antibodies to C2 and C21 in patients with antibodies to the parietal cell antigen

Antibodies to C2 were measured in 20 normal sera and 22 patients with autoimmune diseases which were not thyroidal in origin and who had PCA Ab, none of whom had antibodies to TPO or the thyroid microsomal antigen. Antibodies to C21 were measured in 17 normal sera and 18 of the 22 patients with PCA Ab. Based on the mean + 2SD of the normals, 12/22 (55%) of patients with PCA Ab have C2 Ab and 18/18 (100%) have C21 Ab.

Analysis of PCR products and hybridisation

Following 35 cycles of the PCR and electrophoresis of the PCR products, two bands were visible, an intense band at about 370 base pairs and a weaker band at about 200 base pairs. These are the sizes predicted for the full length and alternatively spliced forms of TPO respectively.

Upon hybridisation with the junction probe, the weaker band at 200 base pairs gave a strong signal whilst the 370 base pair band, despite being considerably more abundant, gave a much weaker hybridisation signal. This is as expected, since the junction probe is homologous to the alternatively spliced TPO over 20 nucleotides but to the full length TPO over only 10 nucleotides.

DISCUSSION

When 10 sera from patients with AITD were affinity purified using nitrocellulose filters saturated either with C2 or control recombinant proteins, only C2 eluates from sera containing antibodies both to TPO and C2 bound to the native enzyme in an RIA. The fact that control eluates were negative, indicates that the binding of C2 eluates to TPO is because C2 antibodies are able to bind to the intact protein and not because of non-specific binding of TPO antibodies, distinct from C2 antibodies.

In a previous study we noted that 6 out of 9 patients with NTAID who had antibodies to the PCA; were positive for C2. PCA has recently been characterized as the $H^+K^+ATPase$ and comparison of its sequence with that of C2 reveals an eleven residue fragment in which 6 amino acids are identical and 3 are conservative substitutions (10) the fragment is found both in C2 and C21 peptides of TPO (11). we have shown that 55% of 22 patients with non thyroidal autoimmunity who are PCA antibody positive bind to C2 and 100% of 18 of these patients bind to C21. this is highly suggestive of an epitope shared between the two tissue specific enzymes, TPO and $H^+K^+ATPase$.

Using the PCR, we have demonstrated the existence of the alternatively spliced form of TPO (which had until now been found only in Graves' thyroid glands) in normal thyroid, thus reducing the likelihood that the shorter form of TPO might be implicated, as an altered self antigen, in the pathogenesis of AITD.

ACKNOWLEDGMENTS

Supported by the Wellcome Foundation and Ministero della Pubblica Istruzione Italiane.

REFERENCES

1. Ludgate, M., Mariotti, S., Libert, F., Dinsart, C., Piccollo, P., Santini, F., Ruf, J., Pinchera, A., Vassart, G. (1989): Antibodies to human thyroid peroxidase in autoimmune thyroid disease : studies with a cloned recombinant complementary deoxyribonucleotic acid epitope. *J. Clin. Endocr. Metab.* 68, 1091-1096.

2. Jemmerson, R. (1987): Antigenicity and native structure of globular proteins : low frequency of peptide reactive antibodies. *Proc. Natl. Acad. Sci. USA.* 84, 9180-9184.

3. Karlsson, F.A., Burman, P., Loof, L., Mardh, G. (1988): Major parietal cell antigen in autoimmune gastritis with pernicious anemia is the acid producing H^+, K^+-adenosine triphosphatase of the stomach. *J. Clin. Invst.* 81, 475-479.

4. Kimura, S., Kotani, T., Bride, O.W., Umeki, K., Hirai, K., Nakayama, T., Ohtaki, S. (1987): Human thyroid peroxidase sequence, chromosome mapping and identification of two alternatively spliced mRNAs. *Proc. Natl. Acad. Sci. USA.* 86, 5555-5559.

5. Barnett, P.S., Banga, J.P., Watkins, J., Huang, G.C., Gluckman, D.R.B., Page, M.J., McGregor, A.M. (1990): Nucleotide sequence of the alternatively spliced human thyroid peroxidase cDNA, TPO-2. *Nucleic Acids Research.* 18, 670.

6. Huynh, T., Young, R., Davis, R. (1984): Constructing and screening cDNA libraries in lambda gt 10 and lambda gt 11. In: "*DNA cloning techniques : a practical approach*", ed. D.M. Glover, pp. 49-78. Oxford: IRL Press Ltd.

7. Saiki, R., Scharf, F., Faloona, S., Mullis, K., Horn, G., Ehmich, H., Anheim, N. (1985): Enzymatic amplification of β-globin genomic sequences and restriction site analysis for diagnosis of sickle cell anemia. *Science.* 230, 1350-1354.

8. Maniatis, T., Fritsch, E., Sambrook, J. (1982): Molecular Cloning : a laboratory marcial. *Cold Spring Laboratory Publications.*

9. Southern, E. (1975): Detection of specific sequences among DNA fragments separated by gel electrophoresis. *J. Mol. Biol.* 98, 503-510.

10. Shull, G.E., Lingrel, J.B. (1986): Molecular cloning of the rat stomach (H$^+$ + K$^+$)-ATPase. *J. Biol. Chem.* 261, 16788-16791.

11. Libert, F., Ruel, J., Ludgate, M., Swillens, S., Alexander, N., Vassart, G., Dinsart, C. (1987): Thyroperoxidase, an autoantigen with a mosaic structure made of nuclear and mitochondrial gene modules. *European Molecular Biology Organisation Journal.* 6, 4193-4196.

Résumé

Le criblage d'une banque de cDNA thyroidiens humains clonés dans le phage lambda gt11 au moyen d'auto-anticorps provenant de patients atteints de maladies thyroidiennes autoimmunitaires a conduit à l'identification de deux peptides de la peroxydase thyroidienne (TPO) qui portent des auto-épitopes: C2 (résidus 590 à 675) et C21 (résidus 655 à 755). C2 se comporte comme un épitope majeur en ce qu'il est reconnu par les deux tiers des patients atteints d'une maladie autoimmunitaire thyroidienne. Les auto-anticorps anti-C2 sont capables de se fixer sur la TPO native. Le peptide C21 est reconnu par 50% de ces mêmes patients. Les patients atteints d'une maladie autoimmunitaire non thyroidienne ne reconnaissent ni C2 ni C21. Font exception à cette règle, les patients qui produisent des auto-anticorps dirigés contre l'antigène des cellules pariétales de l'estomac. Cinquante cinq pourcent d'entre eux sont positifs pour les anticorps anti-C2 et 100% pour les anticorps anti-C21. Les peptides C2 et C21 se chevauchent sur une longueur de 20 acides aminés et présentent dans leur segment commun un peptide (résidus 659 à 669) qui offre une ressemblance frappante avec les résidus 177 à 187 de la H$^+$ K$^+$ ATPase, qui a été identifié comme l'antigène des cellules pariétales.

Par ailleurs, la présence de transcrits correspondant à la forme de TPO engendrée par épissage différentiel a été démontrée dans une thyroide normale au moyen de la réaction en chaîne à la polymérase.

Identification of nine amino acids as the epitope for two monoclonal anti-peroxidase antibodies

R. Finke, P. Seto, M. Derwahl and B. Rapoport

University of California San Francisco, California, VAMC (111T), 4150 Clement Street, San Francisco, California 94121, USA

To determine precisely, at the amino acid level, the epitope(s) in human thyroid peroxidase (TPO) that are recognized by auto-antibodies in the sera of patients with autoimmune thyroid disease, we constructed a Lambda-Zap TPO segment library (3.8×10^6) that contains, exclusively, 200-500bp random fragments of TPO. Expressed as a beta-galactosidase fusion protein in E.coli, innumerous fragments of TPO protein could be immunoscreened using a panel of 13 human sera, known to be strongly positive for antimicrosomal antibodies, or two murine monoclonal antibodies (MAb-2010, MAb-IK4028) generated against denatured purified TPO (kindly provided by Dr. L. DeGroot). The sera were used at different dilutions from 1:200-1:20. The MAb were used at a 1:200 dilution. Detection of fusion proteins containing the antibody's epitope was achieved using peroxidase-coupled goat anti-human or -mouse second antibody.

Using the human sera we could not detect a single positive clone. Only the two MAb yielded positive plaques. The nucleotide sequences of 15 (MAb-2010) and 11 (MAb-IK4028) randomly-selected clones coding for proteins recognized by the respective MAb were determined. All clones recognized proteins coded for by virtually the same region of TPO cDNA. All MAb-2010 clones contained cDNA fragments with overlapping regions from 881-927 bp. All IK-4028 clones contained cDNA fragments with overlapping regions from 839-930 bp. The smallest common region for the Mab-2010 clones codes for an epitope of 15 amino acids, from amino acid positions 266 to 281 in the human TPO protein. Because MAb-2010 was also found to bind to rat TPO expressed in an FRTL5 thyroid cell cDNA library, we compared both the human and the rat TPO cDNA sequences in the epitope region. The first 27bp show a 78% homology and code for the same nine amino acids (NPCFPIQLP). The following six amino acids are all different, and are unlikely to be part of the epitope. This further narrows the boundaries of the epitope.

In conclusion, we have defined the epitope for two monoclonal antibodies against human TPO. Both antibodies recognize either an identical epitope or ones that are very close to each other in the same region of the molecule. Sequence data from 11 MAb-IK4028 clones recognize a common region of 30 amino acid residues, including a tract of 15 amino acids recognized by all MAb-2010 clones. Based on the homology to rat TPO in this region, the epitope may be narrowed to 9 amino acid residues. This is close to the expected size of a B cell epitope (6-8 residues). Natural epitope(s), i.e. the antigenic determinants for anti-TPO auto-antibodies in Hashimoto's thyroiditis, were not detectable with our fragment library approach. Most probably the TPO fragments expressed as bacterial fusion proteins do not resemble the correct three dimensional configuration of the natural epitope(s). It will be very helpful to determine epitopes of other MAb that are known to interfere with binding of autoantibodies to TPO, or with TPO functional activity.

Determination of epitope specificities of monoclonal antibodies to thyroid peroxidase using recombinant antigen preparations

D.L. Ewins, J.P. Banga, R.W.S. Tomlinson, P.S. Barnett and A.M. McGregor

Department of Medicine, King's College School of Medicine, London, SE5 9PJ, UK

The aim of this study was to determine the epitope specificities of monoclonal antibodies (MoAbs) to thyroid peroxidase (TPO) using recombinant antigen preparations.

Six separate MoAbs to TPO were raised by immunising Balb/c mice with human TPO purified by high performance liquid chromatography (HPLC). Each MoAb was purified from ascites by HPLC and shown to bind to human microsomal antigen (TMA) by an enzyme-linked immunosorbent assay (ELISA) with titres up to 1:500,000. One MoAb inhibited oxidation of guaiacol catalysed by TPO suggesting binding to, or close to, the enzymatic site.

Using recombinant DNA technology in conjunction with the polymerase chain reaction (PCR), 7 small fragments (averaging 104 amino acid residues) and 2 large fragments (160 and 269 amino acids) of TPO, encompassing 80% of the extracellular region of the molecule, have been generated. The sequential epitopes on rTPO recognized by these MoAbs were analysed by immunoblotting using the recombinant TPO fragments. rTPO preparation R1b, encompassing residues 70-160, was shown to harbour epitopes recognized by MoAbs A4 and A5. A further MoAb A6 reacts with thyroid microsomes by immunoblotting but does not show any reactivity with rTPO preparations. The inability of the other MoAbs to recognize recombinant fragments under the reducing conditions of the immunoblot, despite binding to TMA by ELISA, suggests they either recognize conformational determinants on the TPO molecule or epitopes not expressed as recombinant preparations.

These MoAbs have been used to affinity purify TPO from crude microsomal preparations.

Effects of TPO autoantibody on the thyroid cell

Effets des auto-anticorps anti-TPO sur la cellule thyroïdienne

Autoantibodies inhibiting thyroid peroxidase enzyme activity : specificities of anti-thyroid peroxidase antibodies in healthy subjects and patients with systemic lupus erythematosus

Y. Kohno, N. Naito*, F. Yamaguchi*, K. Saito, H. Niimi and T. Hosoya*

*Department of Pediatrics, School of Medicine and * Faculty of Pharmaceutical Sciences, Chiba University, Chiba 280, Japan*

INTRODUCTION

Previously, it was reported that sera of patients with chronic thyroiditis contain anti-thyroid peroxidase (TPO) autoantibodies and that the major antigen in the thyroid microsomes is TPO itself (Czarnocka et al., 1985; Portmann et al., 1985; Kohno et al., 1986; Kotani et al., 1986). Furthermore, we found that the anti-TPO autoantibodies in sera of these patients are capable of inhibiting the activity of purified TPO (Kohno et al., 1986).

On the other hand, most patients with chronic thyroiditis had anti-thyroglobulin (Tg) autoantibodies in sera (Shimojo et al., 1987) and the autoantibodies from patients with chronic thyroiditis bound to the antigenic determinants of Tg which were not recognized by anti-Tg antibodies from healthy subjects having no evident symptoms of thyroid diseases (Naito et al., 1990). In addition, the 5-10-kDa tryptic fragments from porcine Tg were able to induce thyroiditis in normal CBA mice (Salamero et al., 1987). These findings suggest that the restricted antigenic determinants of Tg are recognized by autoantibodies and/or T cells in patients with autoimmune thyroid diseases.

Anti-microsome antibodies, i. e. anti-TPO antibodies, show a better correlation with histological thyroiditis than do anti-Tg antibodies (Baker et al., 1983). Thus, the study of the epitopes of TPO recognized by autoantibodies from patients with thyroid disorders seems to be of importance. In the present study, we first examined whether we can detect healthy subjects whose sera contain anti-TPO antibodies and, if any, whether or not these antibodies are able to inhibit the activity of TPO in both guaiacol and iodide assays. In addition, specificities of anti-TPO antibodies in patients with systemic lupus erythematosus (SLE) were studied in comparison with those in patients with thyroid disorders. SLE is known as a typical organ nonspecific autoimmune disease, but autoimmune thyroid disorder is a typical organ specific autoimmune disease. However, anti-Tg and anti-microsome autoantibodies in the SLE group occurred with twice the frequency of controls (Weetman & Walport, 1987). If the autoimmune response against restricted epitopes of TPO occurs characteristically in thyroid disorders, there is the possibility that the fine specificities of anti-TPO antibodies in SLE patients without goiter or suggestive symptoms of thyroid disorders are different from those in patients with thyroid disorders.

MATERIALS AND METHODS

Subjects. In the studies of anti-TPO antibodies of healthy subjects, Japanese patients with chronic thyroiditis (2 males, 15 females, age range 12.9-39.9 years, mean 20.1) and two groups of healthy subjects (group I, 41 males, 37 females, age range 17.3-23.1 years, mean 19.1; group II, 1 male, 3 females, age range 21.3-40.8 years, mean 28.0) were examined. Healthy subjects in group I were tested for the incidence of anti-TPO antibodies detectable in healthy subjects and for the occurrence of inhibition of TPO activities by these antibodies. Healthy subjects in group II were used for the previous experiments of TPO immunoprecipitation by anti-Tg antibodies and all contained anti-Tg antibodies (Naito et al., 1990). They were not included when data concerning the proportion of healthy subjects with anti-TPO antibodies in normal population were analysed. All patients with chronic thyroiditis were histologically confirmed by needle biopsy. Levels of free triiodothyronine (T3), free thyroxine (T4) and thyroid-stimulating hormone (TSH) concentrations in sera of healthy subjects were of normal range. Goiters or suggestive symptoms of thyroid disorders or other autoimmune diseases were absent at the time of experiment. In addition, family histories of healthy subjects were essentially negative for thyroid disorders and other autoimmune diseases.

In the studies of anti-TPO autoantibodies in patients with SLE, randomly selected Japanese patients with SLE (1 male, 23 females, age range 13-37 years, mean 28.2), patients with thyroid disorders (chronic thyroiditis, 1 male, 13 females, age range 16-36 years, mean 25.2; Graves' disease, 1 male, 10 females, age range 17-25 years, mean 21.3), and 21 healthy Japanese subjects (2 males 19 females, age range 20-38 years, mean 27.6), were examined. Age and sex of patients with thyroid disorders and healthy subjects were similar to those of patients with SLE. All patients with SLE fulfilled the 1982 criteria of the American Rheumatism Association for the diagnosis of SLE and most of them were on small doses of corticosteroids. Anti-Tg antibodies measured by ELISA and/or anti-microsome autoantibodies measured by haemagglutination were detected in sera of 7 patients but not in the other 17 patients with SLE. The former were denoted as group A, and the latter as group B when data concerning anti-TPO autoantibodies were analysed. Levels of free T3, free T4 and TSH concentrations in sera of patients with SLE in both group A and group B were, however, in normal range. Goiters and symptoms suggestive of thyroid disorders were absent at the time of experiments.

Purification and determination of thyroid peroxidase activities. Human TPO was purified commencing with thyroids of patients with Graves' disease, as described (Kohno et al., 1986). The Reinheit Zahl (A_{413}/A_{280}) of the TPO preparation was 0.35. Peroxidase activities were determined using guaiacol or iodide as the second substrate, as described (Hosoya et al., 1985; Kohno et al., 1986).

Immunoprecipitation of TPO with antibodies. Immunoprecipitation of TPO with IgG isolated from sera was studied according to the methods described (Kohno et al., 1986). The relative per cent precipitation was calculated according to the equation:

$$\text{relative per cent precipitation} = (1 - \frac{a}{b}) \times 100$$

where a = TPO activities in a supernatant layer from patient or healthy subject, b = mean value of TPO activities in supernatant layers from healthy subjects in group I shown in Table 1 or healthy subjects shown in Table 3. The assay was performed as duplicates per point.

Inhibition of TPO activities by antibodies. Inhibition of TPO activities by IgG isolated from sera was studied according to the reported methods (Kohno et al., 1986). The per cent inhibition of TPO activity by antibodies was obtained using the equation:

$$\text{per cent inhibition} = (1 - \frac{a}{b}) \times 100$$

where a = TPO activities in the mixture from patient or healthy subject, b = mean value of TPO activities in the mixtures from healthy subjects without anti-TPO antibodies. The assay was performed as duplicates per point.

Isolation of IgG fraction of serum by ion exchange chromatography. IgG was obtained from sera of patients or healthy subjects, according to our methods (Kohno et al., 1986).

Statistics. Statistical analysis of the results was performed with Student's t-test. Significant levels of anti-TPO antibodies were taken as over two standard deviations above the mean value for the levels in healthy subjects in group I shown in Table 1 and normal controls shown in Table 3. The standard formula was used to calculate correlation coefficients. $P < 0.05$ was considered significant.

RESULTS

Immunoprecipitation of TPO by IgG from healthy subjects. The levels of anti-Tg autoantibodies and anti-microsome autoantibodies were measured by passive haemagglutination. Sixteen out of 17 patients with chronic thyroiditis had anti-Tg and/or anti-microsome autoantibodies in their sera at high levels. Out of 78 healthy subjects in group I, 2 subjects had anti-microsome antibodies and another 2 subjects had anti-Tg antibodies in their sera at low levels. Three healthy subjects with anti-TPO antibodies detected by immunoprecipitation had positive anti-microsome antibodies (2 subjects in group I and 1 subject in group II) and none of them had anti-Tg antibodies found by haemagglutination.

Immunoprecipitation experiments revealed that distinct precipitation of TPO was caused by IgG isolated by ion exchange column chromatography in sera of patients with chronic thyroiditis (Table 1, C). In contrast, IgG from sera of most healthy subjects did not precipitate TPO (Table 1, A). However, in 5 out of 78 healthy subjects (3 males, 2 females; 6.4 per cent), positive anti-TPO antibodies were evident. The mean value of immunoprecipitation of TPO by IgG from these 5 healthy subjects with anti-TPO antibodies was 32.0 ± 4.7 (SEM) per cent. Furthermore, it was confirmed that healthy subjects in group II had positive anti-TPO antibodies (Table 1, B).

Inhibition of TPO activities by IgG from healthy subjects. In addition to healthy subjects with anti-TPO antibodies in group I, inhibition activities of TPO by IgG from healthy subjects having anti-TPO antibodies in group II were also examined. IgG fractions isolated from sera of healthy subjects with anti-TPO antibodies did not inhibit the activities of the enzyme measured by both iodide and guaiacol assays (Table 2, A), whereas IgG fractions isolated by ion exchange chromatography from sera of the patients with chronic thyroiditis caused a significant reduction in TPO activities (Table 2, B). IgG from healthy subjects without anti-TPO antibodies did not inhibit TPO activities (Table 2, C).

Table 1. Immunoprecipitation of TPO activity with IgG from healthy subjects

Antibodies	Relative % precipitation (mean ± SEM)
A) Healthy subjects in group I (n=78)	0.0 ± 1.2 [b), d)]
B) Healthy subjects in group II (n=4) [a)]	25.7 ± 4.6 [c)]
C) Patients with chronic thyroiditis (n=17)	45.7 ± 3.3

The TPO activities were determined under standard conditions and the percentage of precipitation was calculated as described in Materials and Methods.
a) Healthy subjects in group II were used in the previous experiment and anti-TPO antibodies in them were demonstrated (Naito et al., 1990).
b) and c) $P < 0.01$ vs. patients with chronic thyroiditis.
d) $P < 0.01$ vs. healthy subjects in group II.

Table 2. Inhibition of TPO activities with IgG from healthy subjects

Antibodies	% inhibition (mean ± SEM)	
	Guaiacol assay	Iodide assay
A) Healthy subjects with anti-TPO antibodies (n=9) [a)]	2.7 ± 2.6 [c), d)]	-4.4 ± 6.0 [e), f)]
B) Patients with chronic thyroiditis (n=17)	31.3 ± 4.6	30.8 ± 2.8
C) Healthy subjects without anti-TPO antibodies [b)] (n=16)	0.0 ± 2.1	0.0 ± 2.6

The TPO activities determined under standard assay conditions and the percentage inhibition was calculated as described in Materials and Methods.
a) Healthy subjects with anti-TPO antibodies consisted of 5 subjects in group I and 4 subjects in group II shown in Table 1. b) Healthy subjects without anti-TPO antibodies were included in healthy subjects in group I shown in Table 1. c) and e) $P < 0.01$ vs. patients with chronic thyroiditis.
d) and f) Not significant (NS) vs. healthy subjects without anti-TPO antibodies.

Table 3. Immunoprecipitation of TPO activity with IgG from sera of SLE patients

Antibodies	Relative % precipitation (mean ± SEM)
A) Patients with SLE[a] (n=24)	18.0 ± 2.1 [b), c)]
Group A (n=7)	26.0 ± 4.8 [d)]
Group B (n=17)	14.7 ± 1.7
B) Patients with thyroid disorders (n=25)	66.3 ± 7.1 [e)]
C) Healthy subjects (n=21)	0.0 ± 1.0

These data were taken from Kohno et al. (1989).
a) Patients with SLE in group A had positive anti-Tg and anti-microsome antibodies and patients with SLE in group B had not.
b) $P < 0.01$ vs. patients with thyroid disorders. c) $P < 0.01$ vs. healthy subjects. d) NS vs. group B. e) $P < 0.01$ vs. healthy subjects.

Table 4. Reduction of TPO activities with IgG from SLE patients

Antibodies	% inhibition (mean ± SEM)	
	Guaiacol assay	Iodide assay
A) Patients with SLE (n=18)	3.9 ± 3.6 [a), b)]	1.0 ± 2.2 [e), f)]
Group A (n=4)	-0.6 ± 5.3 [c)]	5.3 ± 5.6 [g)]
Group B (n=14)	5.2 ± 4.4	-0.2 ± 2.4
B) Patients with thyroid disorders (n=25)	18.2 ± 2.2 [d)]	5.7 ± 2.4 [h)]
C) Healthy subjects (n=21)	0.0 ± 0.5	0.0 ± 0.8

These data were taken from Kohno et al. (1989).
a) $P < 0.01$ vs. patients with thyroid disorders. b) NS vs. healthy subjects.
c) NS vs. group B. d) $P < 0.01$ vs. healthy subjects. e) NS vs. patients with thyroid disorders. f) NS vs. healthy subjects. g) NS vs. group B.
h) $P < 0.01$ vs. healthy subjects.

Anti-TPO autoantibodies in patients with SLE. IgG isolated by ion exchange chromatography from sera of SLE patients distinctly precipitated TPO but the mean value of levels of anti-TPO autoantibodies in patients with SLE was lower than that of sera of patients with thyroid disorders (Table 3, A and B). Twenty two out of 24 (91.7 per cent) SLE patients, all patients of group A and 15 out of 17 (88.2 per cent) patients of group B, had positive anti-TPO antibodies, while 24 out of 25 (96 per cent) patients with thyroid disorders had anti-TPO antibodies. The levels of anti-TPO autoantibodies in group A of SLE patients were not significantly different from those in group B.

Inhibition of TPO activity by IgG from patients with SLE. IgG fractions isolated from sera of patients with SLE, either in group A or group B, did not inhibit the activity of the TPO (Table 4, A). The values of inhibition by IgG from patients with thyroid diseases (Table 4, B) were lower than those shown in Table 2 but were statistically different from those of healthy controls.

DISCUSSION

The present study has demonstrated that anti-TPO autoantibodies are present in some healthy subjects and most patients with SLE. However, TPO activities were scarcely inhibited in both guaiacol and iodide assays with IgG from sera of the healthy subjects and patients with SLE (Table 2 and 4). This is quite a contrast to the cases of IgG from sera of patients with thyroid disorders and indicates that the specificities of anti-TPO antibodies in sera of healthy subjects and SLE patients differ from those in sera of thyroid disorders.

The difference in the inhibition of TPO activities with anti-TPO antibodies between healthy subjects and patients with chronic thyroiditis or between SLE patients and patients with thyroid disorders cannot be ascribed to the differences in the levels of anti-TPO antibodies, since titres of anti-TPO antibodies measured by immunoprecipitation did not correlate with the values of per cent inhibition of TPO activities by antibodies measured by guaiacol assay or by iodide assay (data not shown).

The specificities of anti-TPO autoantibodies are reportedly heterogeneous and can be separated into specific subgroups (Kohno et al., 1986; Doble et al., 1988; Ruf et al., 1989). Our previous study of anti-TPO autoantibodies in sera from patients with chronic thyroiditis (Kohno et al., 1986) suggested that epitopes on TPO molecules recognized by anti-TPO autoantibodies in sera of patients may be classified into four groups; (a) epitopes relating to the iodide-combining site; (b) epitopes relating to the tyrosyl residue-combining site; (c) epitopes relating to both combining sites for iodide and tyrosyl residues; (d) epitopes not relating to the substrate-combining sites. From the results described here, main epitopes recognized by anti-TPO antibodies in healthy subjects and SLE patients may be classified in the last group mentioned above. Recently, it has been reported that substrate enzymatic sites on TPO may serve as autoantigenic determinants in autoimmune thyroid diseases (Doble et al., 1988; Ruf et al., 1989). These results are in harmony with our category of epitopes on TPO molecules. However, it is not known whether the inhibition of TPO activities by autoantibodies is correlated with pathophysiology of thyroid diseases. The findings that anti-TPO antibodies in healthy subjects and patients with SLE did not inhibit TPO enzyme activities should provide additional insight into the role of autoantibodies to catalytic sites of TPO in thyroid disorders.

CONCLUSION

We found the different fine specificities of anti-TPO antibodies between normal states or SLE and thyroid disorders. These findings suggest that the mechanisms of induction of anti-TPO antibodies in healthy subjects or patients with SLE are different from those in patients with thyroid disorders.

had anti-TPO antibodies. The levels of anti-TPO autoantibodies in group A of SLE patients were not significantly different from those in group B.

<u>Inhibition of TPO activity by IgG from patients with SLE.</u> IgG fractions isolated from sera of patients with SLE, either in group A or group B, did not inhibit the activity of the TPO (Table 4, A). The values of inhibition by IgG from patients with thyroid diseases (Table 4, B) were lower than those shown in Table 2 but were statistically different from those of healthy controls.

DISCUSSION

The present study has demonstrated that anti-TPO autoantibodies are present in some healthy subjects and most patients with SLE. However, TPO activities were scarcely inhibited in both guaiacol and iodide assays with IgG from sera of the healthy subjects and patients with SLE (Table 2 and 4). This is quite a contrast to the cases of IgG from sera of patients with thyroid disorders and indicates that the specificities of anti-TPO antibodies in sera of healthy subjects and SLE patients differ from those in sera of thyroid disorders.

The difference in the inhibition of TPO activities with anti-TPO antibodies between healthy subjects and patients with chronic thyroiditis or between SLE patients and patients with thyroid disorders cannot be ascribed to the differences in the levels of anti-TPO antibodies, since titres of anti-TPO antibodies measured by immunoprecipitation did not correlate with the values of per cent inhibition of TPO activities by antibodies measured by guaiacol assay or by iodide assay (data not shown).

The specificities of anti-TPO autoantibodies are reportedly heterogeneous and can be separated into specific subgroups (Kohno et al., 1986; Doble et al., 1988; Ruf et al., 1989). Our previous study of anti-TPO autoantibodies in sera from patients with chronic thyroiditis (Kohno et al., 1986) suggested that epitopes on TPO molecules recognized by anti-TPO autoantibodies in sera of patients may be classified into four groups; (a) epitopes relating to the iodide-combining site; (b) epitopes relating to the tyrosyl residue-combining site; (c) epitopes relating to both combining sites for iodide and tyrosyl residues; (d) epitopes not relating to the substrate-combining sites. From the results described here, main epitopes recognized by anti-TPO antibodies in healthy subjects and SLE patients may be classified in the last group mentioned above. Recently, it has been reported that substrate enzymatic sites on TPO may serve as autoantigenic determinants in autoimmune thyroid diseases (Doble et al., 1988; Ruf et al., 1989). These results are in harmony with our category of epitopes on TPO molecules. However, it is not known whether the inhibition of TPO activities by autoantibodies is correlated with pathophysiology of thyroid diseases. The findings that anti-TPO antibodies in healthy subjects and patients with SLE did not inhibit TPO enzyme activities should provide additional insight into the role of autoantibodies to catalytic sites of TPO in thyroid disorders.

CONCLUSION

We found the different fine specificities of anti-TPO antibodies between normal states or SLE and thyroid disorders. These findings suggest that the mechanisms of induction of anti-TPO antibodies in healthy subjects or patients with SLE are different from those in patients with thyroid disorders.

REFERENCES

Baker, B.A., Gharib, H. & Markowitz, H. (1983): Correlation of thyroid antibodies and cytologic features in suspected autoimmune thyroid disease. Am. J. Med. 74, 941-944.

Czarnocka, B., Ruf, J., Ferrand, M., Carayon, P. & Lissitzky, S. (1985): Purification of the human thyroid peroxidase and its identification as the microsomal antigen involved in autoimmune thyroid diseases. FEBS Lett. 190, 147-152.

Doble, N.D., Banga, J.P., Pope, R., Lalor, E., Kilduff, P. & McGregor, A.M. (1988): Autoantibodies to the thyroid microsomal/thyroid peroxidase antigen are polyclonal and directed to several distinct antigenic sites. Immunology 64, 23-29.

Hosoya, T., Sato, I., Hiyama, Y., Yoshimura, H., Niimi, H. & Tarutani, O. (1985): An improved assay method for thyroid peroxidase applicable for a few milligrams of abnormal human thyroid tissues. J. Biochem. (Tokyo) 98, 637-647.

Kohno, Y., Hiyama, Y., Shimojo, N., Niimi, H., Nakajima, H. & Hosoya, T. (1986): Autoantibodies to thyroid peroxidase in patients with chronic thyroiditis: effect of antibody binding on enzyme activities. Clin. Exp. Immunol. 65, 534-541.

Kohno, Y., Naito, N., Saito, K., Hoshioka, A., Niimi, H., Nakajima, H. & Hosoya, T. (1989): Anti-thyroid peroxidase antibody activity in sera of patients with systemic lupus erythematosus. Clin. Exp. Immunol. 75, 217-221.

Kotani, T., Umeki, K., Matsunaga, S., Kato, E. & Ohtaki, S. (1986): Detection of autoantibodies to thyroid peroxidase in autoimmune thyroid diseases by micro-ELISA and immunoblotting. J. Clin. Endocrinol. Metab. 62, 928-933.

Naito, N., Saito, K., Hosoya, T., Tarutani, O., Sakata, S., Nishikawa, T., Niimi, H., Nakajima, H. & Kohno, Y. (1990): Anti-thyroglobulin autoantibodies in sera from patients with chronic thyroiditis and from healthy subjects: differences in cross-reactivity with thyroid peroxidase. Clin. Exp. Immunol. in press.

Portmann, L., Hamada, N., Heinrich, G. & DeGroot, L.J. (1985): Anti-thyroid peroxidase antibody in patients with autoimmune thyroid disease: possible identity with anti-microsomal antibody. J. Clin. Endocrinol. Metab. 61, 1001-1003.

Ruf, J., Toubert, M-E., Czarnocka, B., Durand-Gorde, J-M., Ferrand, M. & Carayon, P. (1989): Relationship between immunological structure and biochemical properties of human thyroid peroxidase. Endocrinology 125, 1211-1218.

Salamero, J., Remy, J.J., Michel-Bechet, M. & Charreire, J. (1987): Experimental autoimmune thyroiditis induced by a 5-10-kDa tryptic fragment from porcine thyroglobulin. Eur. J. Immunol. 17, 843-848.

Shimojo, N., Kohno, Y., Tarutani, O., Sasaki, N. & Nakajima, H. (1987): Enzyme-linked immunosorbent assay (ELISA) for IgG antibodies to thyroglobulin. Clin. Chim. Acta 163, 41-49.

Weetman, A.P. & Walport, M.J. (1987): The association of autoimmune thyroiditis with systemic lupus erythematosus. Br. J. Rheumatol. 26, 359-361.

ABSTRACT

Previously we reported that anti-TPO autoantibodies in sera of patients with chronic thyroiditis inhibited TPO activity measured by guaiacol assay and iodide assay and that by studying the inhibition of TPO by autoantibodies in sera of these patients, at least three or four epitopes of TPO molecule were recognized by autoantibodies. In the present study, we found that antibodies to TPO were detectable in limited healthy subjects and most patients with systemic lupus erythematosus (SLE) whose levels of free T3, free T4 and TSH concentrations were of normal range, and goiter and suggestive symptoms of thyroid disorders were absent at the time of experiments. However, in contrast with IgG from sera of patients with autoimmune thyroid disorders, IgG from sera of healthy subjects and patients with SLE did not inhibit TPO activities both in guaiacol and iodide assays. These findings suggest that the specificities of anti-TPO antibodies in healthy subjects or patients with SLE are different from those in cases of autoimmune thyroid disorders.

Résumé

Nous avons récemment rapporté que les auto-anticorps anti-TPO sériques de patients atteints de thyroïdite chronique, inhibaient l'activité de la TPO mesurée par dosage au guaiacol et à l'iode. L'étude de cette inhibition a révélé qu'au moins 3 ou 4 épitopes de la molécule de TPO étaient reconnus par les auto-anticorps. Dans la présente étude, nous avons trouvé que les anticorps anti-TPO étaient décelables chez quelques sujets sains et chez la plupart des patients atteints de lupus erythémateux (SLE) dont les taux de concentration en T3 et T4 libres et en TSH étaient normaux et exempts de goitre ou de tout symptome caractéristique de maladie thyroïdienne, au moment de l'expérience. Cependant, contrairement aux IgG provenant de sérums de patients atteints de troubles thyroïdiens autoimmunes, les IgG sériques provenant de sujets sains et de patients souffrant de SLE, n'inhibaient pas l'activité enzymatique de la TPO, mesurée à la fois par la méthode au guaiacol et par la méthode à l'iode. Ces résultats suggèrent que la spécificité des anticorps anti-TPO chez les sujets sains, diffère de celle des anticorps anti-TPO de patients souffrant de troubles thyroïdiens autoimmunes.

Is TPO the only thyroid antigen involved in the complement dependent cytotoxicity ?

R. Winand and P. Wadeleux

Tour de Pathologie, B23, CHU, 4000 Sart-Tilman, Liège 1, Belgique

INTRODUCTION

Thyroid microsomal antibodies (Mic ab), recently identified as antithyroid peroxidase antibodies [Czarnocka et al., 1985] are frequently present in patients with autoimmune thyroid disease and have been thought to be implicated in thyroid cells damage observed in autoimmune thyroiditis. In a support of this concept, antibodies which are cytotoxic for thyroid cells in vitro has been evidenced in the sera of patients with autoimmune thyroiditis and exhibiting antimicrosomal antibodies. These cytotoxic antibodies are active both directly in the presence of complement [Pulvertaft et al., 1961; Forbes et al., 1962; Khoury et al., 1981] and in association with K cells [Schleusener & Bogner, 1985].

Most of the clinical laboratories measure microsomal antibodies in the various thyroid diseases and recently a routine assay of antithyroid peroxidase autoantibodies has beeen developed [Ruf et al., 1988]. In a recent report, Wadeleux et al., [1989] have described an assay for the quantitation of the complement dependent thyroid cytotoxic antibodies. In the present study, we have used the same assay to correlate the presence of these antibodies with the presence of antimicrosomal and antithyroid peroxidase antibodies.

MATERIAL AND METHODS

Patients sera

Sera are from patients with various suspected thyroid disorders. They were obtained in the out-patients clinics of the hospital.

In order to test all the sera in identical condition with respect to the complement activity, they were previously heat inactivated (1/2 h. 56°C). This procedure was also shown to destroy some "non specific" cytotoxic activity present in some sera [Garland et al., 1972].

Cytotoxic assay

Cytotoxic assay is performed essentially as previously described [Wadeleux et al., 1989]. Porcine thyroid cells were isolated by using the dispase digestion technique [Bidey et al., 1980] and unless otherwise stated plated in 24 well-plates (0.75 x 10^6 cells/well) and incubated in the presence of test substance in 0.6 ml 199 culture medium containing 1 µCi (L-4-N^3H) leucine (60 Ci/mmol; 1 mCi = 37 megabq). Assays are performed in duplicate. Forty eight hours after platting the cell layer is washed removed, and processed for DNA [Labarca & Paigen, 1980] protein [Bradford, 1976] and [^{3}H] leucine incorporation determination.

As control of specificity, hepatocytes isolated from foetal rats by the technique of Kremers et al. [1981] were treated in strictly identical conditions.

Antimicrosomal antibodies

Antimicrosomal antibodies determination was performed by using the PROMAK assay^R (Henning Berlin GMBH). This test is based on a solid phase technique using tubes coated with microsomal antigen and the ability of ^{125}I labelled protein A to bind to the previously fixed autoantibodies.

Antithyroid peroxidase antibodies

The antithyroid peroxidase antibodies assay was based on autoantibody inhibition of the binding of labelled TPO to a solid phase bound monoclonal antibody to TPO [Ruf et al., 1988].

Miscellaneous procedures

Antibodies titre against thyroglobulin was determined with a commercially available kit (Techland, Belgium).
Gammaglobulins were purified from serum by QAE Sephadex chromatography [Joustra & Lundgren, 1969] or by ammonium sulphate precipitation.

RESULTS

When thyroid cells are incubated in the presence of normal human serum, they form, 48 hours after plating, a monolayer of epithelial cells. In the presence of a cytotoxic serum from a patient with autoimmune thyroiditis, very few cells stick to the bottom of the dish. Quantitation of the cell layer, may be performed by using DNA determination, protein measurement or [^{3}H] leucine incorporation. In the figure 1, we have illustrated the results obtained by using increasing amount of a cytotoxic serum. For these three parameters, the dose-response-curves are identical. Since [^{3}H] leucine incorporation requires less material, this method has been choosen for the presentation of the following results.

As already reported [Wadeleux et al., 1989] this effect requires the presence of complement. It is specific for thyroid cells since no cytotoxic effect could be obtained by using fibroblasts [Wadeleux et al., 1939] or hepatocytes (Fig. 2) instead of thyroid cells. The figure 3 shows that the cytotoxic effect was associated with the gammaglobulin fraction isolated from the cytotoxic sera. A dose-response-curve was obtained analogous to that obtained by addition of unfractionated serum.

We investigated on a large scale the possible correlation between antimicrosomal and cytotoxic antibodies. Figure 4 shows the relation between the cytotoxic antibodies and microsomal antibodies in one representative of 13 experiments. In these 13 experiments, the subjects visited the out-patients clinics for various suspected thyroid disorders. When [^{3}H] leucine incorporation, which decreased proportionaly to the cytotoxic effect, is plotted versus the Mic ab level (on a logarithmic scale) a significant correlation may be obtained ($p<0.05$). For a relation of type $Y = A + B \log x$ the following values are : $A = 176 \pm 40$, $B = -35 \pm 8$ and $r = -0.57 \pm 0.08$. Clearly however, some discrepancies were observed. Some sera with high titre of antimicrosomal antibodies had no cytotoxic effect and sera will low titre had a marked cytotoxic effect. Moreover, in 17/240 (7 %) of these antimicrosomal antibodies negative "all coming" patients, a cytotoxic effect has also been observed. This last effect was also due do a factor copurified with the gammaglobulin fraction, was complement dependent and was not observed with hepatocytes.

We next investigated wether anti TPO antibody could be a better indices of the presence of the cytotoxic antibodies. One hundred and thirty sera of patients with thyroid diseases have been tested in the anti TPO assay. A close correlation was observed when anti TPO was tested both in the absence or in the presence of added thyroglobulin,

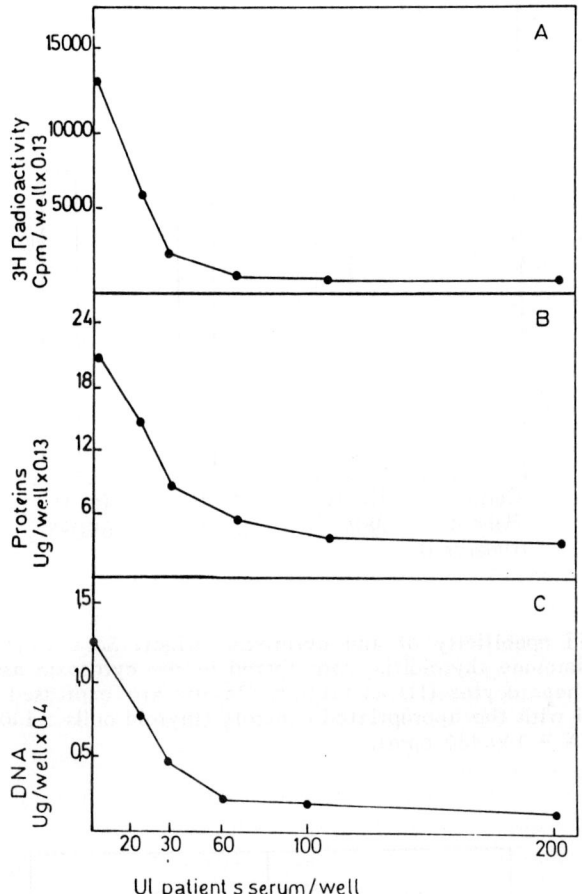

Figure 1 : Cytotoxic assay with increasing amounts of sera from patients with autoimmune thyroiditis. In this experiment, we have used 6 well-plates (3 x 10^{0} cells/9.6 cm^{2}). The total amount of serum is adjusted to 200 µl with normal human serum. After 48 hrs incubation, cell layer is washed and recovered in 1.5 ml of physiological buffer. Cells are homogeneized by a sonicator (30").
A) [^{3}H] leucine incorporation is determined with 200 µl of cell homogenate.
B) Protein test is performed with 200 µl of cell homogenate after solubilization by 100 µl of 0.1 M NaOH (1/2 h; 100°C).
C) DNA content is determined with 600 µl of cell homogenate.

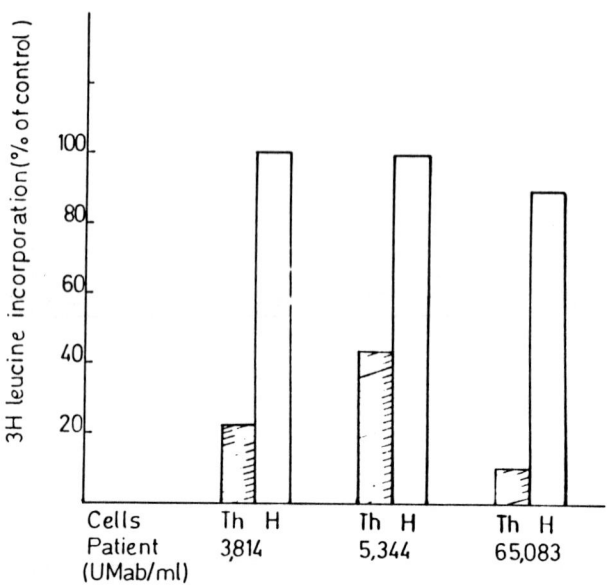

Figure 2 : Thyroid specificity of the cytotoxic effect. Sera from control or from patients with autoimmune thyroiditis were tested in the cytotoxic assay by using thyroid cells (Th) or hepatocytes (H) as targets. Results are expressed as percentage of the values obtained with the appropriated controls (thyroid cells : 100 % = 74,774 cpm; hepatocytes : 100 % = 140,430 cpm).

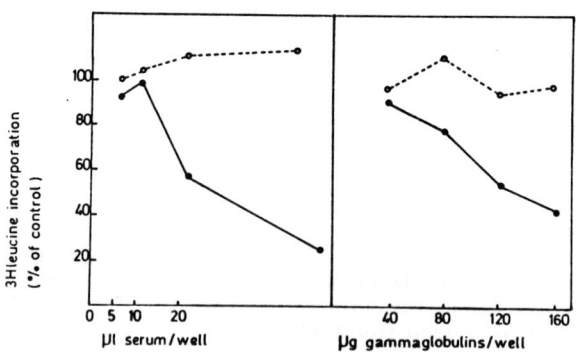

Figure 3 : Left : Thyroid cytotoxic assay with increasing amounts of a control serum (0----0) or of a serum of patient with autoimmune thyroiditis (0   0). Right : Thyroid cytotoxic assay with increasing amounts of the gammaglobulins isolated from the corresponding sera. Results are expressed as percentage of the appropriate controls (for serum 100 % = 85,645 cpm; for gammaglobulins 100 % = 75,751 cpm).

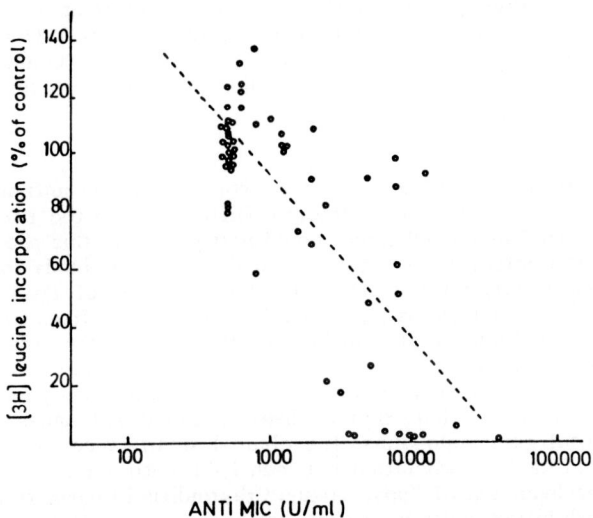

Figure 4 : Correlation between thyroid cytotoxic activity and microsomal antibodies level in various patients visiting the out-patients clinics.

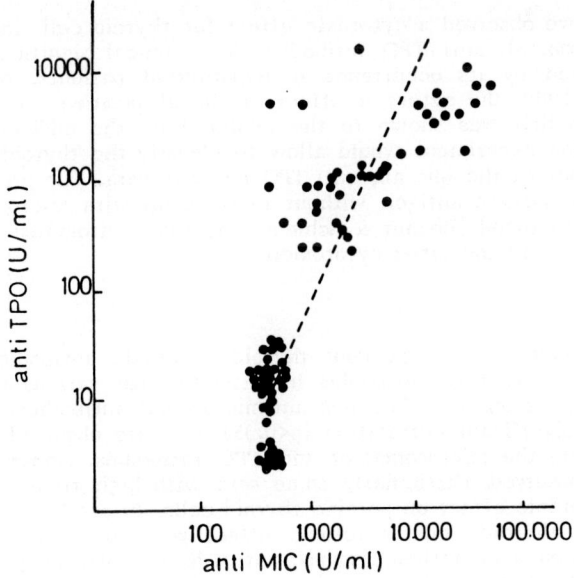

Figure 5 : Correlation between anti TPO titre and anti Mic ab in a series of patients with various suspected thyroid diseases.

confirming that antithyroglobulin antibodies do not interfer in this test (data not shown). Results of antimicrosomal antibodies assay and anti TPO test showed a direct correlation (Fig. 5) except in some cases (2/47) where anti TPO antibodies were detected in the absence of antimicrosomal antibodies (and of cytotoxic antibodies).

DISCUSSION

If a significant relation exists between cytotoxic effect and antimicrosomal antibodies level, some discrepancies were also detected. Differences in the two methods with respect to the implicated immunoglobulins could partly explain this phenomenon. Thus protein A, used for the detection of antimicrosomal antibodies, binds to the various classes of gammaglobulins (IgG1, IgG2, IgG4) with the exception of IgG3 [Kunkel, 1982] but does not bind to immunoglobulins A, M and E. Complement fixes to immunoglobulins M and G. For immunoglobulin G, its binding ability varies in the order Ig3 >Ig1 >Ig2 >Ig4 [Dean et al., 1983]. Several reports indicate that the subclass distribution of antimicrosomal antibodies [McLachlan et al., 1987] and of anti TPO gammaglobulins [Kotani et al., 1986] vary in the various thyroid diseases and is not necessary identical to the distribution of total gammaglobulins. The clinical significance of these subclass distribution is suggested by the association between IgG1 antimicrosomal antibodies (and not IgG4) and the developement of "post partum" thyroiditis in patients which are clinically euthyroid and exhibiting antimicrosomal antibodies positive sera in early pregnancy [Jansson et al., 1986]. An identical phenomenon could explain the "unexpected" high cytotoxic effect that we observed in one case of Hashimoto's thyroiditis.

The direct correlation between anti TPO and antimicrosomal antibodies level confirm the concept that TPO is identical to the microsomal antigen. The lack of cytotoxic effect of several antimicrosomal antibodies positive sera could not be explained by an absence of anti TPO antibody.

In several cases, we observed a cytotoxic effect for thyroid cells in sera from patients without antimicrosomal, anti TPO antibodies. The clinical significance of this phenomenon is suggested by its occurrence in hypothyroid patients. As already reported [Wadeleux et al., 1989] the cytotoxic effect of Mic ab positive sera from patients with autoimmune thyroiditis was shown to the inhibited by the addition of purified TPO. Analogous inhibition experiment would allow to identify the thyroid antigen involved in the cytotoxic effect of the Mic ab, anti TPO negative sera. The presence of antibodies directed against a surface antigen without relationship with microsomal, TPO antigen has already been reported [Bogner & Schleusener, 1988; Hiromatsu et al., 1988] in the antibody-dependent cell mediated cytotoxicity test.

CONCLUSION

We studied the complement dependent thyroid cytotoxic antibodies, the microsomal antibodies and the anti TPO antibodies in patients with various thyroid diseases. A direct correlation was observed between antimicrosomal antibodies level and anti TPO antibody titre. A significant correlation ($p<0.05$) was also observed between the cytotoxic antibodies and the microsomal or anti TPO antibodies. However, some clear discrepancies were observed. Particularly some sera with high titre of microsomal antibodies had no cytotoxic effect on porcine thyroid cells. Inversely, a complement dependent, specific for thyroid cells, cytotoxic effect was observed in some hypothyroid patients in the absence of antimicrosomal, anti TPO or antithyroglobulin antibodies. These data indicate that circulating antimicrosomal or anti TPO antibodies may represent heterogeneous population. Some antibodies may play a role in thyroid cell destruction via the complement dependent cytotoxicity. However, in several cases, the possibility of an identical effect via an antigen without relationship with microsomal or TPO antigen should not be discarded.

Résumé

Nous avons étudié la cytotoxicité thyroïdienne dépendant du complément, les anticorps antimicrosomiaux et les anticorps anti TPO chez des patients avec différentes affections thyroïdiennes. Une corrélation directe a été observée entre les titres en anticorps antimicrosomiaux et en anti TPO. Une corrélation significative ($p<0,05$) a été également obtenue entre les anticorps cytotoxiques et les anticorps microsomiaux ou anti TPO. Cependant, des discordances nettes sont observées, en particulier, certains sera avec un titre élevé en anticorps antimicrosomiaux n'ont pas d'effet cytotoxique. A l'inverse, certains patients hypothyroïdiens présentent un effet cytotoxique dépendant du complément, spécifique pour les cellules thyroïdiennes, en l'absence d'anticorps antimicrosomiaux, d'anticorps anti TPO ou d'anticorps antithyroglobuline. Ces données indiquent que les anticorps antimicrosomiaux et les anticorps anti TPO peuvent représenter une population hétérogène. Certains peuvent jouer un rôle dans la destruction des cellules thyroïdiennes via la cytotoxicité dépendant du complément. Par ailleurs, on ne peut écarter la possibilité d'une action identique par l'intermédiaire d'un antigène sans parenté avec l'antigène microsomial (ou la peroxydase thyroïdienne).

ACKNOWLEDGEMENTS

The authors with to thank Mrs. Ch. Bourdoux, M. Detilloux and L. Wery for their skilfull technical assistance and Mrs. H. Fastré for their help in the preparation of the manuscript. This work was partly supported by a grant from the Belgian Fonds de la Recherche Médicale (N°3.4521.81).

REFERENCES

1. Bidey, S.P., Marshall, N.J. & Ekins, R.P. (1980): Inhibition by normal immunoglobulins of thyrotropin-stimulated production of cyclic AMP in slices of normal human thyroid. J. Endocr. 87, 271-277.
2. Bogner, U. & Schleusener, H. (1988): Cytotoxic and microsomal antibodies are not identical in Hashimoto's thyroiditis. Abstract n°82, 17th Annual Meeting of the European Thyroid Association.
3. Bradford, M.M. (1976): A rapid and sensitive method for the quantitation of microgram quantities of protein using the principle of protein-dye binding. Anal. Biochem. 72, 248-254.
4. Czarnocka, B., Ruf, J., Ferrand, M., Carayon, P. & Lissitzky S. (1985): Purification of the human thyroid peroxidase and its identification as the microsomal antigen involved in autoimmune thyroid diseases. FEBS Lett. 190, 147-152.
5. Dean, B.M., Bottazzo, G.F. & Cudworth, A.G. (1983): IgG subclass distribution in organ specific autoantibodies. The relationship to complement fixing ability. Clin. Exp. Immunol. 52, 61-66.
6. Forbes, I.J., Roitt, I.M., Doniach, D. & Solomon, I.L. (1962): The thyroid cytotoxic autoantibody. J. Clin. Invest. 41, 996-1006.
7. Garland, J.T., Lottes, M.E., Kozak, S. & Daughaday, W.H. (1972): Stimulation of DNA synthesis in isolated chondrocytes by sulfation factor. Endocrinology 90, 1086-1090.
8. Hiromatsu, Y., Fukazawa, H., Guinard, F., Salvi, M., How, J. & Wall, J.R. (1988): A thyroid cytotoxic antibody that cross-reacts with an eye muscle cell surface antigen may be the cause of thyroid-associated ophthalmopathy. J. Clin. Endocrinol. Metab. 67, 565-570.
9. Jansson, R., Thompson, P.M., Clark, F. & McLachlan, S.M. (1986): Association between thyroid microsomal antibodies of subclass IgG-1 and hypothyroidism in autoimmune postpartum thyroiditis. Clin. Exp. Immunol. 63, 80-86.

10. Joustra, M.J. & Lundgren, H. (1969): Preparation of freeze-dried monomeric and immunochemically pure IgG by a rapid and reproducible chromatographic technique. In Protides of Biological Fluids, ed. H. Peters, p 511. Proceedings of the 17th Colloquium, Bruges, Belgium, Pergamon Press, Oxford.
11. Khoury, E.L., Hammond, L., Bottazo, G.F. & Doniach, D. (1981): Presence of the organ specific "microsomal" autoantigen in the surface of human thyroid cells in culture : its involvement in complement-mediated cytotoxicity. Clin. Exp. Immunol. 45, 316-328.
12. Kotani, T., Kato, E., Hirai, K., Kuma, K. & Ohtaki, S. (1986): Immunoglobulin G subclasses of anti-thyroid peroxidase autoantibodies in human autoimmune thyroid diseases. Endocrinol Japon. 33, 505-510.
13. Kremers, P., Goujon, F., De Graeve, J., Van Cantfort, S. & Gielen, J. (1981): Multiplicity of cytochrome P 450 in primary fetal hepatocytes in culture. Eur. J. Biochem. 116, 67-72.
14. Kunkel, H.G. (1982): The Immunoglobulins. In Clinical Aspects of Immunology, ed. P.J. Lackman & P.K Peter, pp. 3-17. Blackwell Scientific Publication Oxford.
15. Labarca, C.& Paigen, K. (1980): A simple, rapid and sensitive DNA assay. Procedure. Analytical Procedure 102, 344-352.
16. McLachlan, S.M., Feldt-Rasmussen, U., Young, E.T., Middleton, S.L., Blichert-Toft, M., Siersboek-Nielsen, K., Date, J., Carr, D., Clark, F. & Rees Smith, B. (1987): IgG subclass distribution of thyroid autoantibodies : a "fingerprint" of an individual's response to thyroglobulin and thyroid microsomal antigen. Clin. Endocrinol. 26, 335-346.
17. Pulvertaft, R.J., Doniach, D. & Roitt, I.M.(1961): The cytotoxic factor in Hashimoto's disease and its incidence in other diseases. Br. J. Exp. Pathol. 42, 496-503.
18. Ruf, J., Czarnocka, B., Ferrand, M., Doullais, F. & Carayon, P. (1988): Novel routine assay of thyroperoxidase autoantibodies. Clin. Chem. 34, 2231-2234.
19. Schleusener, H. & Bogner, U. (1985): Cytotoxic mechanisms in autoimmune thyroiditis. In Autoimmunity and the Thyroid, ed. P.G. Walfish, J.R. Wall & R. Volpe, pp. 95-107. Autoimmunity and the Academic Press.
20. Wadeleux, P., Winand-Devigne, J., Ruf, J., Carayon, P. & Winand, R. (1989): Cytotoxic assay of circulating thyroid peroxidase antibodies. Autoimmunity 4, 247-254.

Thyroid cytotoxic antibodies are not identical with thyroid microsomal/peroxidase antibodies

U. Bogner, H. Peters and H. Schleusener

Endocrine Section of the Department of Medicine, Free University Berlin, Hindenburgdamm 30, 1000 Berlin 45, FRG

INTRODUCTION

Since the detection of microsomal antibodies in Hashimoto's thyroiditis (HT) and the association of cytotoxic antibody activity with the microsomal antibody fraction, it has been generally accepted that the presence of these antibodies is an indicator of thyroid cell destruction (Pulvertaft et al., 1959, 1961; Forbes et al., 1962; Irvine, 1962). Nevertheless, clinical follow-up studies showed that in some patients microsomal antibodies (Mab) are present for many years without development of hypothyroidism (Lazarus et al., 1984; Tunbridge et al., 1981). Preliminary data of our laboratory suggested that no correlation exists between the cytotoxic antibody activity and the titers of Mab (Bogner et al., 1987). In this paper we add further evidence for the diversity of cytotoxic and microsomal/thyroid peroxidase antibodies (TPOab).

PATIENTS AND METHODS

Sixty-seven patients, 57 women and 10 men, aged 21 - 83 years (mean 55 years), with autoimmune thyroiditis were studied. Sixty-one normal subjects, 53 women and 8 men, aged 27 - 64 years (mean 45 years), with no history of thyroid disease were included.

Determination of antibody-dependent cell-mediated cytotoxicity (ADCC)

Thyroid tissue obtained from surgical specimens of patients with multinodular goiter (blood group 0) was finely minced and enzymatically isolated by incubation in 0.5 % collagenase (Boehringer, Mannheim, FRG). After 45 min of incubation at 37 C, the cells were washed and diluted to 5×10^6/mL in

Iscove's medium containing 10 % FCS, antibiotics and 7.5 % dimethylsulfoxide. The cell solution was tranferred to cryovials, frozen and stored in liquid N_2 until used for the experiments.

ADCC was determined as previously described (Bogner et al., 1984). The frozen cells were replated in 75 cm^2 flasks, cultured for three days, transferred in suspension and radiolabelled with 100 /uCi $Na_2{}^{51}CrO_4$ (Behring AG, Marburg, FRG). Fifty /uL radiolabelled cells (5 x 10^3/well) were then incubated in triplicate with 100 /uL 1:10 diluted heat-inactivated serum or 100 /uL IgG (1 mg/mL) in microtiter plates at 37 C and 5 % CO_2 in a water-saturated incubator. Then 100 /uL effector mononuclear cells (1.25 x 10^5) from a normal subject were added, giving an effector:target cell ratio of 25:1. After 18 h of incubation an aliquot of the supernatant was aspirated and the radioactivity was measured in a gamma-counter (cpm_{exp}). Samples for the determination of the 100 % value (cpm_{max}) and nonspecific lysis ($cpm_{nonspec}$) contained medium instead of lymphocytes. Specific lysis was then calculated according to the following formula:

$$\% \text{ specific lysis} = \frac{cpm_{exp} - cpm_{nonspec}}{cpm_{max} - cpm_{nonspec}} \times 100$$

Cytotoxicity was considered positive if the specific lysis of the patient's serum was above the 95th percentile of the control sera determined in the same assay.

Addition of TPO

Fifty /uL serum from patients with HT (n=9), in whom the % specific lysis was previously found to be elevated, was preincubated with purified TPO (final concentration 66 and 100 /ug/mL) at 37 C for 90 min. Then the sera were centrifuged at 6000 x g and the supernatant added into the ADCC assay. The TPOab titers of the sera, determind by TPOab radioimmunoassay, varied between 0 and 10000 U/mL.

IgG preparation

The IgG fraction was isolated from serum samples by means of affinity chromatography on columns of protein A-Sepharose CL-4B (Pharmacia, Uppsala, Sweden).

Effector cells

Fresh mononuclear cells were obtained from heparinized blood of a normal adult by means of Ficoll (Seromed) density centrifugation. The mononuclear cells were washed and diluted with medium to 1.25 x 10^6/mL.

Microsomal/ thyroid peroxidase and thyroglobulin antibodies

Serum microsomal antibodies were determined by passive hemagglutination technique (Thymune M, Wellcome Diagnostics, Kent, UK) and by an enzyme immunoassay in which purified

the Mab/Tab-negative group 36.9 % and 33.6 %, respectively (Fig.1).

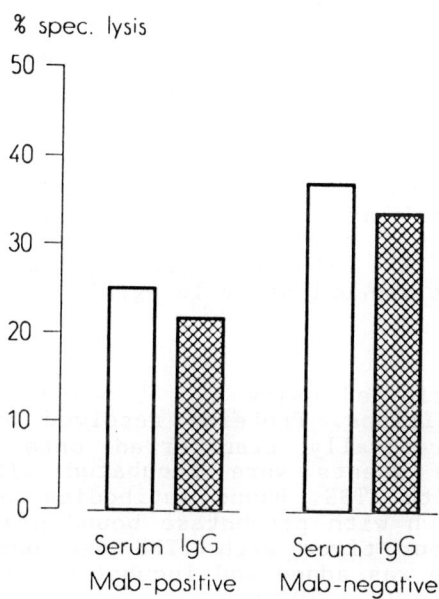

Fig. 1: Cytotoxicity determined by addition of serum and IgG (1 mg/mL) in the ADCC assay. In both groups (Mab-positive and -negative) the cytotoxic activity was found to be located in the IgG fraction, which proves that cytotoxic activity in Mab-negative sera is also mediated by an IgG.

To investigate in more detail whether the cytotoxic antibody is different from the TPO antibodies, sera with positive and negative titers of TPOab, but positive results for cytotoxicity, were preincubated with purified TPO for 2 h and then added to the ADCC assay. Interestingly, the cytotoxic activity remained unchanged in 7 of 9 sera, irrespective of whether they had a positive or negative result for TPOabs (Fig.2). Only 2 cases showed a significant decrease in cytotoxicity after preincubation with TPO, interestingly both, with low (130 U/mL) or undetectable titers for TPOabs.

microsomal antigen was bound to a solid phase (Thyr Mic-IgG EIA, Pharmacia). Thyroid peroxidase antibodies were measured by a radioimmunoassay against solid-phase-bound monoclonal anti-TPO-antibodies (DYNOtest, Henning Co, Berlin, FRG). Mab-titers of > 1:400, > 16 U/mL, >100 U/mL, determined by passive hemagglutination, ELISA, and TPO-ab radioimmunoassay, respectively, were defined as positive.

Thyroid membrane preparation

Thyroid tissuewas minced and homogenized in an Omnimixer (Sorvall Instruments, DuPont, Wilmington, USA). The homogenate was centrifuged with 1000 x g for 5 min. The supernatant was collected and spun with 100000 x g for 1 h at 4 C. The pellets were washed and resuspended in buffer. The suspension was layered on a sucrose gradient and centrifuged at 100000 x g for 2.5 h. The layer at the interface was collected and solubilized at 65 C for 15 min in 0.009 M Tris/HCl buffer containing 2.5 % SDS and 2.25 M urea. The protein concentration was approximately 10 mg/mL.

Immunoblotting

SDS-PAGE was performed using a 5 % polyacrylamide gel under nonreducing conditions. Proteins resolved by electrophoresis were electrophoretically transferred onto a nitrocellulose (nc) sheet. The sheets were incubated with serum samples diluted 1:250 with TTBS. Bound antibodies were visualized by incubation for 1 h with phosphatase bound goat anti-human IgG. After washing four times with TTBS and once with substrate buffer, substrate was added and incubation was continued until bands were visible (2 - 30 min).

RESULTS

ADCC in Hashimoto's thyroiditis (HT)

ADCC was positive in 42 (63 %) of 67 investigated patients with HT. The median of the specific lysis was 20.2 % (range 2.1 - 58.8 %) compared to 8.1 % (range 0 - 19.6 %) in the normal controls (p=0.00001). Values above the 95th percentile (> 15.4 %) were regarded as positive. No correlation could be found between the titers of Mab/TPOab, determined either by passive hemagglutination technique, enzyme immunoassay method or TPOab-Ria technique, and the activity of the cytotoxic antibodies (r=0.2, r=0.16 and r=0.02), respectively. There was likewise no correlation between the cytotoxicity and the titers of thyroglobulin antibodies (r=0.00).

Characterization of the cytotoxic activity

IgGs from 16 sera with positive and 4 sera with negative Mab and Tab titers were simultaneously tested in the ADCC assay. The median specific lysis in the Mab/Tab-positive group was 25 % with addition of serum and 21.6 % with addition of IgG, in

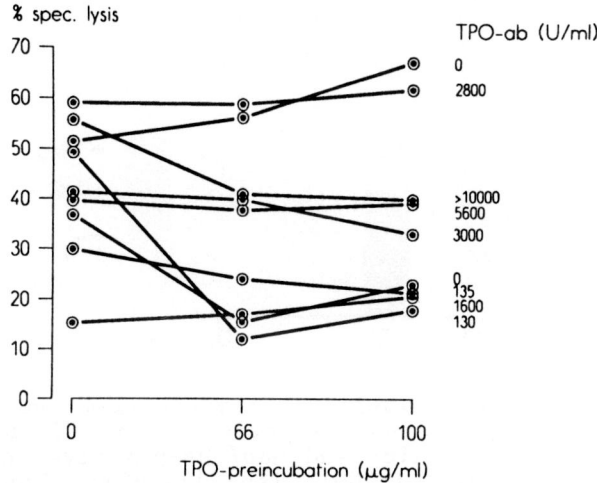

Fig. 2: Influence of preincubation with increasing concentrations of thyroid peroxidase (TPO) for 2 h on % specific lysis in sera of patients with HT. Values at the curves indicate the TPOab levels.

Immunoblotting following SDS-PAGE

Western blot experiments following SDS polyacrylamid gel electrophoresis were performed to show binding of the cytotoxic antibody to human thyroid membranes. Sera of patients with high cytotoxic activity in the ADCC assay and undectable as well as elevated titers of Mab were tested (Fig.3). Cytotoxic positive sera (lane C and D), both negative for Thyroglobulin- and microsomal antibody titers, showed no binding for serum D to the microsomal/TPO antigen fraction or to other components of the thyroid membrane preparation. There was only minimal staining with the serum C, which might be due to a low concentration of microsomal antibodies not detectable by the insensitive passive hemagglutination technique.

DISCUSSION

Earlier data of our laboratory, applying an ADCC assay against cultured human thyroid cells as targets, indicated a simultaneous occurrence of cell lysis and microsomal antibodies (Bogner et al., 1984). Including a higher number of patients, however, we could no longer prove any correlation between cytotoxicity and microsomal antibody activitiy. These results are in aggreement with previously published data in patients with Graves'disease, in whom we also could not find an association between cytotoxicity and microsomal antibody activity (Bogner et al., 1987).

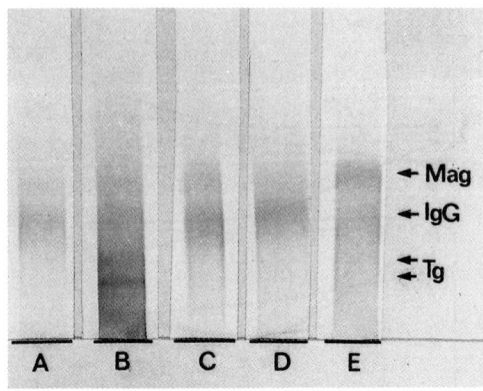

Fig. 3: SDS-Page of solubilized thyroid membrane fractions and immunoblotting with sera from patients with HT. Lane A: normal serum; lane B: Cytotoxic- and Mab/Tab-positive serum (specific lysis 43.6 %; Mab 1:400; Tab 1:2560); lane C and D: Cytotoxic-positive, Mab/Tab-negative sera (specific lysis 33.9 and 32 %, respectively, Mab/Tab negative); lane E: Mab positive control serum (Mab titer 1:25600). Mag=microsomal antigen. Tg=thyroglobulin.

The microsomal antigen has now been identified as the thyroid peroxidase (Czarnocka at al., 1985; Portmann wt al., 1985). To exclude the influence of false-negative Mab determinations by the insensitive passive hemagglutination technique, we measured in the same sera the antibody concentrations by an ELISA technique and a highly sensitive TPOab radioimmunoassay. However, there was still no correlation between cytotoxicity and Mab/TPOab. Our data, presented in this study, clearly demonstrate that cytotoxicity in the microsomal antibody negative sera is mediated by an IgG. Preincubation of TPOab-negative and -positive sera with purified TPO had no influence on the cytotoxic effect in the majority of tested sera. Although we cannot explain, why, in 2 sera, the cytotoxic activity decreased after preincubation with TPO, our data suggest that cytotoxic IgGs and TPO antibodies are induced by and directed against different antigen structures on the thyroid cell surface. In preliminary western blot experiments with solubilized thyroid membrane preparations and immunoblotting of Mab-negative/ cytotoxic positive sera we could not find a binding of the cytotoxic antibody to thyroid membrane fractions, which might be due to the lower sensitivity of the western blot technique in comparison to the ADCC method. Furthermore, sera with high cytotoxic activity did not bind to the TPO antigen, which gives further evidence that cytotoxic antibodies are not identical with TPOabs. This finding supports the hypothesis that TPOabs are not cytotoxic and that the cytotoxic effect will be mediated by an antibody not yet identified.

CONCLUSION

Our data give evidence that besides the well known thyroid autoantibodies a further antibody exists which is responsible for thyroid cell destruction in autoimmune thyroid disease. This antibody can occur simultaneously but also separately with the other autoantibodies and might, in some cases, be the only factor which proves the autoimmune pathogenesis of the disease. Further studies are in progress to support the hypothesis of the diversity of cytotoxic and thyroid peroxidase antibodies.

REFERENCES

Bogner, U. et al. (1987): Cellular and antibody mediated cytotoxicity in autoimmune thyroid diesease. Acta endocrinol. (Copenh).281: 133-38.

Bogner, U. et L (1984): Antibody-dependent cell-mediated cytotoxicity against human thyroid cells in Hashimoto's thyroiditis but not Graves'disease. J. Clin. Endocrinol. Metab. 59: 734-8.

Czarnocka, B. et al (1985): Purification of the human thyroid peroxidase and its identification as the microsomal antigen involved in autoimmune thyroid disease. FEBS Letters 190: 147-52.

Forbes, I.J. et al. (1961): Thy thyroid cytotoxic autoantibody. J Clin. Invest. 41: 996-1006.

Irvine WJ.(1962): Studies on the cytotoxic factor in thyroid disease. Br. Med. J.: 1444-9.

Lazarus, J.H. et al. (1984): The prevalence and progression of autoimmune thyroid disease in the elderly. Acta Endocrinol. (Copenh). 106: 199-202.

Portmann, L. et al. (1985): Anti-thyroid peroxidase antibody in patients with autoimmune thyroid disease: possible identity with anti-microsomal antibody. J. Clin. Endocrinol. Metab. 61: 1001-3.

Pulvertaft, R.J.V. et al.(1959): Cytotoxic effects of Hashimoto serum on human thyroid cells in tissue culture. Lancet 2: 214-6.

Pulvertaft, R.J.V. et al. (1961): The cytotoxic factor in Hashimoto's disease and its incidence in other thyroid diseases. Brit. J. Exp. Pathol.42: 496-503.

Tunbridge, W.M.G. et al. (1981): Natural history of autoimmune thyroiditis. Br. Med. J. 282: 258-62.

ACKNOWLEDGMENT

This work was supported by Deutsche Forschungsgemeinschaft. We would like to thank Dr. Carayon for the generous gift of purified thyroid peroxidase.

Résumé

L'activité cytotoxique dans le sérum de patients atteints de thyroïdite d'Hashimoto a été mesurée par dosage de la cytotoxicité cellulaire dépendante d'anticorps. La cytotoxicité a été déterminée dans un essai de relargage du chrome 51, en utilisant pour cibles des cellules thyroïdiennes humaines incubées dans du sérum inactivé par la chaleur, ou des IgG provenant de thyroïdites d'Hashimoto. Les cellules effectrices provenaient de cellules mononucléaires périphériques de sujets normaux. La cytotoxicité était plus élevée chez les patients atteints de thyroïdite d'Hashimoto (lyses moyennes spécifiques 20.2 %, zone 2.1 - 58.8%) que chez les sujets normaux (lyses moyennes spécifiques 8.1%, zone 0 - 19.5 %; $p < 0.00001$). Le pourcentage de lyses spécifiques n'était pas proportionnel aux titres en anticorps anti-microsomiaux déterminé selon différentes méthodes: technique de l'hémagglutination passive, dosage immuno-enzymatique et dosage radio-immunologique d'anticorps anti-TPO ($r=0.02$). L'activité cytotoxique a été localisée dans la fraction IgG, à la fois pour les sérums Mab positifs et Mab négatifs. La préincubation des sérums Mab/TPO positifs ou négatifs en présence de TPO purifiée, suivie par l'analyse dans le dosage ADCC, a montré une cytotoxicité moindre, dans deux cas seulement, et inchangée dans tous les autres sérums. Des expériences préliminaires de Western blot, utilisant des membranes thyroïdiennes solubilisées et des sérums positifs en cytotoxicité et négatifs en anticorps anti-microsomiaux, n'ont montré aucune fixation sur la TPO. Nos résultats suggèrent que la cytotoxicité dans le sérum des patients atteints de thyroïdite d'Hashimoto n'est pas médiée par les anticorps anti-TPO, mais par des anticorps non encore identifiés.

Cellular immunology and experimental models

Immunologie cellulaire et modèles expérimentaux

Induction of CD[4+] T cells from autoimmune thyroid disease by thyroperoxidase (TPO) *in vitro*

F. Akasu, Y. Kasuga, S. Matsubayashi, P. Carayon* and R. Volpé

*Endocrinology Research Laboratory, Wellesley Hospital, University of Toronto, Toronto, Ontario M4Y 1J3, Canada, and *INSERM U.38 Laboratoire de Biochimie Médicale, Faculté de Médecine, Marseille, France*

INTRODUCTION

Autoimmune thyroid diseases (AITD) are associated with the presence of circulatory autoantibodies reacting with antigens localized to the cell cytoplasm, surface membranes and colloid space (19). One of these autoantigens, the microsomal antigen (TMc) appears to play a major role in the pathogenesis of human AITD (2,11). The nature of TMc has recently been unraveled by studies indicating that the antigen is identical with thyroid peroxidase (TPO) (5,13,16), an organ-specific enzyme which plays a central role in thyroid hormone synthesis (14). It is further well known that there is increased activation of CD4+ cells in vivo in AITD, although the antigen(s) involved in that activation are not yet identified (19). Taking advantage of purified human TPO, we have attempted to determine whether peripheral CD4+ T cells from AITD could be activated by TPO under in vitro conditions.

MATERIALS AND METHODS

Subjects

Patients studied included 26 with Graves' disease (GD; 42.8 ± 15.7 yr.), 15 with Hashimoto's thyroiditis (HT; 41.3 ± 13.2) and 7 with nontoxic nodular goiter (NTNG) diagnosed by the usual criteria. Fourteen normal persons (N; 36.6 ± 10.5) acted as controls.

Antigens and antibodies

Native human TPO was immunopurified on anti-TPO monoclonal antibody (mAb) affinity column from a (NH4)2SO4 precipitate of solubilized human thyroid microsomes as previously described by Czarnocka et al. (5). Purified tuberculin derivative (PPD) was purchased from Cedarlane Laboratories. The murine monoclonal antibodies (mAb) used were FITC-labeled anti CD4, phycoerythrin (PE)-labeled anti HLA-DR; PE-labeled mouse IgG2a was used as a negative control for marker placement. All mAbs were purchased from Becton Dickinson.

Cell Cultures and immunofluorescence

Peripheral blood mononuclear cells (PBMC) were obtained by the standard Ficoll-Hypaque gradient centrifugation. PBMC were finally suspended in RPMI1640 medium containing 10% heat inactivated fetal calf serum (FCS) (Gibco) at 1 million viable cells. Cells were cultured in tissue culture tubes in a 37° C, 5% CO_2 incubator for 7 days in the presence or absence of TPO at final concentrations of 3, 30 and 300 ng/ml. PPD was added at a final concentration of 300 ng/ml. To deplete monocytes (in one study), the cell suspension was added to plastic petri dishes and cultured at 37° C for a period of 2 hours. The monocytes remained adherent to the dishes. Cultured PBMC were washed extensively with PBS containing 0.1% sodium azide and 0.5% BSA, and allowed to react for 30 minutes on ice with 10 ul of FITC-anti CD4 and PE-anti HLA-DR at 1×10^6 cells in a total volume of 20 ul. For negative control, PE-mouse IgG was used instead of anti HLA-DR.

Cells were then washed twice in cold PBS/azide and resuspended in cold 1% paraformaldehyde in PBS, pH 7.4. Samples were stored at 4° C in the dark until analysis.

Flow cytometry and data analysis

Samples were analyzed on a single laser FACScan flow cytometer; a minimum of 10,000 lymphocytes from each sample were analyzed, using a Consort 30 computer system (Becton Dickinson Immunocytometory Systems). Data were presented as two dimensional contour maps. Markers defining activated CD4+ cells (HLA-DR+ CD4+) were positioned to include >98% of the control mAB (PE-mouse IgG). The percentage of activated CD4 + cells was calculated on each sample as the number of DR+CD4+ cells/total CD4+ cells x 100. A stimulation index (SI) was used as a measure of response, defined as the ratio between the percentage of activated CD4+ cells in the presence versus the absence of antigen.

$$SI = \frac{DR+CD4+/total\ CD4\ with\ antigen}{DR+CD4+/total\ CD4\ without\ antigen} \times 100$$

One way or two way analysis of variance (ANOVA) was used to determine the statistical significance between subgroups. A two-tailed paired or unpaired T-test was also employed.

RESULTS

Activated CD4+ cells in the autologous mixed lymphocyte reaction.

Fig. 1 shows the percentage of activated CD4+ cells cultured for 7 days without antigen. Compared to N, CD4+ cells from GD and HT were less activated. However, there was no significant difference between NG and N.

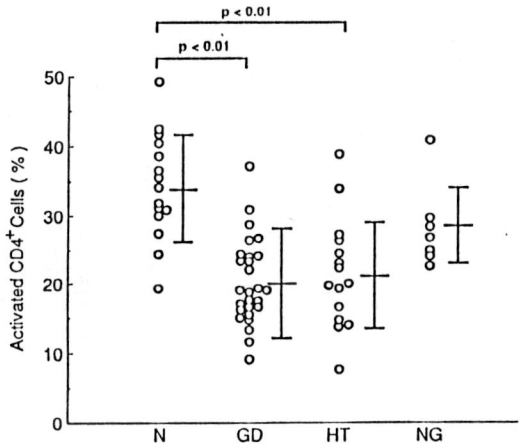

Fig. 1 Activation of CD4+ cells in the autologous MLR. % of activated CD4+ cells represents % of HLA-DR+ CD4+ among total CD4 Cells.
Mean values ± S.D.

TPO SPECIFIC ACTIVATION

As mentioned in Materials and Methods, the optimal concentration of TPO which stimulated the maximal response to CD4+ cells (measured as SI) varied markedly in both patients and normal subjects. It was therefore necessary to compare maximal responses from each subject, rather than selecting a particular TPO concentration. Fig. 2a illustrates that the SI was significantly higher in GD and HT as compared with N. There was no difference between NG and N.

When patients were further subgrouped, as illustrated in Fig. 2b, the SI was significantly higher in both hyperthyroid and euthyroid Graves' disease, as well as in euthyroid HT, as compared with N. The highest mean SI was found in patients with hyperthyroid GD (p<0.01), followed by euthyroid HT, (p<0.05) and euthyroid GD (p<0.05). However, there was no significant difference between hypothyroid HT and N.

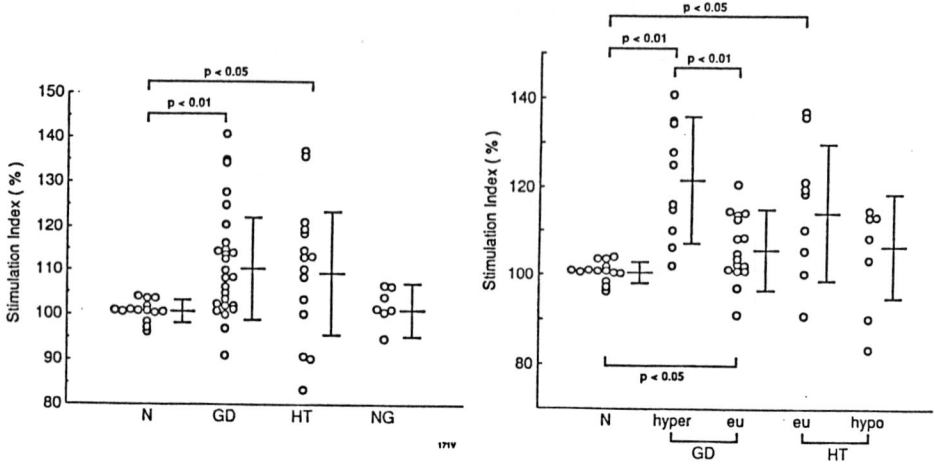

Fig. 2a Activation of CD4+ cells by TPO as measured by the stimulation index (SI). Mean Values ± SD.

2b Patients with AITD in Fig. 2b were further subdivided by thyroid status, i.e., hyperthyroid GD, euthyroid GD, euthyroid HT or hypothyroid HT.

Regression curves for serum T_3 and SI, T_4 and SI in GD, and T_4 and SI in HT, are illustrated in Fig. 3. There was no correlation between SI with other thyroid parameters.

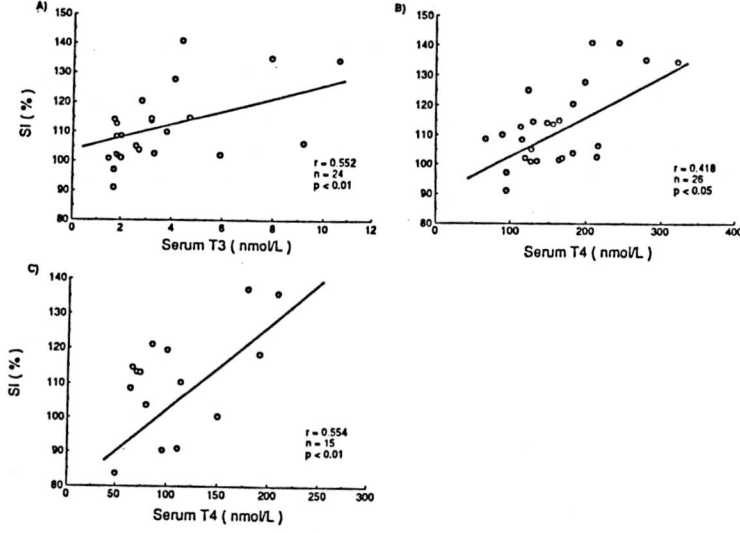

Fig. 3 Relationship between stimulation index (SI) and serum T_3 (A) or serum T_4 (B) in GD, and serum T_4 (C) in HT.

THE ROLE OF MONOCYTES AS AN ANTIGEN PRESENTING CELL

The function of antigen presentation by monocytes was examined in preparations from 3 GD and 5 N who were positive by skin reaction to PPD. TPO in GD and PPD in N were able to activate CD4+ cells more than the antigen free culture, (Fig 4). When monocytes were removed, there was no induction of CD4+ cells from any subjects. Even in antigen free culture, CD4+ cells were less induced without monocytes than with monocytes.

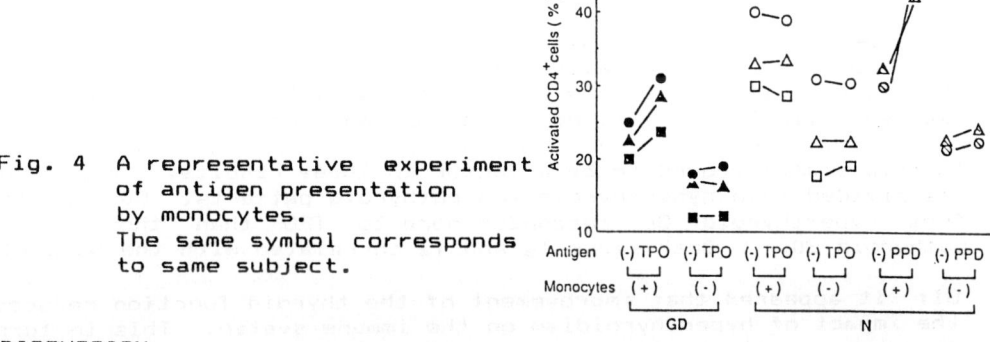

Fig. 4 A representative experiment of antigen presentation by monocytes.
The same symbol corresponds to same subject.

DISCUSSION

This study has demonstrated that TPO acted as an efficient immunogen in activating AITD CD4+ cells, but not normal CD4+ cells. In the process of antigen recognition by CD4+ cells, monocytes were shown to play a crucial role as antigen presenting cells. In contrast with the demonstration of TPO specific activation, it was shown that induction of CD4+ cells in the autologous MLR was impaired in AITD. To measure the activation of T cells, a previously utilized technique has been the (3H) thymidine uptake assay. However we have employed the two-color flow cytometric analysis, because we wished to focus on the CD4+ subset without eliminating other subsets from the culture. When PBMC are cultured in the absence of any known exogenous stimulant, T cells proliferate in response to non-T cells. This reaction is known as the autologous mixed lymphocyte reaction (auto MLR). By flow cytometric analysis, this reaction is demonstrable by increased numbers of DR+ T cells. An impaired response in the auto MLR has been described in several human autoimmune diseases (18). In addition, Canonica et al. (4) have reported a defective response of peripheral T cells in the auto MLR in AITD patients. We have confirmed this impaired reactivity of CD4+ cells in the auto MLR in AITD in this study. CD4+ cells may be subdivided into two functionally distinct populations, namely a helper subset and a suppressor inducer subset. The helper subset proliferates well upon exposure to soluble antigen, while the suppressor inducer subset proliferates well in auto MLR. It thus seems likely that the impairment of CD4+ cells in auto MLR may be due primarily to abnormal reactivity of the suppressor inducer subset (providing there are no abnormalities in the stimulator cells).

It has been suggested that HLA-DR+ thyroid cells in patients with AITD are capable of presenting antigen directly and thus activating intrathyroidal T lymphocytes as a primary inductive phenomenon (3,8). However current evidence indicates that thyrocyte HLA-DR expression is a secondary phenomenon, i.e. secondary to the secretion of interferon gamma by intrathyroidal T lymphocytes (9,12,17), although it may act as an amplification factor in the pathological process. It is thus likely that the initial antigen presenting cell (APC) in AITD is the monocyte/macrophage (17) and/or the dendritic cell (10), and indeed there appears to be synergy between thyroid cells and monocytes in the presentation of antigen (6). We have shown that intact thyroid cells are not necessary to demonstrate a specific CD4+ T cell response to TPO, as long as monocytes are present in the preparation as APC.

Our results indicate that AITD CD4+ cells respond more to TPO when compared to those with those from normal subjects and NG. This is consistent with the view that the AITD PBMC have already been specifically sensitized to thyroid antigen.

Thyroid status proved to be a factor in these results. When GD was divided into hyperthyroid and euthyroid patients, CD4+ cells from hyperthyroid GD responded more to TPO than those from euthyroid GD. Both serum T_3 and T_4 correlated with the maximal

SI: it appeared that improvement of the thyroid function reduced the impact of hyperthyroidism on the immune system. This in turn has been noted to improve generalized suppressor T lymphocyte numbers and function and may consequently reduce thyroid-directed CD4+ cell function in vivo (7,19). There was no significant difference between euthyroid HT and hypothyroid HT, although euthyroid HT tended to respond more than hypothyroid HT. The observation that NG did not respond to TPO was compatible with the previous report by Aguayo et al. (1), who demonstrated that PBMC from NG unlike AITD PBMC, did not stimulate autologous thyrocyte HLA-DR expression. The new data are consistent with the view that NG cannot be considered a primary autoimmune disorder.

REFERENCES

1. Aguayo, J., Sakatsume, Y. et al. (1989): Nontoxic nodular goiter and papillary thyroid carcinoma are not associated with peripheral blood lymphocyte sensitization to thyroid cells . J. Clin. Endocrinol. Metab. 68:145.

2. Banga, J.P., Pryce, G. et al. (1985): Structural features of the autoantigen involved in thyroid autoimmune disease: the thyroid microsomal/microvillar antigen. Mol. Immunol. 22:629.

3. Bottazzo, G.F., Pujol-Borrel, R. et al. (1983): Role of aberrent HLA-DR expression and antigen presentation in induction of endocrine autoimmunity. Lancet 1:1115.

4. Canonica, G.W., Croci, R. et al. (1984): Deficiency of the autologous mixed lymphocyte reaction in patients with autoimmune thyroid disease. Int. Archs. Allergy Appl. Immunol. 73:137.

5. Czarnocka, B., Ruf, J. et al. (1985): Purification of the human thyroid peroxidase and its identification as the microsomal antigen involved in autoimmune thyroid diseases. FEBS Let 190:147.

6. Eguchi, K., Otsubo, T. et al. (1988): Synergy in antigen presentation by thyroid epithelial cells and monocytes from patients with Graves' disease Clin. Exp. Immunol. 72:84.

7. Gerstein, H., Rastogi, R. et al. (1987): The decrease in non-specific suppressor T lymphocytes in female hyperthyroid Graves' disease is secondary to the hyperthyroidism. Clin. Invest. Med. 10:377.

8. Hanafusa, T., Pujol-Borrel, R. et al. (1983): Aberrant expression of HLA-DR antigen on thyrocytes in Graves' disease: relevance for autoimmunity. Lancet 2:1111.

9. Iwatani, Y., Gerstein, H.C. et al. (1986): Thyrocyte HLA-DR expression and interferon-production in autoimmune thyroid disease. J. Clin. Endocrinol. Metab. 63:695.

10. Kabel, P.J., Voorbij, H.A.M. et al. (1988): Intrathyroidal dendritic cells. J. Clin. Endocrinol. Metab. 66:199.

11. Khoury, E.L., Bottazzo, G.F. et al. (1984): The thyroidal microsomal antibody revisited. J. Exp. Med. 159:577.

12. Khoury, E.L., Greenspan, J.S. et al. (1988): Ectopic expression of HLA class II antigens on thyroid follicular cells: induction and transfer in vitro by autologous mononuclear leukocytes. J. Clin. Endocrinol. Metab. 67:992.

13. Kotani, T., Umeki, K. et al., (1986): Detection of autoantibodies to thyroid peroxidase in autoimmune thyroid disease by micro-ELISA and immunoblotting. J. Clin. Endocrinol. Metab. 62:928.

14. Nunez, J. (1980): Iodination and thyroid hormone synthesis. In: *The Thyroid Gland*, p 39, Raven Press, New York, De Visscher M (ed.)

15. Opelz G., Kinch, M. et al. (1975): Autologous stimulation of human lymphocyte subpopulations. J. Exp. Med. 142:1327.

16. Portmann, L., Hamada, N. et al. (1985): Antithyroid peroxidase antibody in patients with autoimmune thyroid disease: possible identity with anti-microsomal antibody. J. Clin. Endocrinol. Metab. 61:1001.

17. Weetman, A.P., Gunn, C. et al. (1985): Thyroid autoantigen-induced proliferation in Graves' disease and Hashimoto's thyroiditis. Clin. Lab. Immunol. 17:1.

18. Weksler, M.E., Moody, C.E. et al. (1981): The autologous mixed lymphocyte reaction. Adv. Immunol. 31:271.

19. Volpé, R. (1990): <u>Autoimmunity and Endocrine Diseases</u>. CRC Press, Boca Raton, Fl. (in press).

Résumé

Nous avons étudié l'activation spécifique d'un antigène des cellules T CD4+ (helper/inducer) par la TPO purifiée. Des cellules mononucléaires sanguines périphériques ont été prélevées sur 26 patients atteints de Basedow, 15 souffrant de thyroïdite d'Hashimoto, 7, présentant un goitre à nodule non-toxique et 14 sujets normaux. Les cellules ont été mises en culture pendant 7 jours en présence ou absence de TPO, à des concentrations finales de 3, 30 et 300 ng/ml. Retirées de la culture, les cellules ont été mises en contact avec des anticorps monoclonaux murins anti-CD4 conjugués au FITC et anti-HLADR conjugués à la PE. Le pourcentage de cellules CD4+ activées HLA-DR positives a été déterminé par fluorocytométrie. Le 7ème jour, les cellules CD4 ont été activées sans aucun stimulant spécifique, par réaction lymphocytaire mixte autologue (AMLR). En AMLR, les cellules CD4+ étaient moins activées chez les malades atteints de Basedow et d'Hashimoto que chez les sujets normaux ou présentant des goitres nodulaires non-toxiques. Les résultats de l'activation spécifique par la TPO ont été exprimés en index de stimulation (SI), défini comme étant le rapport entre le pourcentage des cellules CD4+ activées en présence ou absence de TPO. Les SI maximum des sujets normaux, atteints de thyroïdite de Basedow, d'Hashimoto, et de goitre nodulaire étaient respectivement de 100.7 + 2.3, 111.8 + 12.5**; 110.4 + 14.9* et 102.1 + 4.1 (** $p<0.01$, * $p<0.05$ vs.N). Les cellules hyperthyroïdiennes de Basedow étaient davantage activées par la TPO que les euthyroïdiennes ($p<0.01$). Par contre on ne notait aucune différence significative entre les cellules euthyroïdiennes et hypothyroïdiennes de Basedow.

En conclusion: 1) la réactivité AMLR des cellules CD4+ de Basedow et d'Hashimoto était diminuée.

2) Cependant les cellules CD4 étaient davantage activées par la TPO que celles des sujets normaux.

3) Cette induction dépend en partie de l'état in vivo de la thyroïde.

Localization in tryptic fragments from thyroglobulin of epitope(s) related to Hashimoto's thyroiditis or experimental autoimmune thyroiditis

H. Tang, E. Baudin and J. Charreire

INSERM U.283, Hôpital Cochin, 75664 Paris Cedex 14, France

RESUME

Des autoanticorps anti-thyroglobuline (Tg) sont détectés dans les sérums de patients ou d'animaux atteints de thyroïdites auto-immunes. Cependant, ils sont aussi détectés dans les sérums de sujets normaux ou de sujets souffrant d'autres affections thyroïdiennes auto-immunes (maladie de Basedow) ainsi que dans les sérums d'animaux immunisés par de la Tg mais ne développant pas la thyroïdite auto-immune expérimentale (TAE). Le but de ce travail a consisté à rechercher si des sous-populations d'autoanticorps anti-Tg dirigés contre des fragments tryptiques de la molécule de Tg, induisant la TAE chez la souris CBA/J, pourraient corréler avec l'incidence et l'évolution de cette maladie. Nous avons démontré que des autoanticorps reconnaissant un fragment tryptique de la molécule de Tg de 5-10 kDa corrélaient effectivement avec l'apparition, la phase aigüe et la guérison de la TAE ; de même que chez les patients atteints de thyroïdite de Hashimoto, le pourcentage de ces autoanticorps parmi les autoanticorps anti-Tg est significativement augmenté.

SUMMARY

Autoantibodies to Tg are detectable in sera from patients or animals suffering from autoimmune thyroiditis. However they are also detectable in sera from normal donors, from patients with Graves' disease and in sera from animals immunized by Tg but which do not develop EAT. The aim of this work was to characterize Tg epitope(s) related to thyroiditis through evaluation of subsets of anti-Tg A-Abs in sera from HT patients and from mice with EAT. We demonstrated that such A-Abs specific for a linear 5-10 kDa tryptic fragment from Tg molecule correlate with HT or EAT.

INTRODUCTION

Hashimoto's thyroiditis (HT) and experimental autoimmune thyroiditis (EAT) result in the damage of the thyroid glands. They are characterized by both the production of autoantibodies (A-Abs) to thyroid peroxidase (TPO) and thyroglobulin (Tg) antigens and by the thyroid gland infiltrations by lymphocytes (for review, Charreire, 1989). Whereas murine models of HT have demonstrated (Rose & Witebsky, 1956) that Tg is responsible for the induction of EAT, no relationship was evidenced between anti-Tg A-Ab levels and EAT or HT severity (Vladutiu & Rose, 1971). This discrepancy could be explained if one considers: i) that Tg molecule is a vast continuum of antigenic

determinants, each of which may trigger A-Ab production; ii) Tg epitope(s) related to pathology represent (an) immunodominant population(s).
The aim of this work was to attempt to characterize Tg epitope(s) related to pathology through evaluation of subsets of anti-Tg A-Abs in sera from humans or mice suffering from HT or EAT respectively.

MATERIALS AND METHODS.

Donors and patients. Sera were obtained from patients with clinical diagnosis of Graves' disease (GD) or HT. Moreover GD patients were selected among patients with circulating anti-Tg A-Abs. As negative controls, sera from normal donors without anti-Tg A-Ab were used.

Animals. Six to 8 week-old CBA/J ($H-2^k$) and C57BL/6 ($H-2^b$) were provided by the CSEAL-CNRS (Orléans la Source, France). Fifty µg of porcine Tg emulsified in CFA for priming and in IFA for challenge on day 14 were injected subcutaneously.

Antigens. Human Tg was purified from a human thyroid gland by passage through a Sepharose-4B column. Porcine Tg was from Sigma, st-Louis, MO. Purification of 5-10 kDa human or porcine Tg tryptic fragments was obtained as previously described by Tang et al. (in press). Human TPO was kindly given by P. Carayon (Marseille, France).

Detection of A-Abs by ELISA. Briefly, 96-well polyvinyl microtiter plates (Costar No. 3590, Cambridge, MA) were coated overnight at 4°C with 100 µl of 100 µg/ml native Tg or 2.5 µg/ml 5-10 kDa Tg tryptic fragments or 2 µg/ml TPO, in carbonate buffer pH = 9.6.
After washings in PBS-0.1% Tween-20, the free protein binding sites were blocked by the addition of 1.5% BSA for 2 h at 37°C. Then sera from individual mouse or human, diluted 1:1000 and 1:100 respectively, were incubated for 2 h at 37°C and washed out extensively. Alkaline phosphatase-conjugated goat anti-mouse IgG (Miles-Yeda Laboratories, Israël) (or alkaline phosphatase-conjugated rabbit anti-human IgG (Dakodatts, Denmark)), 1/500 diluted, were deposited as second antibody and then revealed after substrate addition. The results were read after 30 min with a Titertek multiskan spectrophotometer at 405 nm.

Statistics. All data were analyzed for statistical significance by Student's t test.

RESULTS.

Histopathological studies and A-Abs to Tg in CBA/J and C57BL/6 mice. From day 0 to day 70 post-Tg immunization, thyroid glands from CBA/J and C57BL/6 mice were collected for blind histopathological studies. In CBA/J mice, thyroid gland infiltrations by lymphoid cells increased until day 28 post-immunization. At that time, EAT was in acute phase. Thereafter, lymphocytic infiltration decreased and animals recovered from disease (Table 1). In contrast, thyroid glands from Tg-immunized C57BL/6 mice never showed lymphocytic infiltrations, regardless of the day post-immunization on which the thyroid glands were studied (Table 1). In parallel, individual murine sera were simultaneously tested for the presence of A-Abs to Tg. The shape of the responses was similar in both strains of animals. More precisely, on a given day post-Tg immunization, no significant differences in anti-Tg A-Ab titers were noted between the two strains of mice. Briefly, titers represented 45 to 55 per cent of the maximum response as early as day 7, increased and plateaued from day 28-35 until day 56. Then they slowly decreased, still exhibiting titers amounted to 60-70 of the maximum response at the end of the study.

Table 1: Kinetic study of thyroid gland infiltrations and anti-Tg A-Abs following immunization of CBA/J and C57BL/6 mice (mean ± SEM of 7-15 mice per group).

Days post-Tg immunization	CBA/J Thyroid gland infiltrations	CBA/J anti-Tg A-Abs	C57BL/6 Thyroid gland infiltrations	C57BL/6 anti-Tg A-Abs	p values*
7	-	554 ± 78**	-	788 ± 50	NS
14	±	1035 ± 150	-	894 ± 31	NS
21	+	1039 ± 76	-	912 ± 68	NS
28	++	1227 ± 58	-	1133 ± 78	NS
35	++	1251 ± 180	-	1343 ± 43	NS
42	ND	ND	-	1319 ± 48	ND
49	+	1363 ± 96	-	1356 ± 73	NS
56	±	1369 ± 67	-	1337 ± 35	NS
63	-	1131 ± 103	-	991 ± 46	NS
70	-	867 ± 67	-	841 ± 36	NS

* p values between titers of counterpart A-Abs in the two strains of mice.
** o.d. values in ELISA at 405 nm.
ND: not done; NS: not significant.

A-Abs to 5-10 kDa Tg tryptic fragments in CBA/J and C57BL/6 mice. Anti-Tg A-Abs specific for the linear 5-10 kDa Tg tryptic fragments inducing EAT behaved differently than A-Abs to native Tg. They were detected only in EAT-susceptible CBA/J mice whereas they remained at background levels in EAT-non susceptible C57BL/6 mice (Table 2). This difference was attested by significant p values < 0.05 to 0.01 between mean A-Abs titers in the two

Table 2: Kinetic study of A-Abs to 5-10 kDa Tg tryptic fragments in CBA/J and C57BL/6 mice (mean ± SEM of 7-15 mice per group).

Days post-Tg immunization	A-Abs to 5-10 kDa Tg tryptic fragments CBA/J	C57BL/6	p values*
7	126 ± 39**	105 ± 10	NS
14	174 ± 67	122 ± 14	p < 0.05
21	342 ± 36	125 ± 8	p < 0.05
28	420 ± 56	182 ± 24	p < 0.01
35	639 ± 73	199 ± 49	p < 0.01
42	ND	229 ± 49	ND
49	781 ± 121	234 ± 43	p < 0.01
56	667 ± 83	182 ± 65	p < 0.01
63	341 ± 46	167 ± 32	p < 0.01
70	291 ± 23	132 ± 23	NS

* p values between titers of counterpart A-Abs in the two strains of mice.
** o.d. values in ELISA at 405 nm.
ND: not done; NS: not significant.

strains of animals, from day 14 to 70 post-Tg immunization. In CBA/J mice, their levels, which represented 15 per cent of the maximum response as early as day 7, increased with time until day 49 where they reached their maximum titer. However, the high level was transient and as soon as day 56 A-Abs to 5-10 kDa Tg tryptic fragments rapidly decreased to nearly reach background levels at the end of the study.

A-Abs to human Tg in HT and GD patient sera (Table 3). A-Abs to human Tg were evaluated in 1:100 diluted sera from 15 HT and 12 GD patients. It must be noted that GD patients were preselected for the presence of anti-Tg A-Abs in their sera. As shown on Table 3, anti-Tg A-Abs were detected in slighly higher amounts in sera from GD patients than in those from HT donors. However the differences between the mean levels of anti-Tg A-Abs in the two groups of patients were not statistically significant. It must be noted that anti-TPO A-Abs behaved similarly as anti-Tg A-Abs and did not allow to discriminate between the two groups of patients. In parallel, sera from 33 normal donors were tested and found free of anti-Tg A-Abs (114 $\pm$ 7).

Table 3: Anti-Tg and anti-TPO A-Abs in HT and GD patient sera (mean $\pm$ SEM).

Patients	n	anti-Tg A-Abs	anti-TPO A-Abs
Hashimoto's thyroiditis	15	655 $\pm$ 89*	856 $\pm$ 154
Graves' disease	12	849 $\pm$ 91	1134 $\pm$ 106

* o.d. values in ELISA at 405 nm.

A-Abs to 5-10 kDa Tg tryptic fragments in HT and GD patient's sera (Table 4). Anti-Tg A-Abs specific for the linear 5-10 kDa tryptic fragments from human Tg were measured simultaneously as those to native Tg; however, they behaved differently; they were higher in HT than in GD sera. This increase became statistically significant ($p < 0.02$) if one considers their percentages among native anti-Tg A-Abs. They represented 36 $\pm$ 5 versus 19 $\pm$ 6 of total anti-Tg A-Abs in HT and GD sera respectively.

Table 4: A-Abs to 5-10 kDa Tg tryptic fragments in HT and GD patient sera (mean $\pm$ SEM).

Patients	n	A-Abs to 5-10 kDa Tg tryptic fragment	% of anti-Tg A-Ab response	
Hashimoto's thyroiditis	15	221 $\pm$ 39*	36 $\pm$ 5	) **
Graves' disease	12	171 $\pm$ 53	19 $\pm$ 6	) $p < 0.02$)

* o.d. values in ELISA at 405 nm.
** p values evaluated using Student's t test.

DISCUSSION.

A-Abs to Tg in the serum of patients with autoimmune thyroid diseases were shown to recognize a very limited number of epitopes, probably between 4 and 6 (Nye et al., 1980) on the large Tg molecule, but attempts to characterize the epitopes have been unsuccessful so far (Male et al., 1985). However, recently, the IgG subclass was hypothesized to reflect the ability of each patient serum to recognize different autoantigenic epitopes on human Tg (Fukuma et al., 1989). In the past, experimental models of thyroiditis have been useful in elucidating some of the pathogenic mechanisms involved in the triggering and the development of thyroid autoimmune reactivity. Therefore, we took advantage of murine EAT to define some Tg epitopes specifically recognized by A-Abs and related to disease development. Moreover, the use of EAT-susceptible and non-susceptible strains of mice (Vladutiu et al., 1971; Beisel et al., 1982; Salamero & Charreire, 1983a, 1983b) allows us to discriminate between A-Abs to Tg involved in autoimmune thyroiditis from those which are not.

Because in a previous work (Salamero et al., 1987) we demonstrated that linear 5-10 kDa Tg tryptic fragments were able to induce EAT and, more recently, that anti-idiotypic A-Abs representing the internal image of the EAT inducer antigen significantly correlate with the disease (Tang et al., in press), we investigated if such A-Abs could also be detectable in mice or humans suffering from EAT or HT respectively.

The present data demonstrate that whereas anti-Tg A-Ab levels do not allow to discriminate between the mice suffering or not from EAT, anti-Tg A-Abs to 5-10 kDa Tg tryptic fragments can do so: they were only detectable in mice with histological features of EAT.

In humans, our data can be compared to those obtained in mice. Whereas anti-Tg A-Abs are detectable as well in HT as in GD patients and their levels do not allow to discriminate between the two autoimmune thyroid disorders, the percentages of A-Abs to 5-10 kDa human Tg tryptic fragments can do so. They are significantly increased in HT patients' sera only.

Because the complete primary structure of the Tg molecule showed that Tg is a highly conserved glycoprotein (Mercken et al., 1985; Malthiery & Lissitzky, 1987), the presence of one Tg epitope related as well to EAT as to HT in a suspension of 5-10 kDa Tg tryptic fragments could be expected. However it must be reminded that 5-10 kDa is large enough to contain several epitopes and that among them, some would be specific for HT while others would be specific for EAT. Further biochemical studies are needed to solve this question.

REFERENCES

Beisel, K.W., David, C.S. et al. (1982): Regulation of experimental autoimmune thyroiditis: mapping of susceptibility to the I-A subregion of the mouse H-2. Immunogenetics 15: 427-430.
Charreire, J. (1989): Immune mechanisms in autoimmune thyroiditis. Adv. Immunol. 46: 263-334.
Fukuma, N., McLachlan, S.M. et al. (1989): Human thyroglobulin autoantibodies of subclasses IgG2 and IgG4 bind to different epitopes on thyroglobulin. Immunology 67: 129-131.
Male, D.K., Champion, B.R. et al. (1985): Antigenic determinants of human thyroglobulin differentiated using antigen fragments. Immunology 54: 419-427.
Malthiery, Y., and Lissitzky, S. (1987): Primary structure of human thyroglobulin deduced from the sequence of its 8448-base complementary DNA. Eur. J. Biochem. 165: 491-498.
Mercken, L., Simons, M.J. et al. (1985): Primary structure of bovine thyroglobulin deduced from the sequence of its 8,431-base complementary DNA. Nature 316: 647-651.
Nye, L., Pontes de Carvalho, L.C. et al. (1980): Restrictions in the response to autologous thyroglobulin in the human. Clin. exp. Immunol. 41: 252-263.
Rose, N.R., and Witebsky, E. (1956): Studies on organ specificity. V.: Changes in the thyroid glands of rabbits following active immunization with rabbit thyroid extracts. J. Immunol. 76: 417-427.

Salamero, J., and Charreire, J. (1983a): Syngeneic sensitization of mouse lymphocytes on monolayers of thyroid epithelial cells. IV.: Correlation with H-2 haplotypes. Cell. Immunol. 78: 387-391.

Salamero, J., and Charreire, J. (1983b): Syngeneic sensitization of mouse lymphocytes on monolayers of thyroid epithelial cells. V.: The primary syngeneic sensitization in under I-A subregion control. Eur. J. Immunol. 13: 948-951.

Salamero, J., Remy, J.J. et al. (1987): Experimental autoimmune thyroiditis induced by a 5-10 kDa tryptic fragment from porcine thyroglobulin. Eur. J. Immunol. 17: 843-848.

Tang, H., Bédin, C., Texier, B. and Charreire, J. (1990): Auto-antibody specific for a thyroglobulin epitope inducing experimental autoimmune thyroiditis (EAT) or its anti-idiotype correlates with the disease. Eur. J. Immunol., in press.

Vladutiu, A.O., and Rose, N.R. (1971): Autoimmune murine thyroiditis. Relation to histocompatibility (H-2) type. Science 174: 1137-1139.

ACKNOWLEDGMENTS.

This work was supported by the Fondation pour la Recherche Médicale (Paris) and Dr. H. Tang was supported by Immunotech. The authors are indebted to J. Decaix for skill full secretarial work.

Do TPO antibodies play a role in lymphocytic thyroiditis in the BB/Wor rat?

N. Yokoyama, A. Taurog, S. Alex, R. Rajatanavin and L.E. Braverman

The University of Texas Southwestern Medical Center, Dallas, TX and the University of Massachusetts Medical School, Worcester, MA, USA

BB/Wor rats spontaneously develop insulin dependent diabetes mellitus and a form of lymphocytic thyroiditis (LT) which resembles Hashimoto's thyroiditis (HT) in man (Sternthal et al., 1981). The incidence of LT is enhanced by excess iodine and serum auto-antibodies to thyroglobulin (anti-Tg) are usually present in rats with LT (Allen et al., 1986). Although microsomal autoantibodies (anti-M) have also been reported to be present in the serum of BB/Wor rats (Banovac et al., 1988), the method that was used did not exclude the possibility of cross reaction with Tg. Since thyroid peroxidase (TPO) is probably identical to the thyroid M antigen (Czarnocka et al., 1985) and since HT in man is almost always associated with positive serum anti-M and antibodies to TPO (anti-TPO) (Mariotti et al., 1987), we examined serum from BB/Wor rats with and without LT for the presence of anti-TPO Ab by 3 different techniques: ELISA, immunoblotting, and immunoprecipitation.

Materials and Methods

<u>Animals</u> - Two separate experiments were performed with BB/Wor rats, with and without lymphocytic thyroiditis (LT), as outlined in the following table.

Table 1. Experimental Groups.

Exp't	n	Iodide Rx	LT	Anti-Tg(O.D.)	Serum TSH(uU/ml)
I	8	-	-	0.07±0.02 *	nm **
	8	-	+	1.68±0.20	nm
II, A	5	-	-	0.02-0.04	31±11
B	5	+	-	0.02-0.04	73±22
C	5	-	+	0.12±0.03 #	39±13
D	5	+	+	0.31±0.12 #	427±72 +
E	5	+	+	0.10±0.03 #	32±3

* Mean ± SE
** nm=not measured
\# $p<0.02$ vs II A & II B
\+ $p<0.01$ vs other groups

Sprague-Dawley or Simonsen rats were used as normal controls. Lewis rats were used to prepare antibodies to procine TPO, as described below for the immunoprecipitation assay.

Purified porcine TPO: This was prepared from the trypsin-detergent-solubilized particulate fraction of porcine thyroid glands, as previously described (Rawitch et al., 1979). The purified enzyme represents a large tryptic fragment (MW~90,000), lacking amino and carboxy terminal portions of the native enzyme (MW~110,000).

Crude rat TPO: Approx 1 g of rat thyroid tissue (100 pairs of glands) was minced with scissors and homogenized at $0°C$ in Tris-HCl-KI, pH 7.0 in a polytron homogenizer. The 27,000 x g pellet was treated with deoxycholate (0.3%), or in some cases with deoxycholate + trypsin (0.0014%), at $25°C$ for 60 min. After centrifugation at 40,000 x g for 60 min, the supernate was dialyzed and used directly as a source of rat TPO. The specific activity of the crude rat TPO was about 2 guaiacol U/mg protein.

ELISA: Wells of Immulon 2 microtiter plates were coated either with purified porcine TPO or with crude rat TPO. In the assays with crude rat TPO, the rat serum samples were preincubated with rat Tg. Serum was diluted 1:100 with ELISA buffer, and 50 ul were added in duplicate to the washed, coated wells and incubated for 3h at room temperature in a moist chamber. The wells were washed and exposed to alkaline phosphatase conjugated to protein A. This was followed after further washing by the addition of p-nitrophenyl phosphate solution. After 30 min at room temperature, the absorbance at 405 nm was measured with an ELISA scanner.

Immunoblotting: Components that had been separated by SDS-PAGE were electrophoretically transferred to a nitrocellulose membrane in a Bio-Rad Trans Blot Cell overnight at 30V. Nonspecific sites were blocked by soaking the membrane for 2 h at room temperature in a solution containing 5% BSA. The membrane was then briefly rinsed and incubated for 2h at room temperature with rat serum diluted 1:100. After four 15 min washes, the membrane was incubated for 1h with ^{125}I-protein A. The membrane was then washed five times, and bound antibody was visualized by radioautography.

Immunoprecipitation: This procedure was based on the use of ^{125}I-porcine TPO and antibodies to procine TPO prepared in Lewis rats. Lewis rats were injected intradermally with 25 or 100 ug of purified porcine TPO in complete Freund's adjuvant at 4 sites on the back. After 2 weeks they were injected in the same manner with half the initial dose in incomplete Freund's adjuvant. Controls were injected with 100 ug BSA in the same manner. Animals were bled two weeks after the last injection. Binding of serum to ^{125}I-TPO was measured by immunoprecipitation with Pansorbin after overnight incubation at 4C. Binding of a standard volume of BB/Wor rat serum (1.0 ul) was compared with that of an equal volume of Lewis rat anti-TPO serum, which showed about 50% binding of the ^{125}I-TPO.

Serum Anti-Tg: Serum anti-Tg was measured by an ELISA using purified rat Tg as the antigen.

Serum TSH: Serum TSH was measured by RIA using materials kindly supplied by the National Pituitary Agency, NIH, Bethesda, MD.

Results

Anti-TPO Measured by ELISA: Although IgG from BB/Wor rat sera demonstrated slightly increased binding to purified porcine TPO measured by ELISA compared to serum IgG from control rats, this increase was not significant and was similar in BB/Wor rats with and without LT (Table 2).

Table 2. Binding of serum IgG to purified porcine TPO (ELISA).

Exp't.	Rat Strain	n	Treatment	LT	O.D. (1:100 Dil)
I	BB/Wor	8	0	-	0.048 ± 0.012*
	BB/Wor	8	0	+	0.050 ± 0.024
	Simonsen	4	0	nm	0.022 ± 0.002
	Lewis	1	Porcine TPO	-	1.16
II	BB/Wor, A	5	0	-	0.034 ± 0.006
	BB/Wor, B	5	Iodide	-	0.039 ± 0.010
	BB/Wor, C	5	0	+	0.031 ± 0.005
	BB/Wor, D	5	Iodide	+	0.026 ± 0.008
	BB/Wor, E	5	Iodide	+	0.039 ± 0.012
	Simonsen	4	0	nm	0.019 ± 0.009
	Lewis	1	Porcine TPO	nm	1.13

* Mean ± SD

When crude rat TPO was used as the antigen, anti-TPO Ab was only present in the serum IgG from BB/Wor rats with LT (Fig.1). However, when the sera was preincubated with rat Tg to absorb the anti-Tg Ab present in these sera, the anti-TPO Ab titer was not significantly higher in the BB/Wor rats with LT (Fig.1). This finding demonstrated that the crude rat TPO was contaminated with Tg.

Immunoblotting to Detect Anti-TPO Ab: Immunoblots comparing sera from BB/Wor rats to normal rats using crude rat TPO as antigen (Fig.2) or purified porcine TPO as antigen (Fig.3) revealed no differences in binding between sera from BB/Wor rats with LT and sera from BB/Wor rats without LT.

Anti-TPO Measured by Immunoprecipation Using Purified Porcine TPO: This assay proved to be relatively insensitive in detecting anti-M (anti-TPO) in human serum, being positive in human sera with an anti-M titer of 1:25,600 (tanned red cell) but negative in human sera with anti-M titers of 1:1,600 and 1:6400 (Table 3). However, anti-TPO detected by this assay was significantly higher in sera from BB/Wor rats with LT than in sera from BB/Wor rats without LT (Table 3).

Table 3. Binding of BB/Wor rat serum and human serum to ^{125}I-porcine TPO by immunoprecipitation (1 ul serum added).

Source of Serum	n	LT	% Added ^{125}I Bound Minus Non-Specific Binding
Lewis Rat	1	−	53.1
BB/Wor Rat, B	5	−	0.99±0.44*
BB/Wor Rat, D	5	+	1.82±0.16**
Human, anti-M 1:1600	3	NA	0
Human, anti-M 1:6400	3	NA	0
Human, anti-M 1:25,600	2	NA	3.7, 5.1

* Mean ± SD   ** $p<0.01$ vs BB/Wor, no LT.

This experiment was repeated using sera from all 5 groups of BB/Wor rats (Table 4). Again, there was significantly greater binding to ^{125}I-porcine TPO in the BB/Wor rats with LT but anti-TPO was not higher in the presence of hypothyroidism and LT. This finding strongly suggests that anti-TPO is not a major factor in the development of iodine induced hypothyroidism in rats with LT.

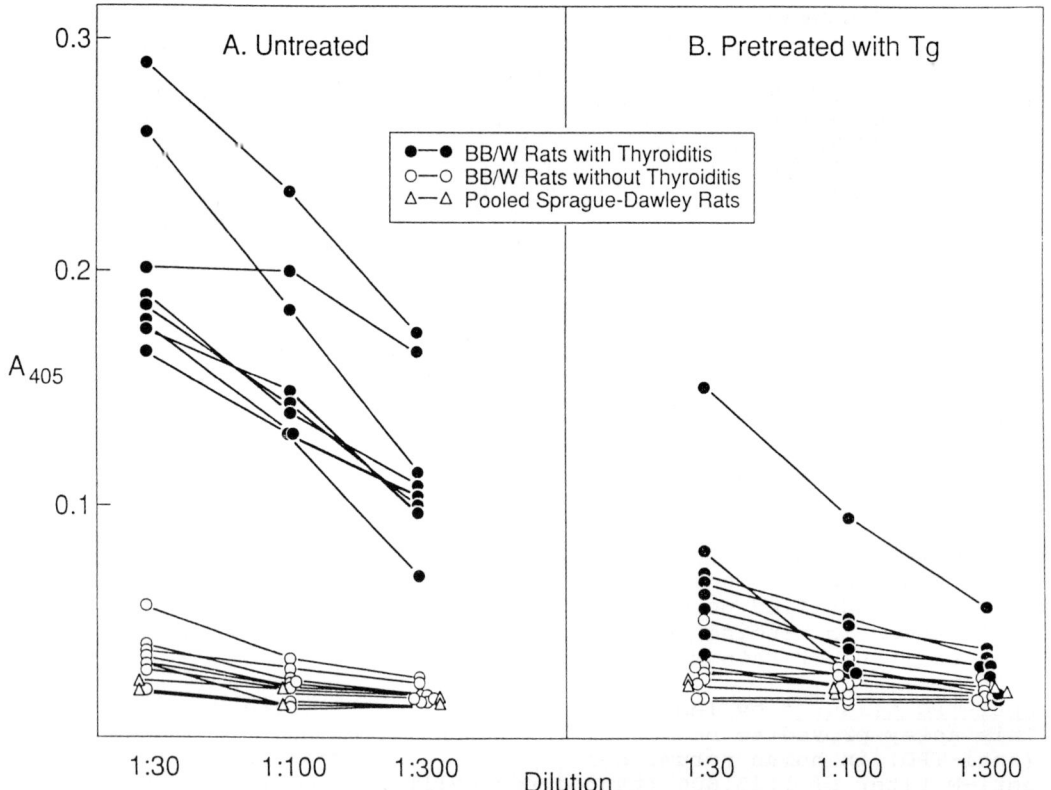

Fig. 1 Effect of Pretreatment with Rat Tg on Binding of Serum IgG from BB/W rats in Exp. 1 to Crude Rat TPO as Determined by ELISA

Table 4. Binding of BB/Wor rat serum and human serum to ^{125}I-porcine TPO by immunoprecipitation (1 ul serum added).

Rat Strain	n	Treatments	LT	TSH	% Added ^{125}I Bound Minus Non Specific Binding
Lewis	1	Porcine TPO	−		44.7
BB/Wor, A	5	0	−	Nor	0.46±0.40*
BB/Wor, B	5	Iodide	−	Nor	0.41±0.44
BB/Wor, C	5	0	+	Nor	1.01±0.23
BB/Wor, D	5	Iodide	+	Elevated	0.93±0.22
BB/Wor, E	5	Iodide	+	Nor	1.08±0.82

*Mean ± SD   LT(+) vs LT(−), $p<0.01$

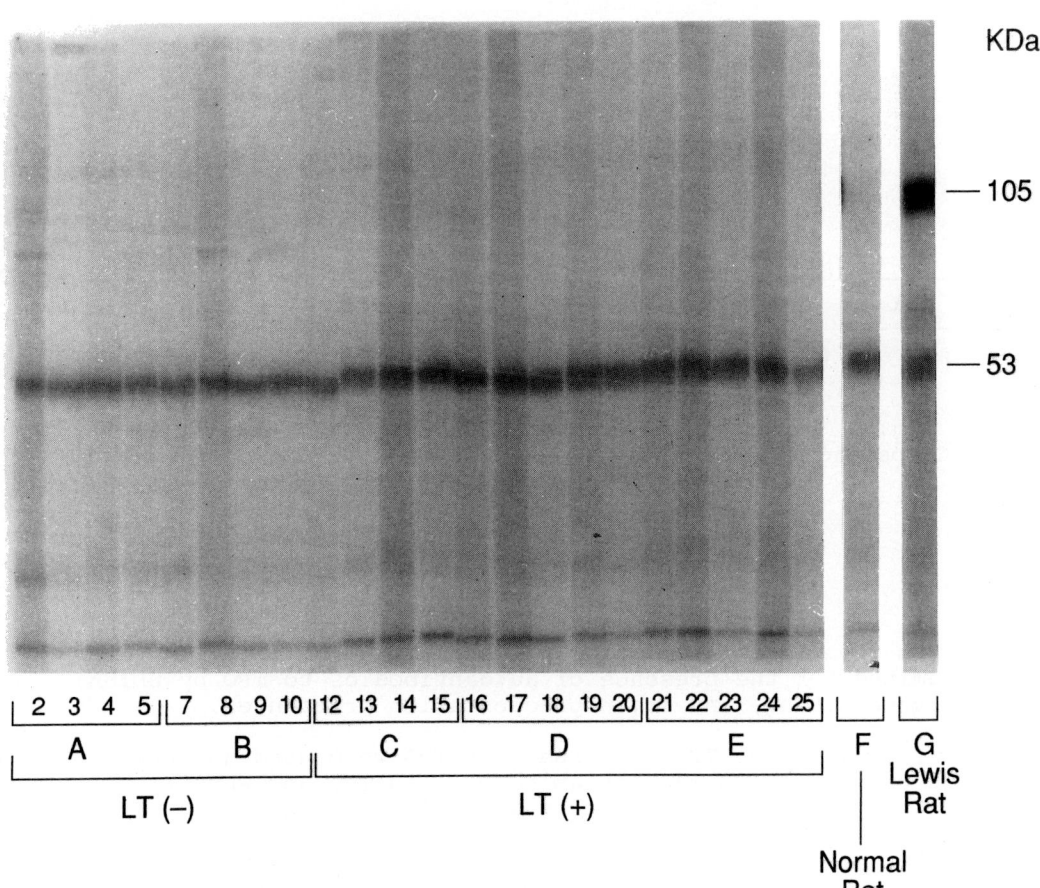

Fig. 2 Immunoblots with Crude, Detergent-Solubilized Rat TPO as Antigen, Comparing Serum from BB/W Rats With and Without Thyroiditis

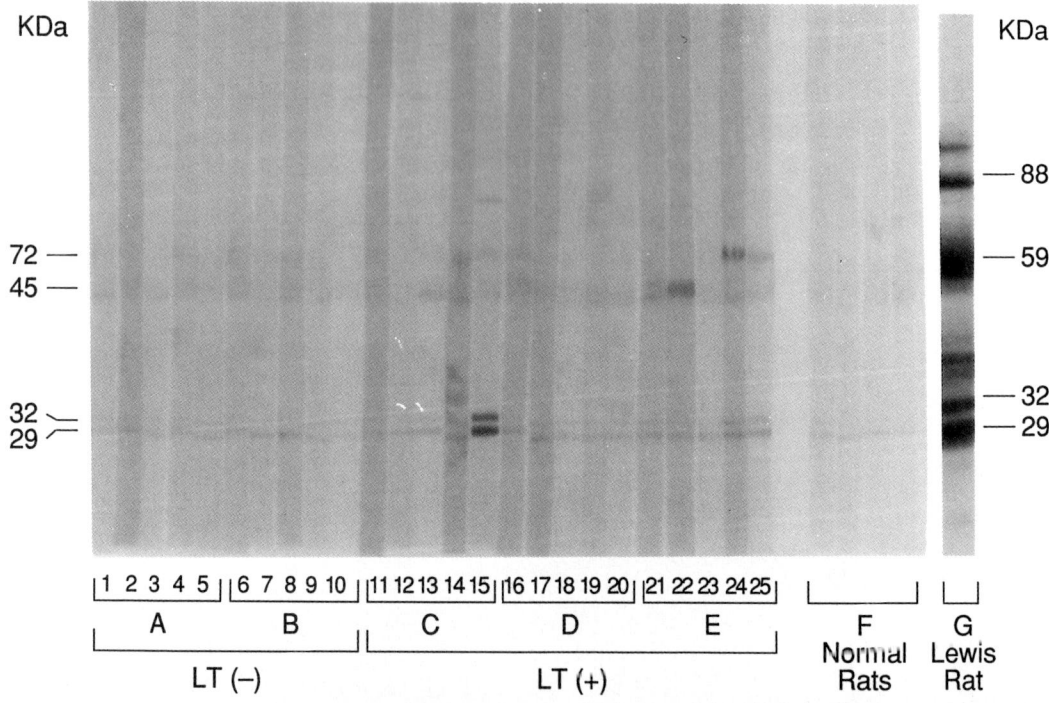

Fig. 3 Immunoblots with Purified Porcine TPO as Antigen Comparing Serum from BB/W Rats With and Without Thyroiditis

Summary and Conclusions

1. Serum from BB/W rats, with and without thyroiditis, was examined for the presence of autoantibodies to TPO by ELISA, immunoblotting, and immunoprecipitation procedures.

2. Purified porcine TPO and crude rat TPO were used as antigens. The crude rat TPO was contaminated with Tg, and when it was used as the antigen, serum samples were first preincubated with rat Tg to absorb Tg autoantibodies.

3. Binding to TPO by IgG in the serum of BB/Wor rats was very low but appeared to be slightly higher than in control rats. With the ELISA or immunoblotting procedures, no differences in binding were observed between BB/Wor rats with and without thyroiditis. However, with the more sensitive ^{125}I-TPO immunoprecipitation technique, a slightly higher binding was observed with serum from rats with thyroiditis. Among the rats with thyroiditis, there was no difference between Group D, with elevated serum TSH concentrations, and Groups C or E, with normal serum concentrations.

4. Our data with a sensitive immunoprecipitation procedure raise the possibility that antibodies to TPO may be present in the circulation of BB/Wor rats with thyroiditis. However, there is no indication that such antibodies are casually related to the thyroiditis or hypothyroidism.

5. Availability of purified rat TPO would help to determine more definitively whether antibodies to TPO are elevated in the circulation of BB/Wor rats with thyroiditis.

References

1. Allen, E.M., Appel, M.C., and Braverman, L.E., (1986): The effect of iodine ingestion on the development of spontaneous lymphocytic thyroiditis in the diabetes-prone BB/Wor rat. Endocrinology 118:1977-1981.

2. Banovac, K., Ghandur-Mnaymneh, L., Zakarija, M., Rabinovitch, A., and McKenzie, J.M., (1988): The effect of thyroxine on spontaneous thyroiditis in BB/Wor rats. Int. Arch. Allergy Appl. Immunol. 87, 301-305.

3. Czarnocka, B., Ruf, J., Ferrand, M., Carayon, P., and Lissitzky, S., (1985): Purification of the human thyroid peroxidase and its identification as the microsomal antigen involved in autoimmune thyroid disease. FEBS Lett. 190:147-51.

4. Mariotti, S., Anelli, S., Ruf, J., et al. (1987): Comparison of serum thyroid microsomal and thyroid peroxidase autoantibodies in thyroid disease. J Clin Endocrinol Metab 65:987-93.

5. Rawitch, A.B., Taurog, A., Chernoff, S.B., and Dorris, M.L., (1979): Hog thyroid peroxidase: Physical, chemical, and catalytic properties of the highly purified enzyme. Arch. Biochem. Biophys. 194:244-257.

6. Sternthal., E., Like, A.A., Sarantis, K., and Braverman, L.E., (1981): Lymphocytic thyroiditis and diabetes in the BB/Wor rat: A new model of autoimmune endocrinopathy. Diabetes 3:1058-1061.

Acknowledgements

Supported in part by Research Grants DK-03612 and DK-18919 from NIDDK, NIH, Bethesda, MD.

ABSTRACT

BB/W rats spontaneously develop insulin-dependent diabetes mellitus and a form of lymphocytic thyroiditis (LT) that resembles Hashimoto's thyroiditis (HT) in man. The incidence of LT is enhanced by excess iodine, and serum autoantibodies to thyroglobulin (anti-Tg) are usually present. Although microsomal autoantibodies (anti-M) have also been reported in the serum of BB/Wor rats, the procedure that was used did not exclude the possibility of cross reaction with Tg. Since HT in man is almost always associated with serum anti-M, we examined serum from BB/Wor rats, with and without LT, for the presence of autoantibodies to thyroid peroxidase (anti-TPO). TPO is very closely related to, if not identical with, the thyroid M antigen. Three different techniques were used to detect anti-TPO in the serum from BB/W rats: ELISA, immunoblotting, and immunoprecipitation. The antigen was either a highly purified preparation of porcine TPO, which had previously been shown to react with thyroid anti-M in serum from patients with autoimmune thyroid disease, or a crude preparation of rat TPO, solubilized with deoxycholate. When crude rat TPO was used as the antigen in ELISA experiments, serum samples were first pretreated with rat Tg to absorb Tg autoantibodies. BB/W rats were grouped as follows: A) No LT, B) Iodide-treated, no LT, C) LT, D) Iodide-treated with LT, E) Iodide-treated with LT and elevated TSH. The latter group had iodide-induced hypothyroidism as observed in patients with HT. Sprague-Dawley rats served as controls. Binding to TPO by serum IgG in the BB/W rats was very low, but appeared to be slightly higher than in control rats. The ELISA and immunoblotting techniques to detect anti-TPO Ab did not differentiate between BB/Wor rats with and those without LT. In contrast, a significantly higher binding of ^{125}I-TPO measured by immunoprecipitation was observed in BB/Wor rats with LT compared to BB/Wor rats without LT. However, anti-TPO Ab were not more elevated in the iodine induced hypothyroid BB/Wor rats with LT than in euthyroid rats with LT. <u>Conclusion</u>: Although the increase is modest, it seems likely that anti-TPO antibodies are present in the sera from BB/Wor rats with LT but that these antibodies are probably not the etiology of iodine induced hypothyroidism in BB/Wor with LT.

Résumé

Les rats BB/W développent spontanément des diabètes insulino-dépendants et une forme de thyroïdite lymphocytaire (LT) qui ressemble à la thyroïdite d'Hashimoto chez l'homme. L'incidence de LT est accrue par excès d'iode, et des anticorps anti-Tg sont habituellement présents. Bien qu'on ait également relevé la présence d'anticorps microsomiaux dans le sérum des rats BB/Wor, il n'est pas exclu, vu le procédé employé, qu'il se produise une réaction croisée avec la Tg. Puisque les thyroïdites d'Hashimoto chez l'homme sont presque toujours associées aux anticorps microsomiaux sériques, nous avons recherché la présence d'anticorps anti-TPO dans le sérum de rats BB/Wor, avec et sans LT. La TPO est apparentée, sinon identique à l'antigène microsomial. Trois méthodes ont été utilisées pour détecter les anti-TPO dans le sérum des rats BB/Wor : l'ELISA, la méthode d'immunoblotting, et celle d'immunoprécipitation. L'antigène était, soit une préparation hautement purifiée de TPO porcine, dont on avait montré précédemment qu'elle réagissait avec les anticorps anti-M sériques de patients atteints de maladies thyroïdiennes auto-immunes, soit une préparation brute de TPO de rat, solubilisée par le déoxycholate. Lorsqu'on a utilisé la TPO brute de rat comme antigène, dans les dosages ELISA, on avait préalablement traité les échantillons de sérum avec de la Tg pour absorber les auto-anticorps anti-Tg. Les rats BB/W ont été groupés comme suit : A) Sans LT, B) Traités par l'iode sans LT, C) LT, D) Traités par l'iode avec LT, E) Traités par l'iode avec LT et présentant un taux élevé de TSH. Le dernier groupe présentait une hypothyroïdie induite par l'iode, comme on l'observe chez les patients atteints d'Hashimoto. Les rats de Sprague-Dawley ont servi de contrôles. La fixation de la TPO par les IgG sériques chez les rats BB/W a été très faible, mais s'est révélée légèrement plus élevée que chez les rats contrôles. La détection des anticorps anti-TPO par ELISA et immunoblotting n'a pas permis de montrer les différences entre les rats BB/W présentant ou non une LT. Par contre, une fixation plus importante de ^{125}I-TPO mesurée par immunoprécipitation a été observée chez les rats BB/Wor avec LT, comparés aux rats BB/Wor sans LT. Cependant, les concentrations d'anticorps anti-TPO n'étaient pas plus élevées chez les rats avec LT chez lesquels avait été induite une hypothyroïdie par l'iode que chez les rats euthyroïdiens avec LT. Conclusion : Quoique leur concentration soit faible, il semble possible que les anticorps anti-TPO soient présents dans le sérum des rats de BB/Wor avec LT, mais que ces anticorps ne soient pas la cause de l'hypothyroïdie induite chez les rats BB/Wor avec LT.

Specific recognition of thyroid peroxidase by thyroid infiltrating T cell clones in human autoimmune thyroiditis

C.M. Dayan, M. Londei, A.E. Corcoran, B. Rapoport* and M. Feldmann

*Charing Cross Sunley Research Centre, Lurgan Ave, London W6 8LW, UK. * Thyroid Molecular Biology Laboratory Veteran's Administration Medical Center, U.C.S.F., San Francisco, USA*

We[1] and others have previously shown that a significant proportion of T cell lines and clones derived independent of antigen from the thyroid infiltrate in Graves' Disease recognise autologous thyroid epithelial cells. However, the antigens involved were not defined. We have used microsomes derived from Chinese Hamster Ovary (CHO) cells transfected with human thyroid peroxidase (TPO) cDNA and synthetic peptides of predicted T cell motifs in the TPO sequence to examine TPO reactivity in thyroid derived T cell clones. 5/24 of OKT3 expanded clones recognised TPO transfected CHO microsomes while showing no response to control microsomes. A further 4 clones recognised a 17 amino-acid peptide (NP-7) derived from the extracellular domain of TPO. Using polyclonal thyroid-derived T cell lines and a panel of different EBV-transformed B cell lines we have shown that the response to NP-7 in this individual is HLA - DP rather than DR or DQ restricted and that at least one further TPO epitope exists (B6) separated from NP-7 by 90 amino acids with a different HLA restriciton requirement.These results show at a molecular level that a high proportion of thyroid infiltrating T cells in Graves' disease are specific for thyroid peroxidase and that this response is not confined to a single epitope or a single HLA restriction element. Further definition of such disease related T cell epitopes may offer the possibility of peptide-based antigen specific immunotherapy as demonstrated recently in an animal model[2,3].

1. Londei,M.,Botazzo,G.F. and Feldmann,M. *Science* 228 85-89 (1985).
2. Wraith,D.C.,Smilek,D.E.,Mitchell,D.J.,Steinman,L. and McDevitt,H.O. *Cell* 59 247-255 (1989).
3. Urban,J.L.,Horvath,S.J. and Hood,L. *Cell* 59 257-271 (1989).

TPO autoantibodies in human

Auto-anticorps anti-TPO chez l'homme

Autoantibodies to thyroid peroxidase and thyroglobulin are inherited as an autosomal dominant characteristic in families not selected for autoimmune thyroid disease

D.I.W. Phillips, L. Prentice, D. Sarsero, S.M. McLachlan, M. Upadhyaya*, P.W. Lunt* and B. Rees Smith

*Endocrine Immunology Unit, Department of Medicine and * Department of Medical Genetics, University of Wales College of Medicine, Heath Park, Cardiff, CF4 4XN, UK*

Introduction

Autoantibodies to the thyroid microsomal antigen (TPO; thyroid peroxidase) and thyroglobulin are associated with the autoimmune process in Graves' hyperthyroidism and Hashimoto's thyroiditis (reviewed in Rees Smith et al 1988). These antibodies are also found in up to 20% of apparently normal women and occur with increased frequency in the relatives of probands with autoimmune thyroid disease (AITD). Recently, using new highly sensitive assays to TPO and Tg in the sera of families with AITD, we have demonstrated that the inheritance of TPO and Tg autoantibodies is consistent with a Mendelian dominant pattern in women but with reduced gene expression in men (Phillips et al 1990). These studies were carried out in a group of pedigrees each ascertained through one or more probands with AITD. Because of the bias inherent in this study, it appeared useful to carry out a study in which the propositi were not selected on the basis of a thyroid disorder. Consequently we have examined the occurrence of antibodies to TPO and Tg in 24 families currently being studied to map the gene for facioscapulohumeral (Landouzy-Déjérine) disease (FSHD) (Upadhyaya et al 1989).

Methods

Sera from a total of 277 FSHD family members (145 men and 132 women) were assayed for TPO and Tg antibody using the highly sensitive direct assays involving ^{125}I-labelled purified TPO or Tg as previously described (Beever et al 1989). In addition, antibodies were measured in sera obtained from 700 female and 100 male blood donors without clinical evidence of thyroid dysfunction. Inheritance patterns were analysed by segregation analysis and significance assessed with X^2 tests.

Results

In the 24 FSHD families TPO antibody was detectable in 6.8% of men and 22% of women, and Tg antibody in 9.8 of men and 20% of women. These figures are comparable with the antibody prevalences obtained in the blood donors (women 20.2% for TPO and 20.1% for Tg; men 10% for TPO and 12% for Tg). Inspection of the pedigrees in the FSHD families suggested that the tendency to produce TPO and Tg antibodies (measured by the direct assay) was dominantly inherited in at least some of the families as shown for two pedigrees in Figure 1.

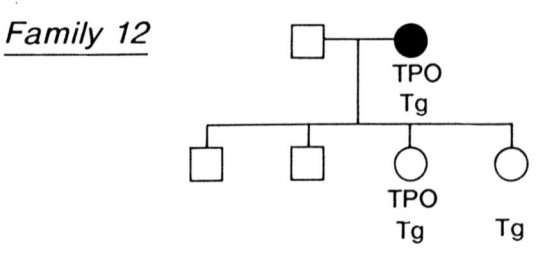
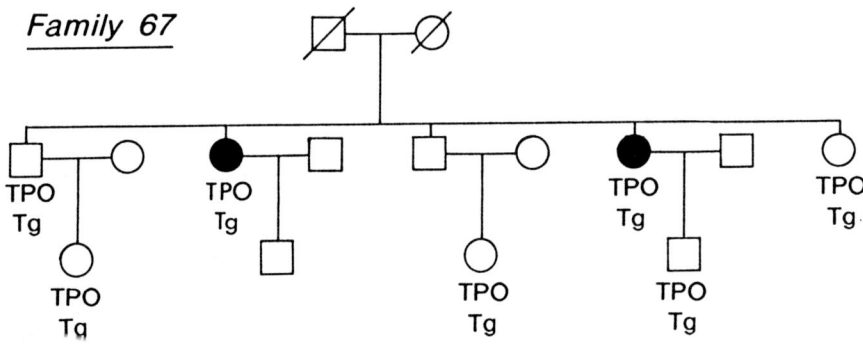

Fig. 1. Autosomal dominant inheritance of TPO and Tg antibody in two FSHD pedigrees. Solid symbols indicate overt autoimmune thyroid disease.

The inheritance patterns of TPO Ab and Tg Ab in the FSHD families were analysed by a segregation analysis (Table 1). Of a total of 41 meioses where one or other parent had TPO Ab, 3 sons were TPO Ab +ve and 19 TPO Ab −ve; 5 daughters were TPO Ab +ve and 15 TPO Ab −ve. These figures are inconsistent with autosomal dominant inheritance ($X^2 = 11.6$ $p< 0.01$ for sons and $X^2 = 5.0$ $p< 0.05$ for daughters). However, the studies among blood donors showed that the prevalence of TPO antibody increased markedly with age from 16% at 15-24 years rising progressively to 27% in the 45+ age group. As these figures suggested that age might interact with our genetic model, we re-examined the FSHD data to see if disease positivity in the offspring of antibody positive parents varied with age. In families where one or other parent was antibody positive, among the 11 daughters aged less than 25, only 1 was TPO Ab +ve which was significantly different from the Mendelian expectation of 50% ($x^2 = 7.4$, $p< 0.01$); in contrast of the daughters aged 25 or over, 4 were TPO Ab +ve and 5 TPO Ab −ve which was not significantly different from the 50% expectation. Similar results were observed for Tg antibody.

Table 1 - Segregation analysis of the tendency to develop TPO antibody and Tg antibody among the 24 families with FSHD.

	TPO Ab		Tg Ab	
	+ve	-ve	+ve	-ve
Sons	3	19	4	20
Daughters (all)	5	15	7	12
Daughters (< 25 years)	1	11	2	8
(> 25 years)	4	5	5	4

Discussion and Conclusions

Early studies suggested that the inheritance patterns of thyroid autoantibodies were consistent with a single gene or gene cluster. For example, Hall et al observed thyroid autoantibodies in 56% of the siblings of probands with AITD and subsequently showed that in 17 of 19 patients with Hashimoto's thyroiditis one or both parents were antibody positive (Hall et al 1960 and 1962). Later, community based studies failed to substantiate this hypothesis suggesting that the tendency to produce the autoantibodies is multifactorial (Hall et al 1972; Howel Evans et al 1967). A major problem of these studies has been the lack of sensitivity in the agglutination assays used to detect thyroid autoantibodies. Our recent results using highly sensitive assays suggested that autoantibodies to TPO and Tg were inherited as an autosomal dominant characteristic in women. We have now extended these studies to a group of families not selected for thyroid disease, and among whom the prevalence of thyroid autoantibodies approximates closely to the prevalence in the normal population. Although based on small numbers, the data obtained in the FSHD families supports the hypothesis of autosomal dominant inheritance of TPO and Tg Ab in women. However, they also indicate that gene expression may be reduced in young women.

References

Beever, K., Bradbury, J., Phillips, D., et al (1989). Highly sensitive assays of autoantibodies to thyroglobulin and to thyroid peroxidase. Clin. Chem. 35:1949-1954

Hall, R., Owen, S. G. and Smart, G.A. (1960). Evidence for a genetic predisposition to the formation of thyroid autoantibodies. Lancet ii:187-188

Hall, R., Saxena, K.M. and Owen, S.G. (1962). A study of the parents of patients with Hashimoto's disease. Lancet ii:1291-1292.

Hall, R., Dingle, P.R. and Roberts, D.F. (1972). Thyroid antibodies: a study of first degree relatives. Clin. Genetics 3:319-324.

Howel Evans, A.W., Woodrow, J.C., McDougall, C.D.M. et al (1967). Antibodies in the families of thyrotoxic patients. Lancet i:636-641.

Phillips, D.I.W., McLachlan, S., Stephenson, A. et al (1990). Autosomal dominant transmission of autoantibodies to thyroglobulin and thyroid peroxidase. J. Clin. Endocrinol. Metab. 70:742-746.

Rees Smith, B., McLachlan, S.M. and Furmaniak, J. (1988). Autoantibodies to the thyrotrophin receptor. Endocrine Reviews 9:106-121.

Upadhyaya, M., Sarfarazi, M., Lunt, P.W. et al (1989). A genetic linkage study of facioscapulohumeral (Llandouzy-Déjérine) disease with 24 polymorphic DNA probes. J. Med. Genet. 26:490-493.

Abstract

The tendency for autoantibodies to thyroid peroxidase (TPO) and thyroglobulin (Tg) to occur in families is well known, but the patterns of inheritance of the autoantibodies has been difficult to clarify. Recently, using highly sensitive assays to measure TPO Ab and Tg Ab in families with autoimmune thyroid disease, we demonstrated that inheritance of TPO Ab and Tg Ab was consistent with Mendelian dominant inheritance in women, but penetrance was reduced in men. As it was possible that the results were biased because the families were ascertained through one or more probands with autoimmune thyroid disease, we have re-examined the inheritance of TPO/Tg Ab in a group of 24 families being studied to map the gene for facioscapulohumeral disease (FSHD) among whom the prevalence of thyroid disease would be expected to approximate to that of the general population. The results of this analysis indicate that our hypothesis concerning autosomal dominant inheritance of TPO Ab/Tg Ab is fundamentally correct but also indicate that gene expression may be reduced in young women.

Résumé

La tendance des anticorps anti-TPO et anti-thyroglobuline à apparaître dans certaines familles est bien connue, mais il a été jusqu'ici difficile de clarifier le mécanisme de l'hérédité des anticorps. Récemment, en utilisant des dosages ultra-sensibles pour mesurer les anticorps anti-TPO et les anticorps anti-thyroglobuline, nous avons démontré que la transmission héréditaire selon les lois mendéléiennes était dominante chez les femmes, mais réduite chez les hommes. Comme les résultats risquaient d'être faussés parce que ces familles présentaient toutes une maladie thyroïdienne auto-immune, nous avons réexaminé la transmission héréditaire des anticorps anti-TPO anti-Tg dans un groupe de 24 familles, étudiées pour localiser le gène de la maladie facioscapulohumérale (FSHD). Dans ces familles, la prévalence de maladies thyroïdiennes devait être approximativement celle de la population en général. Les résultats de cette analyse indiquent que notre hypothèse concernant une transmission autosomale dominante des anticorps anti-TPO/TG est fondamentalement correcte, mais montre également que l'expression du gène peut être réduite chez les femmes jeunes.

Serum anti-thyroid peroxidase autoantibody in autoimmune thyroid disease

S. Mariotti, P. Caturegli, G. Barbesino and A. Pinchera

Istituto di Endocrinologia, University of Pisa, Viale del Tirreno 64 I-56018, Tirrenia-Pisa, Italy

SUMMARY

Thyroid microsomal antibodies (anti-M Ab) have been recently proven to be directed to thyroid peroxidase (TPO). Methods to detect anti-TPO antibodies (anti-TPO Ab) employing purified antigen have been developed, but the available information on the clinical usefulness of this technique is still limited. We have recently evaluated the clinical usefulness of anti-TPO Ab measurements by a newly developed monoclonal antibody-assisted RIA in a large number of subjects including normal controls and patients with different autoimmune (AITD) or non-autoimmune (N-AITD) thyroid diseases. Anti-TPO Ab were detected in 134/181 (74%) patients with Graves' disease, in all but one (99.3%) 144 patients with Hashimoto's thyroiditis or idiopathic myxedema, in 20/188 (10.6%) with miscellaneous N-AITD, in 16/83 (19.2%) patients with differentiated thyroid carcinoma and in 10/119 (8.4%) normal healthy controls. The highest anti-TPO Ab concentrations were found in untreated hypothyroid Hashimoto's thyroiditis, but no simple relationship between anti-TPO Ab levels and thyroid function was observed. Anti-TPO Ab significantly decreased in patients with Graves' disease after treatment with methimazole and in those with hypothyroid Hashimoto's thyroiditis or idiopathic myxedema during L-T4 administration. A highly significant positive correlation ($r=0.979$, $p<0.001$) was found between anti-M Ab titers by passive hemagglutination (PH) and the corresponding average anti-TPO Ab by RIA; discrepant results were almost exclusively limited to sera with negative or low (1/100-1/400) anti-M Ab titers. Absorption studies showed that interference of anti-Tg Ab was responsible for anti-M Ab positive tests in occasional anti-TPO Ab negative/anti-M Ab positive sera from AITD patients. Comparison of the diagnostic accuracy by Galen and Gambino's analysis showed higher specificity and sensitivity for AITD of anti-TPO Ab RIA tests when compared to anti-M Ab by PH, when cut-offs near to the detection limits of the assays were selected. Anti-TPO Ab determination by RIA was unaffected by circulating thyroglobulin concentrations, up to >10,000 ng/ml.

INTRODUCTION

In thyroid autoimmune disorders are frequently detected circulating autoantibodies (anti-M Ab) reacting with the thyroid microsomal antigen (Khoury et al., 1984, Pinchera et al., 1987), recently identified as thyroid peroxidase (TPO) (Czarnocka et al, 1985a,b, Protmann et al., 1985, Kotani et al., 1986, Mariotti et al., 1987, Libert et al., 1987, Seto et al., 1987). The availability of purified TPO provided the basis for the development of radioimmunoassays (RIA) (Czarnocka et al., 1986, Mariotti et al., 1987, Ruf et al., 1988, Beever et al., 1989) and enzyme-liked immunosorbent assays (ELISA) (Kotani et al., 1986) for anti-TPO autoantibody (anti-TPO Ab) detection. The clinical usefulness of these techniques, however, has not yet fully established.

In the last 3 years, we developed several specific radioimmunoassays (RIA) for anti-TPO autoantibodies (anti-TPOAb). (Mariotti et al., 1987, Mariotti et al., 1988). We report here our experience on the usefulness of anti-TPO Ab measurements in autoimmune thyroid diseases (AITD).

MATERIALS AND METHODS

Patients

Control sera were obtained from 119 normal healthy subjects. Pathological sera were obtained from 325 patients with AITD and 271 with several miscellaneous non-AITD (N-AITD). AITD patients included: 181 with Graves' disease, 98 with Hashimoto's thyroiditis, 46 with idiopathic myxedema.

TPO and anti-TPO monoclonal antibody

The monoclonal anti-TPO antibody and TPO used in this study were obtained as detailed elsewhere (Czarnocka et al., 1985b). TPO was iodinated by the chloramine-T method (Hunter & Greenwood, 1962) to a specific activity ranging between 20-40 µCi/µg.

RIA for anti-TPO Ab

The assay is based on the competitive inhibition of [^{125}I]-TPO binding to an anti-TPO monoclonal antibody coated on microtiter plates (Cook Engineering Co. Alexandria, Va.) (Mariotti et al. 1988). Anti-TPO Ab was expressed in International Units (U)/ml using a standard curve calibrated against a positive serum provided by National Institute for Biological Standards and Control (Hamstead, London, U.K.). The minimum detectable amount in the test sera ranged between 5-10 U/ml. Anti-TPO Ab were undetectable by this RIA in several autoimmune sera containing different types of organ- and nonorgan-specific autoantibodies except in those also showing positive anti-M Ab tests. Thyroglobulin (Tg) up to 100,000 ng/ml did not interfere with the binding of ^{125}I-TPO in the RIA.

Thyroid antibody assays by passive hemagglutination (PH)

In the large majority of cases (650 sera), anti-M Ab and anti-thyroglobulin antibody (anti-Tg Ab) measurements by passive hemagglutination (PH) were also available.

PH tests were carried out using commercial kits (Fujizoki Pharmaceutical Co., Tokyo, Japan). Titers ≥1/100 were considered as positive.

Serum Tg assay

This was performed in all patients with thyroid carcinoma by a solid-phase-immunoradiometric assay (TgK Sorin Biomedica S.p.A., Saluggia, Italy).

RESULTS

Assay of anti-TPO Ab in thyroid diseases

For the purpose of the present study any clearly detectable anti-TPO Ab levels (i.e. >10 U/ml) was considered as positive antibody test. As summarized in Fig. 1, anti-TPO Ab were detected in 10/119 (8.4%) (range: 11-210 U/ml) normal controls, in 134/181 (74%) (range: 11-74.000 U/ml) patients with Graves' disease, in all but one patients (range: 11-90.000 U/ml) with Hashimoto's thyroiditis or idiopathic myxedema, in 16/83 (19.2%) (range: 11-6.600 U/ml) patients with differentiated thyroid carcinoma and in 20/188 (10.6%) (range: 11-6.700 U/ml) with miscellaneous N-AITD.

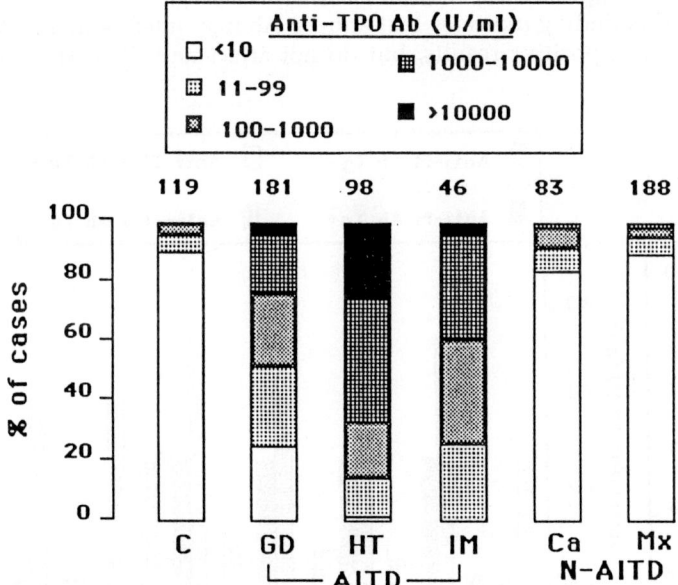

Fig. 1. Prevalence of anti-TPO Ab in normal controls (C), in patients with autoimmune (AITD: GD=Graves' disease, HT=Hashimoto's thyroiditis, IM=idiopathic myxedema) and non-autoimmune (N-AITD: Ca: thyroid carcinoma, Mx: miscellaneous thyroid diseases) thyroid diseases.

Of the 69 untreated hyperthyroid patients with Graves' disease, 55 (79.7%) had serum anti-TPO Ab levels >10 U/ml, with a mean±SE of 4680±1468 U/ml. Anti-TPO Ab tests were found in a lower proportion (74/112=66.1%) of Graves' sera obtained when the patients were euthyroid during or after different forms of treatment. The mean±S.E. antibody titer of this group was lower (2060±932 U/ml) than that found in untreated sera. Positive anti-TPO Ab were found in all 73 untreated patients with hypothyroid or euthyroid goitrous Hashimoto's thyroiditis and in those with idiopathic myxedema. The highest anti-TPO Ab titers (mean±SE: 27970±9188 U/ml) were found in hypothyroid Hashimoto's patients, while significantly lower levels (by Student's t test) were found in euthyroid Hashimoto's (mean±SE 3780±1797, p<0.05) and in idiopathic myxedema (mean±SE: 2389±677, p<0.05). Anti-TPO Ab levels were lower during L-T4 administration in patients with Hashimoto's thyroiditis (mean±SE: 6950±3011) or idiopathic myxedema (mean±SE: 649±257, p<0.05).

Comparison of anti-TPO Ab by RIA and anti-M Ab by PH

A highly significant positive correlation (r=0.979, p<0.001) was found between mean anti-TPO Ab levels by RIA and anti-M Ab titers by PH in the 650 patients available for this analysis. Discrepancies between anti-TPO Ab and anti-M Ab were almost exclusively limited to sera with negative or low (1/100-1/400) titers of anti-M Ab by PH. In sporadic cases, high anti-M Ab were found in sera from patients with AITD and with consistently low or undetectable anti-TPO Ab by RIA. In these samples (Fig. 2) the addition of excess Tg (50 µg/ml) substantlially or completly inhibited hemagglutination reaction, while no change of anti-TPO Ab levels was observed. This finding indicates that anti-Tg Ab may intefere in anti-M Ab assay by PH giving false positive results, but do not affect anti-TPO Ab determination by RIA.

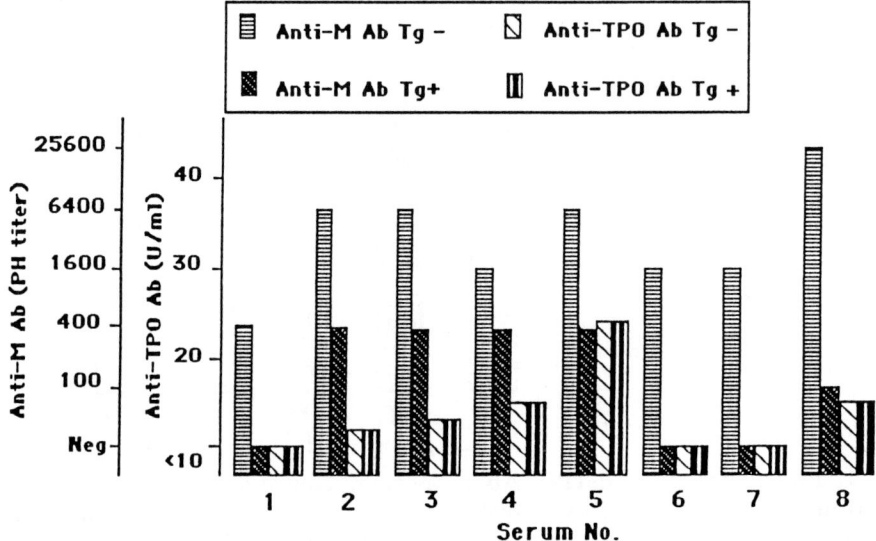

Fig. 2. Effect of preabsorption with Tg on anti-M Ab and anti-TPO Ab measurements in 8 selected sera with high anti-M Ab by PH and low or undetectable anti-TPO Ab by RIA.

Diagnostic accuracy for AITD of anti-TPO Ab versus anti-M Ab

We then compared the diagnostic accuracy for AITD of anti-TPO Ab and anti-M Ab according to the Galen and Gambino's criteria (1975). To this purpose we considered "true positive" any positive antibody assay observed in patients with AITD, while antibody found in normal subjects or in patients with N-AITD was considered "false positive". Conversely, negative antibody tests were considered as "true negative" when found in normal subjects and in patients with N-AITD and "false negative" when observed in AITD. The results of this analysis (Fig. 3) showed a better efficiency of anti-TPO Ab measurements in the diagnostic evaluation of AITD only when the lowest cut-offs were considered.

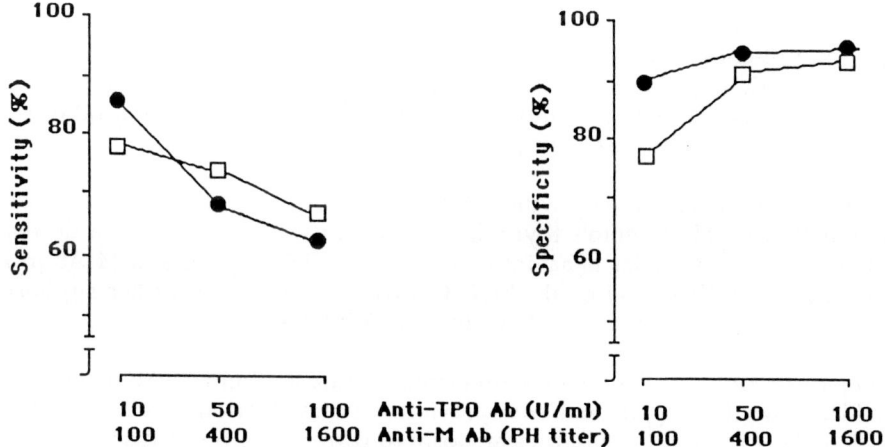

Fig. 3. Diagnostic sensitivity (left panel) and specificity (right panel) for AITD of anti-TPO Ab measuraments by RIA (●——●) and anti-M Ab tests by PH (□——□), evaluated at different cut-offs levels.

Anti-TPO Ab determination by RIA is not affected by serum Tg

The existence of cross-reacting epitopes between Tg and TPO has been recently suggested (Kohno et al., 1988). To verify the relevance of this phenomenon in anti-TPO Ab assays, anti-TPO Ab observed in patients with differentiated thyroid carcinoma were subdivided according to the Tg concentrations observed in the same serum samples. No correlation was found between anti-TPO Ab titers and serum Tg concentrations, up to >10,000 ng/ml.

DISCUSSION

In the present study we report our recent experience on the determination of serum anti-TPO Ab in a large series of normal subjects and patients with autoimmune and non-autoimmune thyroid diseases using a monoclonal antibody assisted solid-phase RIA. The results obtained showed the presence of anti-TPO Ab in most subjects with Graves' disease and in all but one patients with

Hashimoto's thyroiditis and idiopathic myxedema. Anti-TPO Ab were also found, although generally at lower levels, in a minority of patients with several N-AITD (including thyroid carcinoma), and in 8.4% of apparently normal healthy subjects. The highest concentrations of circulating anti-TPO Ab were found in untreated hypothyroid goitrous Hashimoto's thyroiditis, while lower antibody levels were observed in Graves' disease, euthyroid Hashimoto's thyroiditis and idiopathic myxedema. The functional relevance of this finding cannot be derived from our data, since the RIA employed detects all anti-TPO Ab able to bind TPO, independently from their capacity to interfere with the enzymatic activity. Using different experimental approaches, *in vitro* inhibition of TPO enzymatic activity by anti-TPO positive sera or IgG has been reported by some (Khono et al., 1986, Doble et al., 1988, Okamoto et al., 1989, Yokoyama et al., 1989) but not by other investigators (Czarnocka et al., 1985, Portmann et al., 1985). In all these studies, however, no clear relationship was observed between the functional thyroid status and the presence and/or the titer of serum anti-TPO Ab blocking the enzymatic activity. It should also be stressed that high anti-TPO Ab titers may merely be expression of a more active autoimmune reaction involving several other cellular and humoral immune mechanisms (Mariotti et al., 1989).

Treatment of Graves' disease with anti-thyroid drugs and of idiopathic myxedema or hypothyroid Hashimoto's thyroiditis with L-T4 was associated to a decrease of anti-TPO Ab. The similar behavior of serum anti-TPO Ab and anti-M Ab in AITD after treatment (Marcucci et al., 1982, Chiovato et al., 1986) further supports the concept for the identity of anti-M Ab and anti-TPO Ab.

Comparison of anti-TPO Ab measurements by RIA and anti-M Ab determinations by PH, showed, in agreement with previous studies (Mariotti et al., 1987, Mariotti et al. 1988, Ruf et al., 1988), a clear positive correlation. Some discordant results were observed, almost exclusively in sera with undetectable or low levels of either antibody. In a minority of sera from AITD patients the presence of high apparent anti-M Ab titers with low or undetectable anti-TPO Ab levels was due to the interference of anti-Tg Ab in anti-M Ab assays by PH, as previously reported (Mariotti et al., 1978). A higher sensitivity and specificity for AITD of anti-TPO Ab measurements when compared to anti-M Ab by PH was suggested by the comparison of the respective diagnostic accuracies calculated according to the criteria of Galen and Gambino (1975). This phenomenon was evident only when antibody levels corresponding to detection limits of the two assays were considered as cut-offs between "negative" and "positive" tests. At higher cut-off levels both assays showed a marked reduction in sensitivity, preventing a satisfactory clinical use.

It has been recently suggested that TPO and Tg may share common epitopes (Khono et al., 1989). Any significant interference of Tg in anti-TPO Ab RIA was ruled out by the demonstration that Tg did not inhibit the binding of ^{125}I-TPO and by the lack of correlation between serum anti-TPO Ab and Tg levels in patients with thyroid carcinoma.

CONCLUSIONS

In conclusion, the results of the present study carried out in a large series of patients with and without different thyroid disorders are in keeping with the concept of the identity of anti-TPO Ab and anti-M-Ab. Most importantly, the assay of anti-TPO Ab by monoclonal antibody-assisted RIA has substantial advantages in terms of sensitivity and specificity when compared to anti-M Ab determinations by PH. These characteristics should allow its rapid diffusion in the clinical routine for the diagnostic evaluation of thyroid autoimmune diseases.

REFERENCES

Beever K, Bradburry J, Phillips D, et al. Highly sensitive assays of autoantibodies to thyroglobulin and thyroid peroxidase. Clin Chem 1989;35:1949-1954.

Chiovato L, Marcocci C, Mariotti S, Mori A, Pinchera A. L-Thyroxine therapy induces a fall of thyroid microsomal and thyroglobulin antibodies in idiopathic myxedema and in hypothyroid, but not in euthyroid Hashimoto's thyroiditis. J. Endocrinol Invest 1986;9:299-305.

Czarnocka B, Ruf J, Ferrand M, Carayon P, Lissitzky S. Purification of the human thyroid peroxidase and its identification as the microsomal antigen involved in autoimmune thyroid diseases. FEBS Lett 1985a;190:147-152.

Czarnocka B, Ruf J, Ferrand M, Carayon P. Parenté antigénique entre la peroxidase thyroidienne et l'antigène microsomial impliqué dans les affections auto-immunes de la thyroide. C R Acad Sc Paris 1985b;300:577-580.

Czarnocka B, Ruf J, Ferrand M, Lissitzky S, Carayon P. Interaction of highly purified thyroid peroxidase with anti-microsomal antibodies in autoimmune thyroid diseases. J Endocrinol Invest1986;9:135-138.

Doble ND, Banga P, Pope R, Lalor E, Kilduff P, McGregor AM. Autoantibodies to the thyroid microsomal/thyroid peroxidase antigen are polyclonal and directed to several distinct antigenic sites. Immunology. 1988;54:23-29.

Galen RS, Gambino SR. The predictive value and efficiency of medical diagnosis. John Wiley & Sons, New York, 1975.

Hunter WM, Greenwood FC. Preparation of iodine-131 labelled human growth hormone of high specific activity. Nature 1962;194:495-496.

Khoury EL, Bottazzo GF, Roitt I. The thyroid microsomal antibody revisited: its paradoxical binding in vitro to the apical surface of the follicular epithelium. J Exp Med 1984;159:577-591.

Kohno Y, Hiyama Y, Shimojo N, Niimi H, Nakajima H, Hosoya T. Autoantibodies to thyroid peroxidase in patients with chronic thyroiditis: effect of antibody binding on enzyme activities. Clin Exp Immunol 1986;65:534-541.

Kohno Y, Naito N, Hiyama Y, et al. Thyroglobulin and thyroid peroxidase share common epitopes recognized by autoantibodies in patients with cronic autoimmune thyroiditis. J Clin Endocrinol Metab 1988;67:899-907.

Kotani T, Umeki K, Matsunaga S, Kato E, Ohtaki S. Detection of autoantibodies to thyroid peroxidase in autoimmune thyroid diseases by micro-ELISA and immunoblotting. J Clin Endocrinol Metab1986;62:928-933.

Libert F, Ruel J, Ludgate M, et al. Thyroperoxidase, an auto-antigen with a mosaic structure made of nuclear and mithocondrial gene modules. EMBO J, 1987;6: 4193-4196.

Marcocci C, Chiovato L, Mariotti S, Pinchera A. Changes of circulating thyroid autoantibody levels during and after therapy with methimazole in patients with Graves' disease. J Endocrinol Invest 1982;5:13-19.

Mariotti S, Pinchera A, Vitti P, et al. Comparison of radioimmunoassay and haemagglutination methods for anti-thyroid microsomal antibodies. Clin Exp Immunol 1978;34:118-125.

Mariotti S, Anelli S, Ruf J, et al. Comparison of serum thyroid microsomal and thyroid peroxidase autoantibodies in thyroid diseases. J. Clin. Endocrinol. Metab. 1987;65:987-993.

Mariotti S, Anelli S, Piccolo P, et al. New monoclonal antibody radioimmunoassay (RIA) of anti-thyroid peroxidase autoantibodies. In: Nagataki S, Torizuka K Eds. The Thyroid 1988, Amsterdam. Elsevier Science Publishers B.V.; 1988;121-124.

Mariotti S, Chiovato L, Vitti P, et al. Recent advances in the understanding of humoral and cellular mechanisms implicated in thyroid autoimmune diseases. Clin Immunol Immunopathol 1989;50:S73-S84.

Okamoto Y, Hamada N, Saito H, et al. Thyroid peroxidase activity-inhibiting immunoglobulins in patients with autoimmune thyroid disease. J Clin Endocrinol Metab 1989;68:730-734.

Pinchera A, Mariotti S, Chiovato L, et al. Cellular localization of the microsomal antigen and the thyroid peroxidase antigen. Acta Endocrinol (Copenh) 1987;Suppl. 281:57-62.

Portmann L, Hamada N, Heinrich G, DeGroot LJ. Anti-thyroid peroxidase antibody in patients with autoimmune thyroid disease: possible identity with anti-microsomal antibody. J Clin Endocrinol Metab 1985;61:1001-1003.

Ruf J, Czarnocka B, Ferrand M, Doullas F, Carayon P. Novel routine assay of thyroperoxidase autoantibodies. Clin Chem 1988;34:2231-2234.

Seto P, Hirayu, Magnusson RP, et al. Isolation of a complementary DNA clone for thyroid microsomal antigen. Homology with the gene for thyroid peroxidase. J Clin Invest 1987;80:1205-1208.

Yokoyama N, Taurog A, Klee GG. Thyroid peroxidase and thyroid microsomal autoantibodies. J Clin Endocrinol Metab 1989;68:766-773.

Acknowledgements

This work was supported in part by the National Research Council (C.N.R., Rome, Italy), Target Project "Preventive Medicine and Rehabilitation", Subproject "Mechanisms of aging, Grant 87.00403.556 and by Ente Nazionale per lo sviluppo della Energia Nucelare e delle Energie Alternative (E.N.E.A., Rome, Italy), to A.P.

Résumé

Il a été récemment prouvé que les anticorps microsomiaux thyroïdiens étaient dirigés contre la thyropéroxydase. Des méthodes pour détecter les anticorps anti-TPO, utilisant des antigènes purifiés avaient été développées, mais l'information disponible sur l'utilité clinique de cette technique demeurait jusqu'ici limitée. Nous avons récemment évalué l'utilité clinique de l'anti-TPO par RIA utilisant un anticorps monoclonal, récemment mis au point, sur un grand nombre de sujets, comprenant des sujets normaux et des patients atteints de maladies thyroïdiennes auto-immunes et non autoimmunes. Les anticorps anti-TPO ont été détectés chez 134 patients souffrant de thyroïdite de Basedow sur 181 (74%), chez tous les patients moins 1 (99.3%) des 144 patients souffrant de thyroïdite d'Hashimoto ou de myxédème idiopathique, chez 20 patients sur 188 (10.6%) présentant diverses maladies thyroïdiennes non autoimmunes, chez 16 sur 83 (19.2%) de ceux atteints d'un carcinome thyroïdien différencié, et chez 10 des 119 (8.4%) sujets sains de contrôle. Les plus fortes concentrations d'anticorps anti-TPO ont été trouvées chez des patients souffrant de thyroïdites hypothyroïdiennes d'Hashimoto non traitées, mais aucune relation simple entre le taux d'anticorps anti-TPO et la fonction thyroïdienne n'a été observée. Les anticorps anti-TPO diminuent de façon significative chez les malades atteints de Basedow, après traitement au méthimazole, et chez les hypothyroïdiens souffrant de thyroïdites d'Hashimoto ou de myxédème idiopathique, durant leur traitement à la T4 libre. Une corrélation positive significative ($r=0.979$, $P<0.001$) est apparue entre les titres d'anticorps anti-microsomiaux déterminés par hémagglutination passive et les titres d'anticorps anti-TPO déterminés par RIA. Les résultats discordants étaient presque exclusivement limités aux sérums dont la concentration en anticorps anti-microsomiaux était négative ou très basse (1/100 - 1/400). Les études d'absorption ont montré que l'interférence des anticorps anti-thyroglobuline était responsable de la positivité en anticorps anti-microsomiaux dans certains sérums de patients atteints de maladies thyroïdiennes auto-immunes. La comparaison de la valeur diagnostique par l'analyse de Galen et Gambino a révélé une spécificité et une sensibilité du test RIA dosant les anticorps anti-TPO plus grande que celle de l'hémagglutination passive dosant les anticorps microsomiaux, pour les patients présentant une maladie thyroïdienne autoimmune, lorsque le seuil de positivité choisi était situé au niveau des limites de détection. La détermination des anticorps anti-TPO par RIA n'était pas faussée par des concentrations en thyroglobuline circulante pouvant aller jusqu'à < 10.000 ng/ml.

Autoantibodies to thyroperoxidase in various thyroid and autoimmune diseases

F. Doullay, J. Ruf, P. Carayon and J.L. Codaccioni

Service d'Endocrinologie et Maladies Métaboliques, Hôpital de la Conception (FD, JLC) et INSERM U.38 Laboratoire des Hormones Protéiques, Faculté de Médecine (FD, JR, PC), Marseille, France

Introduction

Thyroperoxidase (TPO) is a thyroid specific enzyme responsible for thyroglobulin (Tg) iodination and thyroid hormones synthesis. TPO has been recently identified as the thyroid microsomal antigen (MIC) (1). Discovered almost 30 years ago, autoantibodies (aAb) to MIC were found to be the most frequent aAb present in patients with autoimmune disease of the thyroid (2). It was also shown that these aAb bound to complement and participated in the destruction of the thyroid cells (3). Anti-MIC aAb were, thus, considered of major importance in the pathogeny of autoimmune thyroid disease.

The methods currently in use to measure anti-MIC aAb rely on thyroid membrane preparations contaminated by other antigens, notably Tg which is also involved in thyroid autoimmunity (2). Taking advantage of highly purified TPO and of a carefully selected monoclonal antibody to it, we recently developped the very first anti-TPO aAb assay suitable for routine clinical testing (4).

The present work was aimed to assess the prevalence of aAb to TPO in a large serie of patients with various thyroid and autoimmune diseases. As compared to the test for anti-MIC aAb, our anti-TPO aAb assay appears far more specific and sensitive which strongly support the view that specific anti-TPO aAb testing should replace anti-MIC aAb assays.

Materials and Methods

Serum samples

Sera (n = 262) were obtained from patients with Graves'disease (n=34), Hashimoto's thyroiditis (n=24), euthyroid goiter (n=28), thyroid adenoma (n=12), thyroid cancer (n=3), insulin-dependent diabetes (n=47), myasthenia gravis (n=11), pernicious anemia (n=3), rheumatoid arthritis (n=33), mixed connective tissue disease (n=19), hepatitis and biliary cirrhosis (n=7), Sjögren's syndrom (n=4) or referred for reproductive disease with indication of in-vitro fertilization (n=37). All patients were investigated for clinical and biochemical evidence of morphological and functional alteration of the thyroid gland. The prevalence of thyroid dysfunction in the various groups of patients is presented in Table 1.

Table 1. PREVALENCE OF THYROID DYSFUNCTION IN THE VARIOUS GROUPS OF PATIENTS

	Total	Patients with thyroid dysfunction
Autoimmune thyroid disease	58	58[a] (100)[b]
thyroid disease	43	3 (7.0)
Organ specific autoimmune disease	61	7 (11.5)
Non-organ specific auto-immune disease	63	14 (22.2)
Reproductive disease	37	2 (5.4)

a : number
b : %

Anti-MIC and anti-Tg aAb were assayed by passive hemagglutination test (Thymune-M and Thymune-T, Wellcome Diagnostics, Dartford, UK). TSH-receptor aAb were tested using a commercial kit (TRAK-ASSAY, Henning, Berlin, FRG) based on the inhibition by aAb of labelled TSH binding to thyroid membranes.

Assay for autoantibodies to TPO

Anti-TPO aAb concentration was measured using a method previously published (4,5). Briefly, the assay is based on competitive inhibition by aAb of the binding of radioiodinated TPO to a carefully selected anti-TPO monoclonal antibody coated onto plastic tubes. To further increase the sensitivity of the assay, the duration of the incubation was prolonged from 2 hours to one night. The normal range was reassessed in this condition with sera from 32 normal healthy subjects. Using TPO-affinity purified aAb as standard, the normal range extends from 0.36 to 2.70 mg/L with $p<0.05$ and from 0 to 3.07 mg/L with $p<0.01$. In the present work, concentration equal to or higher than 3.1 mg/L were considered abnormal.

Results

Relationship between anti-TPO and anti-MIC antibodies levels :

Sera of the 262 patients were assayed for anti-MIC aAb by passive hemagglutination and for anti-TPO aAb by radioimmunoassay. Sera from 115 patients were negative in both assays. A good correlation ($r=0.835$, $p < 0.001$) was observed with the 147 remaining sera. However, there were some widely discrepant values. One serum from a patient with euthyroid goiter was very potent (1/25600) in the passive hemagglutination test and normal (2.11 mg/L) in the anti-TPO radioimmunoassay. As the level of anti-Tg aAb was very high in this serum, a false positive result due to anti-Tg aAb could be anticipated. Effectively, preincubation of the serum with 1 g/L Tg completely inhibited aAb binding to thyroid microsomes. This serum was further considered negative in term of anti-MIC aAb. In six other cases, sera with anti-TPO levels ranging between 10.7 to 40.7 mg/L were negative in the hemagglutination test. Five sera were taken from patients with overt Graves'disease ; in four of these sera, aAb to the TSH receptor were also detected. The sixth sera came from a patient with Hashimoto's thyroiditis. Slightly discrepant values were also observed in 62 sera with weakly elevated concentration of anti-TPO aAb (3 to 10 mg/L) which proved negative in the anti-MIC assay.

Anti-TPO aAb in the normal range were found in three sera weakly positive (1/100) by passive hemagglutination test. One serum with 0.94 mg/L anti-TPO aAb, came from a patient with insulin dependent diabetes and no evidence of thyroid dysfunction. The two other sera with anti-TPO aAb levels in the upper limit of the normal range (2.55 and 2.92 mg/L) were taken from one patient with Graves'disease, and another one with myasthenia gravis and thyroid dysfunction. Repeatidly assayed by both tests, these sera were consistently normal by RIA and alternatively normal and abnormal by passive hemagglutination.

Prevalence of aAb to TPO in patients with thyroid dysfunction

In the 84 patients with clinical and/or biochemical evidence of thyroid dysfunction, abnormal levels of anti-TPO aAb were more frequently oberved than anti-MIC aAb (88.1 % vs 70.2 %) whereas anti-Tg aAb were detected in only 32.1 % of the patients (Table 2). As anticipated, aAb to the TSH receptor were essentially found in sera from Graves'patients. In Hashimoto's patients both anti-TPO and anti-MIC assays detected aAb in almost all patients. In contrast, the hemagglutination test appeared clearly less effective than the radioimmunoassay in patients with Graves'disease (64.7 % and 82.4 % positive patients respectively) and non-thyroid related autoimmune disease (57.1 % and 85.7 %). Interestingly, the respective prevalences of aAb to TPO, MIC and Tg were similar among these groups of patients

Table 2. PREVALENCE OF THYROID AUTOANTIBODIES IN PATIENTS WITH ABNORMAL THYROID FUNCTION

Diagnosis	n	Autoantibodies to			
		TPO	MIC	Tg	TSHr
AUTOIMMUNE THYROID DISEASE	58	52[a] (89.7)[b]	44 (75.9)	17 (29.3)	21 (36.2)
Graves' disease	34	28 (82.4)	22 (64.7)	8 (23.5)	19 (55.9)
Hashimoto's thyroiditis	24	24 (100)	22 (91.7)	9 (37.9)	2 (8.3)
PATIENTS REFERRED FOR VARIOUS DISEASES	26	22 (84.6)	15 (57.7)	10 (38.4)	nd
Nodular Goiter	3	2 (66.6)	2 (66.6)	2 (66.6)	0 (0)
Benign nodule	2	1 (50.0)	1 (50.0)	1 (50.0)	0 (0)
Malignant nodule	1	1 (100)	1 (100)	1 (100)	0 (0)
Non-thyroid autoimmune disease	21	18 (85.7)	12 (57.1)	8 (38.1)	9
Organ specific	7	5 (71.4)	4 (57.1)	3 (42.8)	1
Non-organ specific	14	13 (92.8)	8 (57.1)	5 (35.7)	1
Reproductive Disease	2	2 (100)	1 (50.0)	0 (0)	nd[c]
ALL PATIENTS	84	74 (88.1)	59 (70.2)	27 (32.1)	nd

a : number
b : %
c : not done

Table 3. PREVALENCE OF THYROID AUTOANTIBODIES IN PATIENTS WITH NORMAL THYROID FUNCTION

Diagnosis	n	Autoantibodies to		
		TPO	MIC	Tg
GOITER	40	22[a] (55.0)[b]	6 (15.0)	4 (10.0)
Diffuse goiter	28	17 (60.7)	4 (14.3)	4 (14.3)
Nodular Goiter	12	5 (41.6)	2 (16.6)	0
Thyroid adenoma	10	3 (33.3)	1 (10.0)	0 0
Cancer	2	2 (100)	1 (50.0)	0 (33.3)
NON-THYROID AUTOIMMUNE DISEASE	103	43 (41.7)	9 (8.7)	3 (2.9)
Organ Specific Autoimmune Disease	54	18 (33.3)	7 (12.9)	2 (3.7)
Insulin-dependent diabetes	42	10 (23.8)	5 (11.9)	1 (2.4)
Myasthenia gravis	10	6 (60.0)	1 (10.0)	1 (10.0)
Pernicious anemia	2	2 (100)	1 (50.0)	0 (0)
Non-Organ Specific Autoimmune Disease	49	25 (51.0)	2 (4.2)	1 (2.1)
Rheumatoid arthritis	27	12 (44.4)	0 (0)	0 (0)
Mixed connective tissue disease	16	11 (68.8)	2 (12.5)	0 (0)
Hepatitis and biliary cirrhosis	3	0 (0)	0 (0)	1 (33.3)
Sjögren's syndrome	3	2 (66.6)	0 (0)	0 (0)
REPRODUCTIVE DISEASE	35	4 (11.4)	4 (11.4)	0 (0)

a : number
b : %

(Table 2). As compared to anti-MIC and, obviously anti-Tg aAb, anti-TPO appeared as a very sensitive index of thyroid alteration in patients with autoimmune disease causative of or concomitant to thyroid dysfunction.

Prevalence aAb to TPO in patients with normal thyroid function

The remaining 178 patients referred for diffuse and nodular goiter, organ-specific and non organ specific autoimmune diseases and reproductive diseases, were not presenting any clinical and biochemical sign of thyroid dysfunction. In patients with goiter the prevalence of aAb to TPO (55.0 %) was higher than that of anti-MIC aAb (15.0 %). The same situation prevailed in patients with organ specific and non-organ specific autoimmune disease (Table 3). In contrast, the women referred for reproductive disease and indication of in-vitro fertilization presented the same low occurence (11.4 %) of aAb to TPO and MIC.

Discussion

The assay used in this study is based on competitive inhibition by aAb of radioiodinated TPO binding to a carefully selected anti-TPO monoclonal antibody coated onto plastic tubes. The design of the assay ensures its specificity which has been documented previously by testing autoimmune sera depleted in anti-TPO aAb by affinity chromatography onto TPO column (4). The assay also appears far more sensitive than the commonly used passive hemagglutination test and allows to detect anti-TPO aAb in all the sera tested. That physiologically healthy individuals and animals could present low levels of antibodies to self-antigens has been proposed previously (6-8). More recent studies have clearly established the presence in healthy people of aAb called "natural" as opposed to pathogenic aAb specific of patients with autoimmune disease (9,10). A high prevalence of anti-Tg aAb was effectively shown in healthy subjects (11). Using our method, normal levels of anti-TPO aAb in healthy women have been shown to decrease during pregnancy and return to original normal levels after delivery (12).

A potential criticism directed to the design of the assay would be that aAb could react with a portion of TPO not probed by the monoclonal antibody. This would ensue in false negative results in the anti-TPO aAb assay and widely discrepant values with the anti-MIC aAb test. Such a situation was not observed with any of the 262 sera tested. Apparent false negative results in the anti-TPO aAb assay were found in three sera but anti-MIC aAb levels were afternatively positive and negative in all cases and anti-TPO aAb borderline negative in two cases. This absence of wide discrepancy confirms the attention paid to the study of the immunological structure of TPO and to the fine specificity of anti-TPO aAb using monoclonal antibodies (13).

A main consequence of the high sensitivity of the anti-TPO aAb radioimmunoassay is to detect these aAb in a large majority of patients with overt autoimmune thyroid disease. Nevertheless, 10 % of these patients did not show abnormal levels of anti-TPO aAb despite the presence, in few cases, of aAb directed to Tg or the TSH receptor. This is in keeping with previous reports of patients with documented autoimmune thyroid disease and negative aAb to some or all thyroid autoantigens. This situation may be explain by variation of thyroid aAb during the course of the disease (5).

The presence of abnormal levels of thyroid aAb in patients with diffuse or nodular goiter has been already described by other groups: 50% of 20 patients operated for non-toxic goitre with high lymphocytic infiltration had detectable levels of anti-MIC and/or Tg aAb (14) ; 69% of 62 patients with sporadic euthyroid goiter were found positive for the presence of serum thyroid growth-stimulating immunoglobulins (15) ; thyroid-stimulating immunoglobulins were also detected in 100% of 10 patients with hyperthyroidism due to single autonomously functioning thyroid nodule (16).

Numerous studies have dealt with the prevalence of thyroid aAb in patients with various non-thyroid autoimmune diseases. These aAb were found in 11-16% of groups of patients without clinical evidence of thyroid disorders but who either had or were at risk for autoimmune diseases (17). Depending on the selection of patients, the prevalence of anti-MIC aAb was found to vary between 10 to 50% in patients with organ specific autoimmune diseases such as type I diabetes mellitus (18), myasthenia gravis (19) and pernicious anemia (20). Anti-MIC were also found in 30-40% of patients suffering from non-organ specific autoimmune diseases such as rheumatoid arthritis (21), biliary cirrhosis (22) and Sjögren's syndrome (23). In our study, the prevalence of positive anti-MIC aAb in non-thyroid autoimmune diseases is only 8.7% of patients without thyroid dysfunction. This low prevalence could be explained by the strict selection of patients without any sign of thyroid dysfunction. Nevertheless, abnormal level of anti-TPO aAb were found in 41.7% of the cases. In contrast, the level of anti-TPO and anti-MIC aAb were abnormal in the same number of patients referred for reproductive diseases. This further suggests that anti-TPO aAb are specifically elevated in patients with autoimmune diseases as compared to patients representative of the general population.

Taken together, our data indicate that anti-TPO aAb are more frequently present than expected from anti-MIC testing. Taking into consideration that the presence of abnormal levels of thyroid aAb is generally concomitant to lymphocytic infiltration of the gland, the result of this study would suggest that autoimmune thyroid disease is more often associated than generally believed with diffuse or nodular goiter and non-thyroid autoimmune diseases. Accordingly, anti-TPO aAb assay would appear more helpful than anti-MIC and anti-Tg aAb assays to anticipate the evolution of thyroid alteration.

Acknowledgements :

This work was supported in part by a grant from the Association pour la Recherche en Biologie Cellulaire. We are indebted to Prs B. Vialettes, J.R. Weiller, P.C. Acquaviva and J. Pouget and to Drs J.M. Durand and J.P. Mattei for providing several of the sera tested in this work. Pr J.F. Henry is gratefully acknowledged for providing the human thyroid tissue used for the preparation of thyroperoxidase. The expert technical assistance of C. Sylvestre is much appreciated.

References

1. Czarnocka B, Ruf J, Ferrand M, Carayon P, Lissitzky S. Purification of the human thyroid peroxidase and its identification as the thyroid microsomal antigen involved in autoimmune thyroid diseases. FEBS Lett. 1985 ; 190 : 147-52

2. Pinchera A, Fenzi GF Vitti P, Chiovato L, Macchia E, Mariotti S. Significance of thyroid autoantibodies in autoimmune thyroid diseases. In : Walfish PG, Wall JR, Volpé R, eds. Autoimmunity and the Thyroid. Academic Press, New-York. 1985 ; 139-51.

3. Khoury EL, Hammond L, Bottazzo GF, Doniach D. Presence of the organ specific "microsomal" autoantigen in the surface of human thyroid cells in culture : its involvement in complement mediated cytotoxicity. Clin Exp Immunol. 1981 ; 45 : 316-28

4. Ruf J, Czarnocka B, Ferrand M, Doullais F, Carayon P. Novel routine assay of thyroperoxidase autoantibodies. Clin Chem. 1988 ; 34 : 2231-4

5. Codaccioni JL, Orgiazzi J, Blanc P, Pugeat M, Roulier R, Carayon P. Lasting remissions in patients treated for Graves'hyperthyroidism with propranolol alone : a pattern of spontaneous evolution of the disease. J. Clin Endocrinol Metab. 1988 ; 67 : 656-62

6. Besredka M. Les antihémolysines naturelles. Ann. Inst. Pasteur. 1901 ; 15 : 785-807

7. Kennedy WP. The production of spermatoxins. Quart J Exp Physiol. 1924 ; 14 : 279-83

8. Boyden SV. Natural antibodies and the immune response. Adv Immunol. 1963 ; 5 : 1-28

9. Guilbert B, Dighiero G, Avrameas S. Naturally occuring antibodies against nine common antigens in human sera. I. Detection, isolation, and

characterization. J Immunol 1982 ; 128 : 2779-87

10. Ruf J, Carayon P, Lissitzky S. Various expressions of a unique anti-human thyroglobulin antibody repertoire in normal state and autoimmune disease. Eur J Immunol. 1985 ; 15 : 268-72

11. Ericson UB, Christensen SB, Thorell JI. A high prevalence of thyroglobulin autoantibodies in adults with and without thyroid disease as measured with a sensitive solid-phase immunosorbent radioassay. Clin Immunol Immunopathol. 1985 ; 37 : 154-62

12. Lejeune B, Connart D, Carayon P, Servais G, Kinthaert J, Glinoer D. Antithyroid peroxidase antibodies (TPO-Ab) in normal pregnancy. 18th Annual Meeting of the European Thyroid Association. 1989 ; 39 (Abstract)

13. Ruf J, Toubert ME, Czarnocka B, Durand-Gorde J, Ferrand M, Carayon P. Relationship between immunological structure and biochemical properties of human thyroid peroxidase. Endocrinol. 1989 ; 125 : 1211-8

14. Bang U, Blichert-Toft M, Petersen PH, Nielsen BB, Hage E, Diederichsen H. Thyroid function after resection for non-toxic goitre with special reference to thyroid autoantibodies. Acta Endocrinol. 1985 ; 109 : 214-9

15. Van Der Gaag RD, Drexhage HA, Wiersinga WM, Brown RS, Docter R, Bottazzo GF, Doniach D. Further studies on thyroid growth-stimulating immunoglobulins in euthyroid nonendemic goiter. J Clin Endocrinol Metab. 1985 ; 60 : 972-9

16. Grubeck-Loebenstein B, Derfler K, Kassal H, Kapp W, Krisch K, Liszka K, Smyth PPA, Waldhaüsl W. Immunological features of nonimmunogenic hyperthyroidism. J. Clin Endocrinol Metab. 1985 ; 60: 150-5

17. Betterle C, Callegari G, Presotto F, Zanette F, Pedini B, Rampazzo T, Slack RS, Girelli ME, Busnardo B. Thyroid autoantibodies : a good marker for the study of symptomless autoimmune thyroiditis. Acta Endocrinol (Copenh) 1987 ; 114 : 321-7

18. Frasier SD, Penny R, Snyder R, Goldstein I, Graves D. Antithyroid antibodies in hispanic patiens with type I diabetes mellitus. AJDC 1986 ; 140 : 1278-80

19. Garlepp MJ, Dawkins RL, Christiansen FT, Lawton J, Luciani G, McLeod J, Bradley J, Genkins G, Teng CS. Autoimmunity in ocular and generalized myasthenia gravis. Journal of Neuroimmunology. 1981 ; 1 : 325-32

20. Whittingham S, MacKay IR. Pernicious anemia and gastric atrophy. In : Rose NR, MacKay IR eds. The autoimmune diseases. Academic Press, New-York. 1985 ; 243-66

21. Thomas DJB, Young A, Gorsuch AN, Bottazzo GF, Cudworh AG. Evidence for an association between rheumatoid arthritis and autoimmune endocrine disease. Annals of the Rheumatic Diseases 1983 ; 42 : 297-300

22. Elta GH, Sepersky RA, Goldberg MJ, Connors CM, Miller KB, Kaplan MM. Increased incidence of hypothyroidism in primary biliary cirrhosis. Digestive Diseases and Sciences. 1983 ; 28 : 971-5

23. Karsh J, Pavlidis N, Weintraub BD, Moutsopoulos M. Thyroid disease in Sjögren's syndrome. Arthritis and Rheumatism. 1980 ; 23 : 1326-9

Résumé

Un dosage radioimmunologique original destiné au dosage des auto-anticorps (aAc) anti-TPO a été récemment mis au point et s'est avéré bien adaptée à une utilisation de routine hospitalière. La présente étude a été réalisé dans le but d'évaluer la prévalence des aAc dirigés contre la TPO chez des patients présentant des affections thyroïdiennes et auto-immunes variées et, à titre de comparaison, chez des sujets normaux et des patientes présentant des troubles de la fonction de reproduction indiquant la fécondation in-vitro.

Les aAc anti-TPO ont été mesurés dans le sérum de 262 patients chez qui ont été soigneusement recherchées d'éventuelles anomalies morphologiques et fonctionnelles de la glande thyroïde. Les aAc anti-TPO et anti-MIC ont été trouvés normaux chez 115 patients. Chez les 147 autres patients, une corrélation hautement significative ($r = 0.835$, $p<0.001$) a été trouvé entre les taux d'aAc anti-TPO et anti-MIC. Des discordances ont été observées dans quelques cas et attribuées à un manque de spécificité et de sensibilité du dosage des aAc anti-MIC. Chez 84 patients présentant une anomalie de la fonction thyroïdienne, la prévalence des aAc anti-TPO (88.1%) était supérieure à celle des aAc anti-MIC (70.2 %) et ne différait guère parmi les différents groupes de patients. En l'absence de dysfonctionnement thyroïdien, la prévalence des aAc anti-TPO était de 55.0 % chez les patients présentant un goitre euthyroïdien diffus ou nodulaire, 51.0 % chez les patients atteints d'une maladie autoimmune non spécifique d'organe et 33.3 % chez les patients atteints d'une maladie autoimmune spécifique d'organe. Dans ces trois groupes 36.4 % des patients présentaient un taux normal d'aAc anti-MIC (< 1/100) et un taux faiblement anormal (3.1 à 10.0 mg/L d'aAc anti-TPO. Par contre, les femmes présentant des troubles de la fonction de reproduction présentaient la même prévalence faible (11.4 %) de taux anormaux d'aAc anti-TPO et anti-MIC.

Ces données montrent que les aAc dirigés contre la TPO/MIC sont plus fréquemment détectés en utilisant un immunodosage spécifique et sensible que la classique méthode par hemaglutination passive. De plus, la prévalence élevée d'aAc anti-TPO trouvée chez des patients présentant un goitre ou une maladie auto-immune suggère que ces affections sont plus souvent associées à une agression auto-immune de la thyroide que cela avait été montré précédemment. De ce fait, le dosage des aAc anti-TPO apparait d'un intérêt certain dans l'exploration des goitres euthyroidiens et des maladies auto-immunes et peut permettre de prévoir l'émergence d'un trouble de la fonction thyroidienne chez ces patients.

Anti-TPO antibodies in non-thyroid autoimmune diseases

U. Feldt-Rasmussen, M. Hoier-Madsen, K. Bech, L. Hegedüs, H. Perrild,
H. Bliddal, B. Danneskiold-Samso, B. Rasmusson, N.J. Kriegbaum,
K. Müller, A. Schouboe and E. Hippe

Dept of Med F, Herlev Univ Hosp, Autoimmune Lab, State Serum Inst, Steno Memorial Hosp, Dept of Med C, Bispebjerb Hosp, Dept of Rheumatol, Kommunehosp, Dept of Oncol, Odense Hosp, Dept of Rheumatol, State Hosp and Dept of Med C, Gentofte Hosp, Denmark

INTRODUCTION

Presence of thyroid autoantibodies is a frequent phenomenon in autoimmune diseases compared to a control population. The aim of the present investigation was to study the presence of anti thyroid peroxidase antibodies (anti-TPO) by a recently developed commercial method in non-thyroid autoimmune diseases. Furthermore, we wanted to compare the results of anti-TPO measurements with results obtained by immune fluorescence for microsomal antibodies (MAb), a method which is generally considered rather specific, but only semiquantitative.

MATERIAL AND METHODS

Subjects
Normal subjects. Eighty-eight normal subjects (38 men and 50 women) with a median age of 52 years (range: 17-88 years) were studied. None of them had previous or present history of thyroid diseases. They all had a normal thyroid gland volume as determined by ultrasound (Hegedüs et al. 1983) and normal values for triiodothyronine (T_3), thyroxine (T_4), T_3-uptake test, free thyroid hormone indices, and TSH, none received any medication with known influence on thyroid gland function.
Hashimoto's thyroiditis. Fifty-two (51 women and 1 man, median age 63 years, range 25-90 years) with goitre, elevated serum TSH level (in some cases associated with low thyroid hormones) and significantly elevated levels of MAb and/or TgAb.
Patients with non-thyroid diseases: These groups consisted of 34 patients (18 males, 16 females) with insulin dependent diabetes mellitus (IDDM) with a median age 42 years (range 16-72 years), 41 patients (15 males, 26 females) with autoimmune pernicious anaemia with a median age 69 years (range 37-89), 38 patients (6 males, 32 females) with Sjögren's syndrome (53 years (29-79 years)), 19 patients (4 males, 15 females) with rheumatoid arthritis (65 years (39-78)), 9 patients (2 males, 7 females) with primary biliary cirrhosis (65 years (52-77)), and finally 81 patients (56 years, 27-80) with mammary carcinoma.

All patients gave informed consent and the projects had been approven by the local regional ethical committee.

Methods

Serum was stored at $-20^{\circ}C$ and analyzed in consecutive assays. Measurement of serum TSH, total T_4 as well as free thyroid hormone indices were performed as previously described (Kirkegaard et al. 1987). TgAb were analyzed by radiocoprecipitation (Date et al. 1980), MAb by indirect immune fluorescence both undiluted and at a dilution of 1/10 (Weller & Coons 1954) and anti-TPO by a commercial radioimmunological method (DYNOtest , Firma Henning, Berlin). The method was based on a principle described by Ruf et al. (1988). The within assay precision was at a level of 1600 U/ml 6-8%, and at a level of 170 U/ml 12.5-19% (duplicate determinations of 2 control sera in 28 consecutive assays over a 5 month period.

Statistical analyses were performed using Mann-Whitney's U-test, the Chi Square test, and Spearmann's rank correlation.

RESULTS

Six of the 88 control subjects had MAb in serum diluted 1/10, four of them also strongly positive for TgAb. Upper 95%-reference limit was calculated both including all 88 controls (95 U/ml) and when excluding the 4 persons with both positive MAb and TgAb in serum, since they were considered having asymptomatic autoimmune thyroiditis (190 U/ml). The anti-TPO values of these 4 persons ranged from 96-4700 U/ml. The values in the control persons were shown to follow a logarithmic normal distribution.

The percentage of patients in each group positive for anti-TPO in relation to the cut-off level of positivity is shown in Table 1 with values from control persons for comparison. Only few of the patients with non-autoimmune thyroid disease were positive for anti-TPO, except for pernicious anaemia, of whom more than 50% of the patients were positive for anti-TPO (P<0.001, Chi Square test). All patients with Hashimoto's thyroiditis were positive, but one with a level of 32 U/ml. However, also patients with mammary carcinoma had an increased frequency (P<0.01). Quantitative comparison of the anti-TPO values showed significantly higher anti-TPO in patients with Hashimoto's thyroiditis compared with all the other groups. In patients with IDDM, rheumatoid arthritis, and primary biliary cirrhosis the anti-TPO values were not significantly different from controls, in contrast to both those of pernicious anaemia, mammary carcinoma and Hashimoto's thyroiditis.

Comparison between anti-TPO and MAb positive patients showed only true discrepancy in 3 cases with borderline positive level for MAb and unmeasurable anti-TPO. Four patients with mammary carcinoma, 3 patients with primary biliary cirrhosis, and 1 patient with Sjögren's syndrome with negative anti-TPO and ++ for MAb had mitochondrial antibodies which blurred the evaluation of MAb. The correlation between the quantitative anti-TPO values and the semiquantitative measurement of MAb showed an overall significant correlation when combining values from all groups (n=272, Rho=0.81, P<0.001).

Table 1. Percentage positive for anti-TPO in each patient group studied in relation to two different cut-off levels of positivity. Numbers in brackets indicate 95%-confidence limits.

Patients groups	n	Per cent positive at two levels of anti-TPO 95 U/ml	190 U/ml
Controls	88	7 (2.5-14)	2.3 (0.3-8)
Rheumatoid arthritis	19	5 (0-26)	5 (0-26)
IDDM	34	18 (7-35)	15* (5-31)
Sjögren	38	11 (2.9-25)	8 (2-21)
Pernicious anaemia	41	56*** (40-71)	51*** (35-67)
Prim biliary cirrhosis	9	22 (3-60)	22 (3-60)
Mammary carcinoma	81	17 (10-27)	16** (9-26)
Hashimoto	52	98*** (90-100)	98*** (90-100)

*<P0.05, ** P<0.01, *** P<0.001 compared to controls (Chi-Square test)

DISCUSSION

Anti-TPO has in previous clinical studies of thyroid diseases been shown to correlate well with MAb, and is considered a more specific method (Mariotti et al. 1987). In the present study a new commercial method for anti-TPO was evaluated in comparison with MAb by immune fluorescence. Anti-TPO exhibited low values in normal persons without clinical or biochemical evidence of thyroid disease except in 6 persons with positive MAb who in four of cases also were positive for TgAb. Raising the cut-off point for positive results from 95 to 190 U/ml did not significantly change the frequency of patients positive for anti-TPO in the various groups. The anti-TPO method was able to distinguish clearly high levels in Hashimoto's thyroiditis with a good correlation to MAb. Among the non-thyroid autoimmune diseases only patients with pernicious anaemia had a very high incidence of anti-TPO (>50%) in agreement with previous studies of MAb and TgAb (Feldt-Rasmussen et al. 1983). These patients differ from the others by having a closer genetic linkage to Hashimoto's thyroiditis, probably through the HLA system (Feldt-Rasmussen et al. 1983). In the other autoimmune non-thyroid diseases and in mammary carcinoma, previously shown to have evidence of thyroid autoimmunity (Rasmusson et al 1987) the number of patients positive for both anti-TPO and MAb was lower, and without a clear correlation between values of the two methods in the middle range. The reason for this discrepancy is not quite clear. Possible explanations might be differences in sensitivity, different epitopes recognized by the two methods or interference in the immune fluorescence assay from other autoantibodies, e.g. mitochondrial antibodies as shown in the present study.

CONCLUSION

The presence of anti-TPO was comparable to MAb in non-thyroid diseases, but with a higher specificity when evaluating patients with presence of some other autoantibodies. Anti-TPO showed a good agreement with MAb by immune fluorescence when evaluating very high and low values, but with some discrepant results in the middle range of both methods.

ACKNOWLEDGEMENTS

The excellent technical assistance of Bente Friss Mikkelsen, Lisbeth Kirkegaard and Lene overgaard is gratefully acknowledged. Firma Henning, Berlin is thanked for providing the anti-TPO kits.

REFERENCES

Date, J., Feldt-Rasmussen, U., Hyltoft Petersen, P.,and Bech, K. (1980): An improved coprecipitation assay for determination of thyroglobulin antibodies. Scand. J. Clin. Lab. Invest. 40: 37-44.

Feldt-Rasmussen, U., Bech, K., Bliddal, H. et al. (1983): Autoantibodies, immune complexes and HLA-D in thyrogastric autoimmunity. Tissue Antigens 22: 342-347.

Hegedüs, L., Perrild, H., Poulsen, L.R., Andersen, J.R., Holm. B., Schnohr, P., Jensen, G.,and Hansen, J.M. (1983): The determination of thyroid volume by ultrasound and its relationship to body weight, age and sex in normal subjects. J.Clin. Endocrinol. Metab. 56: 260-263.

Kirkegaard, C., Bech, K., Bliddal, H., Danneskiold-Samsoe, B., and Feldt-Rasmussen, U. (1987): Thyroid stimulating antibodies in rheumatoid arthritis: An in vitro phenomenon. J. Endocrinol. Invest. 10: 495-498.

Mariotti, S., Anelli, S., Ruf, J. et al (1987) Comparison of serum thyroid microsomal and thyroid peroxidase autoantibodies in thyroid diseases. J.Clin. Endocrinol. Metab. 65: 987-993.

Rasmusson, B., Feldt-Rasmussen, U., Hegedüs, L., Perrild, H., Bech, K. and Høier-Madsen, M. (1987): Thyroid function in patients with breast cancer. Eur. J. Cancer Clin. Oncol. 23: 553-556.

Ruf, J., Czarnocka, B., Ferrand, M., Doullais, F., and Carayon, P. (1988): Novel routine assay of thyroperoxidase autoantibodies. Clin. Chem. 34: 2231-2234.

Weller, T.H., and Coons A.h. (1954): Fluorescent antibodies with agent of varicella and herpes propagated in vitro. Proc. Soc. Exp. Biol. Med. 85: 789-794.

Résumé

Le but de la présente recherche était d'étudier la présence des anticorps anti-thyropéroxydase (anti-TPO) dans les maladies autoimmunes non-thyroïdiennes et de comparer les concentrations d'anti-TPO et d'anticorps microsomiaux à l'aide de l'immunofluorescence. Nous avons étudié 88 sujets normaux, 52 patients atteints de thyroïdite d'Hashimoto, 34 souffrant de diabète insulo-dépendant, 41, d'anémie pernicieuse, 38 présentant le syndrome de Sjögren, 19, atteints d'arthrite rhumatoïde, 9 de cirrhose biliaire primitive, et enfin, 81 de carcinome mammaire. La limite de référence supérieure à 95% fut calculée en incluant les 88 contrôles (95 U/ml) et en excluant 4 personnes dont le sérum présentait à la fois des anticorps anti-microsomiaux positifs et des anticorps anti-thyroglobuline, signe d'une thyroïdite autoimmune assymptomatique (190 U/ml). Plus de 50% des patients atteints d'anémie pernicieuse présentaient un taux d'anti-TPO positif ($P < 0.001$, Chi Square test). Chez seulement quelques patients atteints de maladie thyroïdienne non-immune, on décelait des anti-TPO, tandis que tous les patients atteints d'Hashimoto étaient positifs (à l'exception d'un seul qui présentait une concentration de 32 U/ml). Chez les patients souffrant de carcinome mammaire, la fréquence des anti-TPO était également élevée ($P < 0.01$). La comparaison quantitative des concentrations d'anti-TPO révélait une teneur significativement plus élevée chez les patients atteints de thyroïdite d'Hashimoto que chez les autres groupes. Chez les patients atteints de diabète insulo-dépendant, d'arthrite rhumatoïde et de cirrhose biliaire primitive, les taux d'anti-TPO n'étaient pas significativement différents de ceux du groupe de contrôle, contrairement aux sujets présentant une anémie pernicieuse, un carcinome mammaire ou une thyroïdite d'Hashimoto. La corrélation entre les valeurs quantitatives d'anti-TPO et les mesures semi-quantitatives d'anticorps anti-microsomiaux s'est révélée surtout significative lorsqu'étaient prises en considération les valeurs de tous les groupes ($n=272$, $Rho=0.81$, $P < 0.001$). Dans 8 cas, cependant, la présence d'anticorps anti-mitochondriaux gênait l'évaluation d'anticorps anti-microsomiaux.

En conclusion, la présence d'anti-TPO était comparable à celle des anticorps anti-microsomiaux dans les maladies non-thyroïdiennes, mais avec une spécificité plus grande chez les patients présentant d'autres auto-anticorps. Une bonne corrélation entre le dosage des anticorps anti-TPO et celui des anticorps anti-microsomiaux par immunofluorescence a été trouvée dans les valeurs très hautes ou faibles, avec quelques discordances pour les valeurs moyennes.

Antithyroid peroxidase antibodies in normal pregnancy

D. Glinoer*, P. de Nayer**, B. Lejeune*, J. Kinthaert*, J. Ruf***, G. Servais* and P. Carayon

*University Hospital Saint-Pierre Brussels, Belgium, ** University Clinics Saint-Luc Louvain-en-Woluwe, Belgium. *** INSERM U.38, Faculté de Médecine, Marseille, France

INTRODUCTION

During the course of a prospective cohort study of thyroid function in pregnant women, antithyroid peroxidase antibodies (TPO-Ab) were determined using a highly specific and sensitive commercially available radioassay, based on the technique recently described by Ruf et al. (1988). The aims of the study were a) to evaluate the usefulness of this new tool during pregnancy; b) to analyze the possible correlations between TPO-Ab and underlying thyroid disorders in mothers; and c) to investigate the presence of TPO-Ab in the neonates.

PATIENTS AND DESIGN OF STUDY

Seven hundred and thirty two consecutive pregnant women were enrolled between January and November 1988, after giving informed consent to the study. The ages ranged between 15 and 49 yrs, with a mean of 28 ± 6 (S.D.) yrs. The mean gestational age at booking was 17 ± 8 wks, with more than 70 % of pregnancies enrolled during the first half of gestation. At booking, a detailed history of thyroid-related past events was recorded, the thyroid gland was carefully palpated and thyroid function tests were carried out as well as thyroid ultrasonography and determination of thyroid auto-antibodies. In women under 29 wks of gestation at booking, a second blood sample was requested during late gestation (30-33 wks). The third series of determinations were performed on the 3rd day after delivery and the fourth series 6 months post partum (in 20 % of the cohort). Cord serum was also obtained at delivery. Were excluded from the study 31 cases who did not complete gestation because of miscarriage.

METHODS

Determinations of "classical" auto-antibodies included TG-Ab (radioassay) and MIC-Ab (indirect immunofluorescence). TPO-Ab was determined using the "DYNOtest anti-TPO" kit (Henning). Serum samples were measured in duplicate, in random order. Statistical analyses were carried out using the Statistical Package for Social Sciences (SPSS) programme on a Elite-PC AT computer (Nie et al. 1975).

RESULTS

Based on the initial clinical and biological informations, women were classified as either "NEGATIVE", i.e. in the absence of any detectable clinical, biochemical, immunological or echographic thyroid abnormality, or "POSITIVE" if one or more of the following criteria were present : a) past history of thyroid disorder; b) palpable goiter or nodularity; c) thyroid dysfunction; d) positive TG-Ab and/or MIC-Ab; e) thyroid abnormalities detected by echography alone (enlargment : > 21 ml and/or nodules).

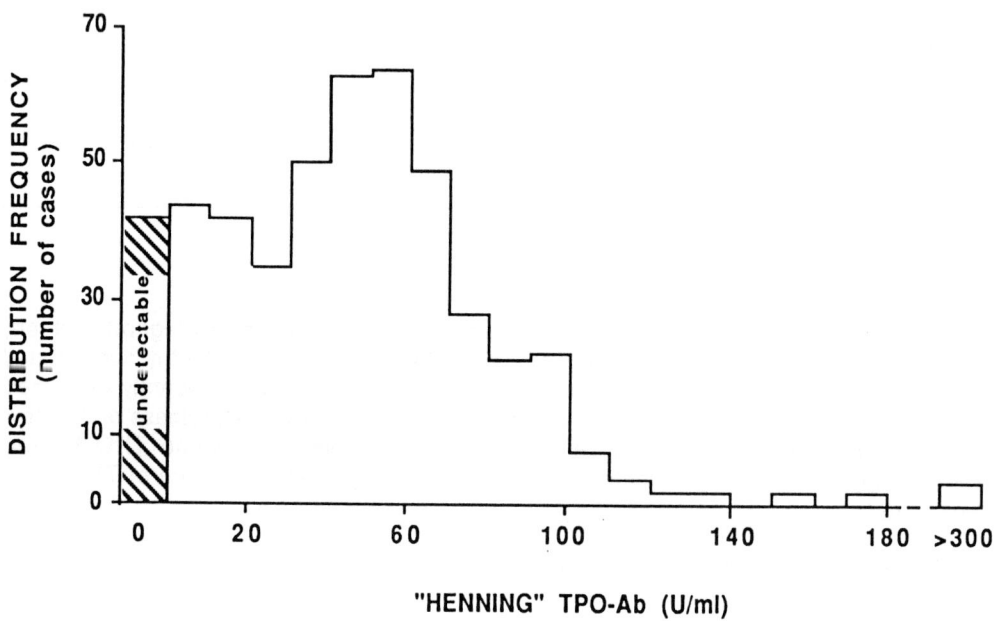

Figure 1 : TPO-Ab AT BOOKING IN "NEGATIVE" PREGNANCIES

Figure 1 shows the distribution frequency of TPO-Ab titers, determined at booking in 480 "negative" pregnant women. The distribution was asymmetrical : TPO-Ab up to 20 U/ml corresponded to 26 % while TPO-Ab up to 100 U/ml (the upper limit of normality provided by the manufacturer) corresponded to 95 % of "negative" pregnancies. TPO-Ab titers above 100 U/ml were found in 23 women (5 %). In 17/23 cases, elevated TPO-Ab was an isolated finding and was not confirmed during later gestation or during post partum. However, in the 6 remaining cases, TPO-Ab titers initially ranged between 128 and 3912 U/ml and elevated titers were confirmed during later gestation, at delivery and in one neonate in cord serum (Table 1).

During gestation, normal TPO-Ab titers decreased in healthy subjects from 45 ± 1 (mean $\pm$ S.E.) U/ml at booking to 37 ± 2 U/ml at 30-33 wks ($p < 0.001$ by paired t-test and by Wilcoxon non parametric test). Thereafter, there was no further significant change in TPO-Ab titers : at delivery 34 ± 2 U/ml and 6 months post partum 32 ± 2 U/ml (with 100 %

of women below 100 U/ml), indicating the absence of rebound during post partum. In neonates born to "negative" mothers, TPO-Ab titers were undetectable in cord serum in 64 % and below 75 U/ml in all cases but one (illustrated in Table 1).

TABLE 1 : ELEVATED TPO-Ab IN "NEGATIVE" PREGNANCIES

Case N°	Booking	Late Gestation	Delivery	Cord Serum
1	128 (a)	nd (b)	nd	10
2	160	217	129	46
3	351	87	132	39
4	479	149	nd	75
5	541	146	136	54
6	3 912	nd	nd	1 120

(a) individual TPO-Ab titers in U/ml; (b) not determined.

We next analyzed the results obtained in pregnant women "positive" for thyroid abnormalities. A first group consisted of 31 mothers with past history of thyroid disorders and/or palpable goiter or thyroid nodularity and/or dysfunction but without detectable TG-Ab or MIC-Ab. Among them, normal TPO-Ab titers were found throughout gestation in 27 mothers and their neonates, while elevated TPO-Ab titers (> 100 U/ml) were found in 4 women (13 %) (Table 2, cases 1-4).

TABLE 2 : ELEVATED TPO-Ab IN "POSITIVE" PREGNANCIES
(non autoimmune thyroid disorders)

Case N°	P.H. (a)	G/N (a)	Dysf. (a)	TG/MIC-Ab (a)	US (a)	Booking (b)	Late Gestation (b)	Cord Serum (b)
1	+	-	-	-	-	400	213	139
2	-	+	-	-	+	179	42	28
3	+	-	+	-	-	409	74	22
4	+	-	-	-	-	153	65	103
5	-	-	-	-	+	880	453	403
6	-	-	-	-	+	135	42	0
7	-	-	-	-	+	108	88	3

(a) criteria for positivity : P.H. = past history of thyroid disorder; G/N = goiter/nodularity; Dysf. = dysfunction; TG/MIC-Ab = classical thyroid-Ab; US = ultrasonographic abnormalities; + = present; - = absent.   (b) individual TPO-Ab titers in U/ml.

A second group consisted of 43 mothers who presented only thyroid abnormalities disclosed by ultrasonography (glandular enlargment and/or nodularity). Among them, normal TPO-Ab titers were found throughout gestation in 40 mothers and their neonates. Elevated TPO-Ab titers were found in 3 women (8 %) (Table 2, cases 5-7).
Three important features deserve a comment. First, TPO-Ab titers decreased significantly during gestation (in average by 59 %). Therefore, 5/7 cases would have been missed if screening for TPO-Ab had been performed only during the last part of gestation or at delivery. Second, TPO-Ab was detectable in 6/7 neonates. Furthermore, TPO-Ab titers in cord serum were slightly elevated in 2 and markedly elevated in 1 neonate. Third, in case n° 3, there was a dramatic rebound in TPO-Ab titers during post partum (5640 U/ml 6 months after delivery) and the patient developed hypothyroidism.

A third group consisted of 17 mothers who presented underlying autoimmune thyroid disorder and were considered positive for TG-Ab and/or MIC-Ab. Among them, TPO-Ab titers were normal in 7. It should be noted that these women presented only positive TG-Ab titers and were negative for MIC-Ab. Elevated TPO-Ab titers were observed in 10/17 women from this group (59 %) (Table 3).

TABLE 3 : ELEVATED TPO-Ab IN "POSITIVE" PREGNANCIES
(autoimmune thyroid disorder)

Case N°	TG-Ab (a)	MIC-Ab (a)	Booking (b)	Late Gestation or Delivery (b)	Cord Serum (b)
1	70	0	383	197	122
2	0	1/10	1658	628	450
3	104	0	959	372	202
4	0	1/40	3052	860	473
5	0	1/40	5050	2434	3043
6	0	1/80	5998	209	nd
7	0	1/10	1758	33	23
8	0	1/10	2729	1200	nd
9	0	1/10	513	239	166
10	>1000	1/320	9999	6991	9463

(a) TG-Ab and MIC-Ab determined at booking. TG-Ab titers are expressed in U/ml and considered positive for titers > 50 U/ml. MIC-Ab titers are expressed in dilution of serum and considered positive for dilutions ≥ 1/20 (1/10 dilution represents the limit of sensitivity).   (b) individual TPO-Ab titers in U/ml; nd = not determined.

At booking, TPO-Ab titers were markedly elevated in the majority (above 1000 U/ml in 70 %). As for the other cases scrutinized above, there was a clearcut trend towards a decrease in TPO-Ab titers during gestation, but TPO-Ab remained elevated up to delivery in most cases. Moreover, elevated TPO-Ab titers were found in 7/8 neonates in whom it was measured. Finally, comparing TPO-Ab positivity to classical thyroid auto-Ab, it was apparent that markedly elevated TPO-Ab titers were observed in several cases for whom MIC-Ab was negative (or at the limit of detection) or only TG-Ab moderately positive.

Figure 2 summarizes the findings. In the present cohort of healthy women with normal pregnancies, subtle thyroid abnormalities (detected clinically, by ultrasonography or by classical determinations of thyroid auto-Ab) were disclosed in 13 % of pregnancies. Among them, elevated TPO-Ab titers were significantly more frequent (19 %) than in their negative counterparts (1 %) (chi-square value = 72.7; $p < 0.001$).

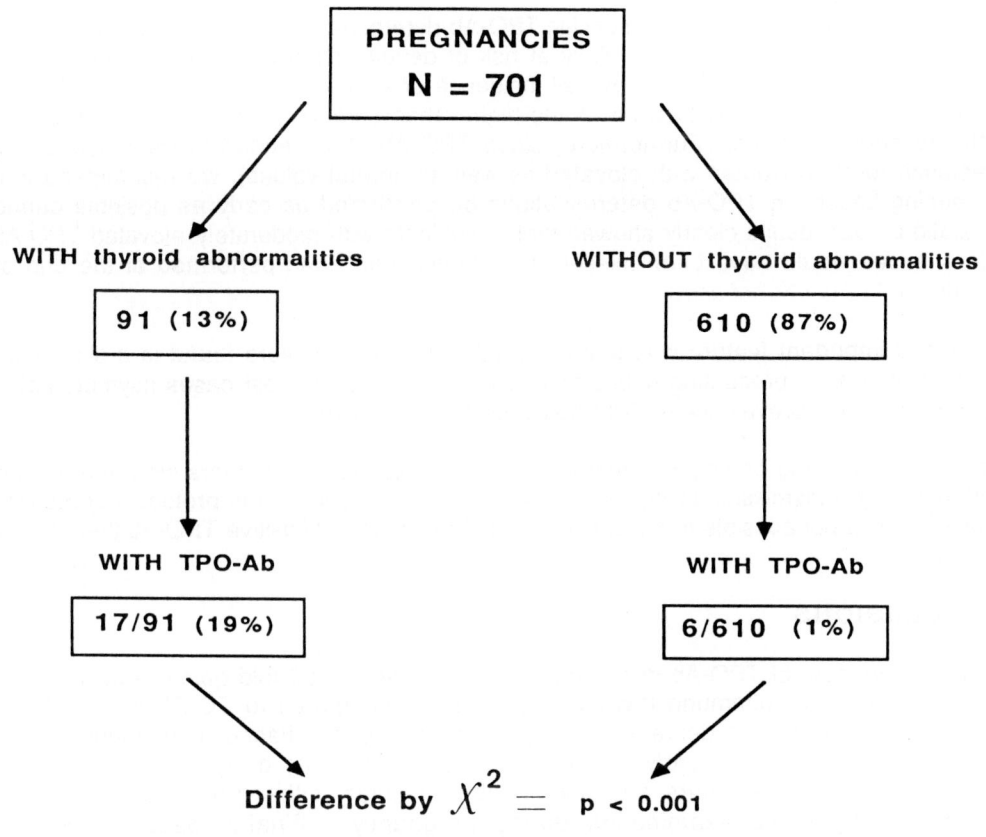

Figure 2 : S U M M A R Y   O F   F I N D I N G S

DISCUSSION

Since the recent discovery of the identity between TPO and the microsomal antigen of human thyroid follicular cells, the purification of human TPO and the development of monoclonal antibodies against TPO epitopes, it has become possible to assay directly the presence of TPO-Ab in patients with thyroid autoimmune processes (Ruf et al. 1988). Recent work has underlined the close relationship between MIC-Ab and TPO-Ab (Mariotti et al. 1988).

This report presents the results of the first study of TPO-Ab in pregnancy. During pregnancy, most antibody titers tend to decrease and this decrease certainly stands true for thyroid auto-Ab as well (Fung et al. 1988; Jansson et al. 1984; Hardisty et al. 1983; d'Armiento et al. 1980). On the other hand, postpartum thyroiditis usually occurs during the first year after delivery and is classically associated with a rebound in auto-Ab titers (Ramsay 1986; Nikolai et al. 1987; Amino et al. 1982; Editorial 1987).

The present results indicate that specific TPO-Ab determination represents a powerful tool for the detection of women potentially at risk of developing thyroid disturbances during post partum. In our hands, the overall incidence of elevated TPO-Ab titers was 3 % of otherwise normal pregnancies, i.e. 2 fold higher than screening based on TG-Ab and/or MIC-Ab determinations. Furthermore, since TPO-Ab titers tended to decrease during gestation (both in women with elevated as well as normal values), we recommend that screening based on TPO-Ab determinations be performed as early as possible during gestation. Our results clearly showed that in subjects with moderately elevated TPO-Ab titers, cases would have been missed if screening had been performed at the end of gestation.

A second important feature was that elevated TPO-Ab titers were found in a significant fraction of women presenting subtle thyroid abnormalities, in most cases asymptomatic. Among them, the prevalence of TPO-Ab positivity reached 19 %.

The third interesting finding was that elevated TPO-Ab titers in mothers were associated with antibody transmission to the neonates. Unfortunately, within the protocole of present studies, it was not possible to assess the clinical relevance of positive TPO-Ab titers in the children.

CONCLUSIONS

The measurement of TPO-Ab during pregnancy allowed for a 2 fold gain in sensitivity for the detection of autoimmune thyroid processes, as compared to TG-Ab and MIC-Ab. TPO-Ab titers tended to decrease during gestation and it is hence recommended that screening be carried out early during gestation. There was a significant correlation between high TPO-Ab titers and thyroid abnormalities, either previously known or discovered by close examination during pregnancy. Finally, passive TPO-Ab transmission from mother to child was evidenced but the relevance of this finding remains speculative. Present studies suggested that specific TPO-Ab measurement, using a highly sensitive technique, is the ideal tool for the screening of pregnant women with an increased potential risk of post partum thyroiditis.

ANNEX

We had the opportunity to determine TPO-Ab with the "SORIN" kit in 320 serum samples selected from the same cohort. Basically, similar results were obtained and the same conclusions can be drawn. There were, however, quantitative differences in absolute titers between "HENNING" and "SORIN" TPO-Ab determinations. They are illustrated in Figure 3.

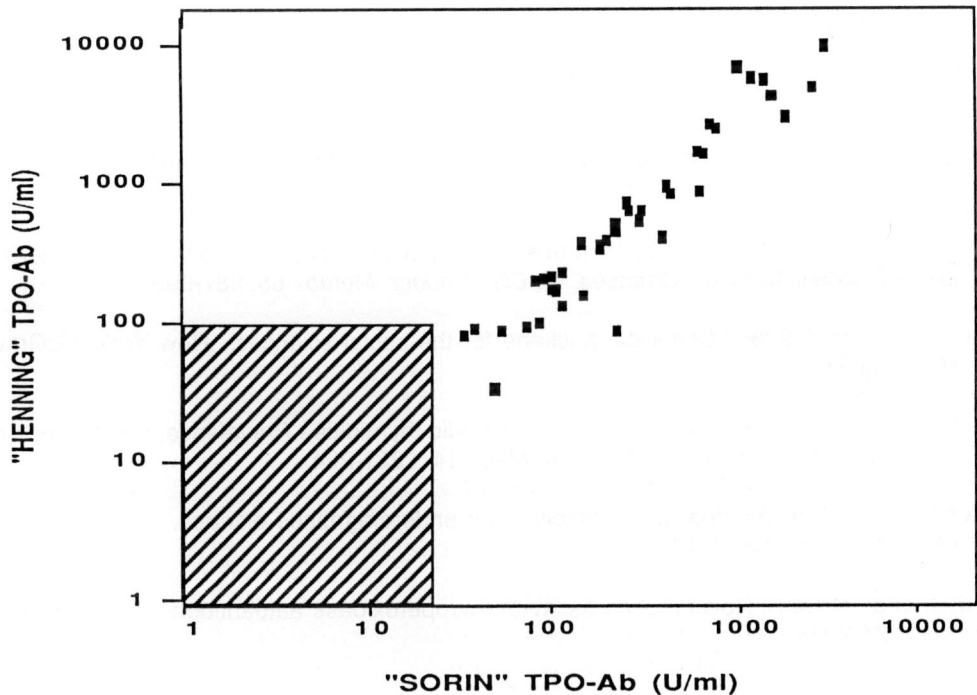

Figure 3 : comparison between TPO-Ab determinations with the "HENNNING" kit (ordinate) and the "SORIN" kit (abscissa).

The hatched area shows the reference ranges of the assays. An excellent correlation was found ($Y = 3.1X - 61$; r= 0.94; $p < 0.001$) but on a quantitative basis, TPO-Ab titers determined with the "HENNING" kit yielded values 3 fold greater than with the "SORIN" kit.

REFERENCES

Amino, N. et al. (1982) : High prevalence of transient post-partum thyrotoxicosis and hypothyroidism. *New Engl. J. Med.* 306: 849-852.

Anonymous (Editorial) (1987) : Postpartum thyroiditis. *Lancet* i: 962.

D'Armiento, M. et al. (1980) : Decrease of thyroid antibodies during pregnancy. *J. Endocrinol. Invest.* 4: 437-438.

Fung, H.Y.M. et al. (1988) : Postpartum thyroid dysfunction in Mid Glamoran. *Brit. Med. J.* 296: 241-244.

Hardisty, C.A. et al. (1983) : Serum long acting thyroid stimulator protector in pregnancy complicated by Graves' disease. *Brit. Med. J.* 286: 934-935.

Jansson, R. et al. (1984) : Autoimmune thyroid dysfunction in the postpartum period. *J. Clin. Endocr. Metab.* 58: 681-687.

Mariotti, S. et al. (1988) : Comparison of serum thyroid microsomal and thyroid peroxidase autoantibodies in thyroid diseases. *J. Clin. Endocr. Metab.* 65: 987-993.

Nio, N.H. et al. (1975) · Statistical package for the social sciences. New York: McGraw Hill. (2nd Edition).

Nikolai, T.F. et al. (1987) : Postpartum lymphocytic thyroiditis - Prevalence, clinical course, and long-term follow-up. *Arch. Intern. Med.* 147: 221-224.

Ramsay, I. (1986) : Postpartum thyroiditis : an underdiagnosed disease. *Brit. J. Obstet. Gynaecol.* 93: 1121-1123.

Ruf, J. et al. (1988) : Novel routine assay of thyroperoxidase autoantibodies. *Clin. Chem.* 34: 2231-2234.

ACKNOWLEDGMENTS

The authors express their gratitude to all colleagues who have manifested interest and have been of considerable help in the realization of this study, in particular to Drs. C. Beckers, G. Copinschi, F. Delange, A.M. Ermans, H. Ham, H. Kleiner and P. Wilkin.

The authors wish to acknowledge the invaluable help of the nursing staff of the department of Gynecology and Obstetrics and the Blood Sampling Center of Hospital Saint-Pierre, the technicians in the laboratories of Nuclear Medicine and Gynecology, particularly Mr. D. Connart and the secretarial staff of the outpatient clinic of Gynecology. The authors greatly acknowledge the secretarial expertise of Mrs. C. Guérit in the preparation of the manuscript. The technical and financial supports of HENNING BERLIN (Fed. Rep. Germany) and SORIN/BIOMEDICA (Italy) are gratefully acknowledged.

Present studies have been reported in part at the 8th Joint Meeting of the British Endocrine Societies (Manchester, April 1989) and the 18th Annual Meeting of the European Thyroid Association (Copenhagen, June 1989).

Résumé

Au cours d'une étude prospective de 701 femmes enceintes, les anticorps antithyroperoxydase (TPO-Ab) ont été déterminés séquentiellement au cours de la grossesse chez la mère et au cordon chez le nouveau-né. Par comparaison avec les anticorps antithyroïdiens "classiques" (TG-Ab et MIC-Ab), la sensibilité de la détection d'un processus thyroïdien auto-immunitaire chez la mère est doublée grâce à l'utilisation de TPO-Ab. Les titres de TPO-Ab tendent à diminuer au cours de la gestation suggérant l'intérêt de réaliser un dépistage le plus tôt que possible au cours de la grossesse. Une corrélation significative a également été démontrée entre la positivité de TPO-Ab et la présence d'anomalies thyroïdiennes discrètes, le plus souvent ignorées et asymptomatiques. Enfin, ce travail a permis de démontrer la transmission passive de TPO-Ab de la mère à l'enfant, mais l'importance clinique de cette découverte demeure spéculative. En conclusion, le présent travail démontre que la mesure spécifique des anticorps antithyroperoxydase, utilisant des techniques très sensibles récemment devenues disponibles, représente un outil idéal pour le dépistage de femmes enceintes présentant un risque potentiel accru de thyroidite du post partum.

Investigation of thyroid autoimmunity

Exploration de l'auto-immunité thyroïdienne

Evaluation of anti-TPO antibody determination in various clinical situations

H. Bornet[1], A.M. Madec[2], P. Rodien[2], R. Latter[3], P. Haond[3], H. Allannic[4] and J. Orgiazzi[2]

[1] *Laboratoire de Biophysique, Faculté Grange-Blanche, Lyon;* [2] *INSERM U.197, Faculté de Médecine Alexis Carrel, Lyon;* [3] *Hôpital des Charpennes, Lyon;* [4] *Hôpital Sud, Rennes, France*

INTRODUCTION

Thyroid peroxidase (TPO), a glycosylated hemoprotein, has been unequivocally identified as the major antigenic component of the thyroid "microsomal antigen" involved in thyroid autoimmunity (Czarnocka et al, 1985). TPO is a 100 kD glycoprotein and the complete gene and aminoacid sequences of human and porcine TPO have recently been determined (Libert et al, 1987; Kimura et al, 1987; Magnusson et al, 1987). Clinical studies have subsequently confirmed identity between TPO and microsomal antigen (M)(Mariotti et al, 1987). However, recently, attempts to trigger experimental thyroiditis in mice, through immunization against TPO, have not been successful indicating that the presence of TPO antibody alone is not sufficient to lead to thyroiditis (McLachlan, 1990). Using a recently available commercial method of anti-TPO antibody (TPOAb) determination, we have tested subjects and patients in various clinical conditions and compared TPOAb titers with the results of conventional antimicrosomal antibody (MAb) assays.

SUBJECTS AND PATIENTS

Four different groups were studied :
- A normal population of 129 elderly subjects (29 men, 100 women) aged 60-70 (n=28), 70-80 (n=41) and over 80 (n=60), involved in an ambulatory follow-program and clinically euthyroid ; thyroid hormone and TSH values were available for each ;
- Lymphocytic thyroiditis patients : 11 patients had atrophic and 9 goitrous thyroiditis ; patients were euthyroid on treatment, most of them having been referred earlier for hypothyroidism ; thyroid lymphocytic infiltration had been documented, in the goitrous patients, by fine needle aspiration biopsy.
- Graves' disease patients : 30 patients are included in this study ; they were part of a prospective randomized study of the long term efficiency of carbimazole treatment of Graves' disease (Allannic et al, 1990) ; patients were subgrouped according not to treatment duration but to post-antithyroid drug outcome; both remission and relapse groups comprised 15 patients, each of them having been followed up for 2 years after treatment completion ; TPOAb, as well as MAb, were determined before treatment and at drug withdrawal.
- Thyroid cancer patients : 60 patients with operated differentiated thyroid cancers were studied ; follow-up ranged between 1-10 years ; the patients were sequentially tested for thyroglobulin (Tg) levels and presence of thyroglobulin antibodies (TGAb) ; they were selected for this study because of occurrence, at least at one occasion, of TGAb.

METHODS

Kits for the determination of MAb (Promak-assay; immunoradiometric assay) and TPOAb (Dynotest anti-TPO; competitive radioimmunoassay) were obtained from Henning Berlin through Behring. TGAb were determined by a personal radioassay according to Lefort et al (1981). In the absence of international standards, antibody titers were expressed in units/liter (U/l) by reference to MRC standards (66/387 for MAb and TPOAb and A 65/73 for TGAb). Thresholds of positivity for MAb, TPOAb and TGAb values were 500, 100 and 50 U/l, respectively. TSH concentrations were measured with a sensitive immunoradiometric assay (ELSA 2-TSH-cis international; normal range : 0.2-4 mU/l).

RESULTS AND DISCUSSION

1. Elderly population

In this population of ambulatory elderly subjects, prevalence of TPOAb is shown in figure 1. Overall prevalence was 13.7 %; it was uneven with a maximum between 70-80 at 22 %. Female predominance was obvious (overall : 16 % vs 3-4 %) in each age group. TPOAb titers ranged between 101 and 9476 U/l. As shown in figure 2, highly significant correlation was found between TPOAb and MAb ($r=0.96$; $p<0.001$).

Thyroid function was assessed in each subject. TSH values were not different in TPOAb positive and negative subjects. However, when the log n of the TSH values were compared, TSH were significantly by greater in the TPO positive 70-80 age subgroup (mean TSH : 4.47 vs 2.12 mU/l ; $p<0.02$). Individual TSH values did not exceed 8.24 mU/l. It should be noted, however, that the only two patients with high TSH (29.3 and 13.5 mU/l) were TPOAb negative.

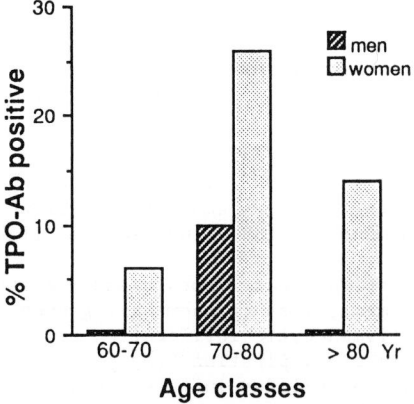

Fig. 1. Prevalence of TPOAb in a normal population of 129 subjects (29 men, 100 women) aged sixty or more.

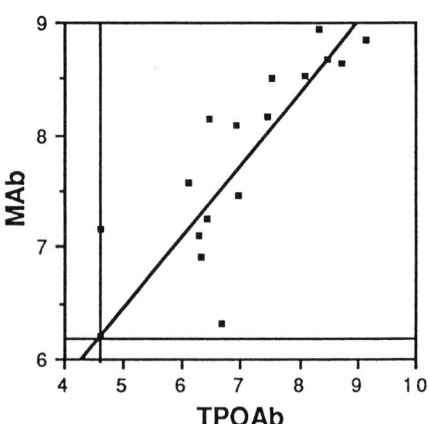

Fig. 2. Correlation between MAb and TPOAb, expressed as ln of U/l, in 129 normal subjects aged sixty or more ($r=0.96$; $p<0.001$).
— Thresholds of positivity of antibody titers.

2. Lymphocytic thyroiditis

In this group of patients, the purpose of the study was to evaluate both TPOAb and MAb in two different forms, atrophic or goitrous, of the disease. The overall correlation between TPO- and MAb was strong (r=0.94 ; p<0.001) with no outlayer. In the atrophic group, TPOAb titers ranged from undetectable (3/11) to 10000 U/l, and in the goitrous going from 2309 to >10000 U/l. As illustrated in fig. 3, antibody titers were significantly greater in the hypertrophic than in the atrophic group (p<0.007) ; the same was observed with MAb. This observation could be related to an antigen availability phenomenon and militates against a direct cytotoxic effect of TPOAb.

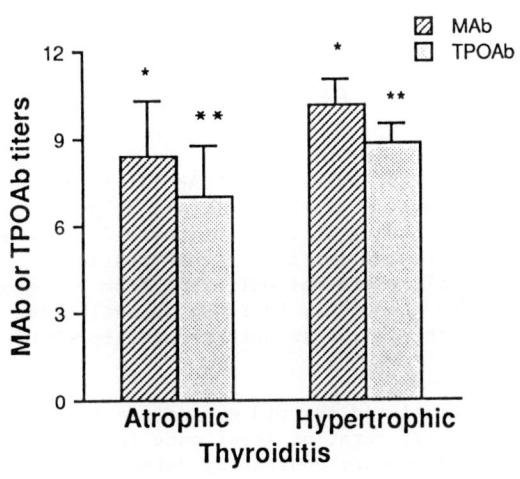

Fig. 3. Comparison of the titers of MAb or TPOAb in subgroups of patients with lymphocytic thyroiditis, either atrophic (n=11) or hypertrophic (n=9). Antibody titers are expressed as ln of U/l.
*:p<0.02 ; **:p<0.007.

3. Graves' disease patients

In this population of patients with Graves' disease sampled before treatment and at the end of an antithyroid drug course of either 6 or 18 months, the concordance between TPOAb and MAb was 0.92 (p<0.001) (figure 4). Figure 5 shows that there was no difference in initial TPOAb titers between the group of patients who relapsed and the group of patients who went into remission. The same lack of difference was observed at the end of the drug course. However, TPOAb at diagnosis was positive in every patient of the relapse group and in only 9/15 of the remission group. A significant trend towards a decrease in TPOAb titers was evident during treatment, as already known (fig. 5) but this decrease was not different between the two groups. Therefore, TPOAb significance appears to be different from that of thyroid stimulating antibodies, the level of which is predictive of relapse when greater than 300 % at the end of treatment (Madec et al, 1984). This discrepancy suggests a different modulation of antithyroid auto-antibody production.

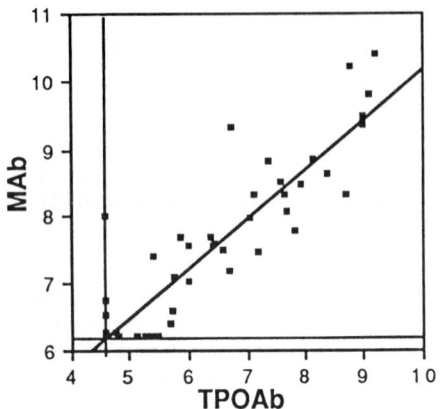 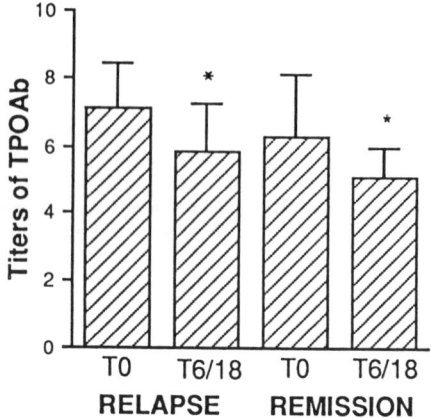

Fig. 4. Correlation between MAb and TPOAb in samples from 30 patients with Graves' disease. r=0.92 ; p<0.001.

Fig. 5. Values of TPOAb titers in Graves' disease patients subgrouped according to post-antithyroid treatment outcome. Initial or end-treatment values are not different from one group to the other. Decrease in antibodies was similar in both groups.*:p<0.02.

4. Cancer patients

In a previous study on TGAb in differentiated thyroid cancer, we found that 32 % of patients had such antibodies in their sera, at least once in a follow-up of 10 years, and in 13 %, these antibodies were constantly detectable (Bornet, 1989). To know whether this presence reflects a more complete auto-immune phenomenon or is just generated by a thyroglobulin secretion, we measured MAb and TPOAb in TGAb positive sera of thyroid cancer patients. We also compared serum antibodies with the tumor outcome to detect an eventual protective or worsening effect.

As shown in figure 6, the levels of MAb and TPOAb were strongly correlated in 134 samples. These data favour the narrow relationship in thyroid cancer between thyroid peroxidase and thyroid microsomal antigens without excluding the existence of other microsomal antigens. By opposition, the correlation between TGAb with either MAb or TPOAb was very poor and not significant (r=0.30 and 0.32, respectively). Pointing out that TPOAb determinations were made on sera of cancer patients with TGAb, it is impossible to appreciate the incidence of TPOAb versus TGAb in a general population (Pacini et al, 1988). However, it appears that TGAb can occur without TPOAb or MAb and are related with the antigen itself. The comparison between antibody titers in patients with or without recidive of their disease is in agreement with this conclusion (figure 7). Patients in remission, whose serum Tg concentrations were low or even nil had TGAb titers significantly lower than patients with metastases. But the evolution of the disease cannot be predicted by anyone of the auto-antibodies since they existed in both situations.

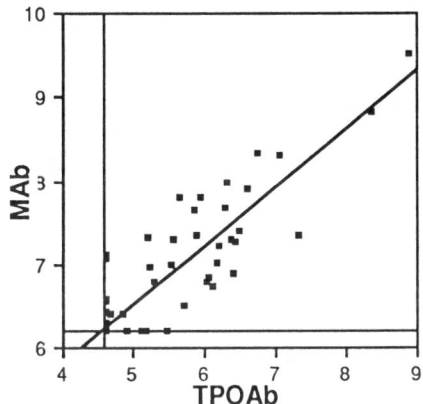
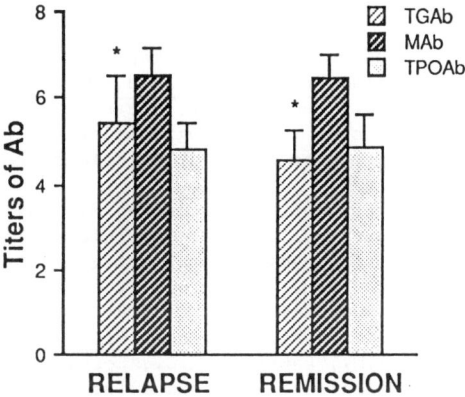

Fig. 6. Correlation between titers of MAb and TPOAb in 134 samples from 60 patients with differentiated thyroid cancer (r=0.91 ; p < 0.001).

Fig. 7. Comparison of antithyroid antibody titers in 56 patients with differentiated thyroid cancer, subgrouped according to evolution. "Relapse" patients (n=21) are characterized by the presence of metastases. The only significant difference was observed for TGAb (*:p< 0.001). Titers of antibody as U/l are expressed as the corresponding ln.

CONCLUSION

Our results confirm the concept that TPO accounts for virtually all the antigenic determinants reacting with the autoantibodies commonly termed antimicrosomal antibodies. This conclusion is based on the positive, close correlation between TPOAb and MAb titers, found in each group studied : normal elderly subjects, patients with autoimmune thyroid disorders-lymphocytic thyroiditis or Graves' disease- and patients with operated differentiated thyroid cancers. This finding indicates that this strict correlation is a general phenomenon, apparently independent from the nature of underlying autoimmune thyroid disease.

The functional implications of TPOAb remain to be elucidated but it is of interest that the identified thyroid autoantigens Tg, TSH receptor and TPO are strictly related to the function of the thyroid cell.

REFERENCES

Allannic, H., Fauchet, R., Orgiazzi, J., Madec, A.M., Genetet, B., Lorcy, Y., Le Guerrier, A.M., Delambre, C., and Derennes, V. (1990): Relapse rate in patients with Graves' disease treated with antithyroid drugs. A prospective randomized study of treatment duration. J. Clin. Endocrinol. Metab. 70: 675-680.

Bornet, H. (1989): Le dosage de la thyroglobuline. Dix ans d'expérience. Comptes-rendus Symposium Behring, pp. 233-239.

Czarnocka, B., Ruf, J., Ferrand, M., Carayon, P., and Lissitzky, S. (1985): Purification of the human thyroid peroxidase and its identification as the microsomal antigen involved in autoimmune thyroid diseases. FEBS Lett. 190: 147-152.

Kimura, S., Kotani, T., McBride, O.M., Unicki, K., Hirai, K., Nakeyama, I., and Ohtaki, S. (1987): Human thyroid peroxidase : complete cDNA and protein sequence, chromosome mapping and identification of two alternately spliced mRNA's. Proc. Natl. Acad. Sci. USA 84: 5555-5559.

Lefort, G., Lanet, M.J., Ducassou, D., and Latapie, J.L. (1981): Dosage des anticorps antithyroglobuline par une méthode radioimmunologique utilisant la protéine A staphylococcique comme agent de séparation. Pathol. Biol. 29: 285-291.

Libert, F., Ruf, J., Ludgate, M., Swillens, S., Alexander, N., Vassart, G., and Dinsart, C. (1987): Complete nucleotide sequence of the human thyroid peroxidase-microsomal antigen cDNA. Nucl. Acids Res. 15: 6735-6739.

McLachlan, S.M., Atherton, C., Nakajima, Y., Napier, J., Jordan, R.K., Clark, F., and Rees Smith, B. (1990): Thyroid peroxidase and the induction of auto-immune thyroid disease. Clin. Exp. Immunol. 79: 182-188.

Madec, A.M., Laurent, M.C., Lorcy, Y., Le Guerrier, A.M., Rostagnat-Stefanutti, A., Orgiazzi, J., and Allannic, H. (1984): Thyroid stimulating antibodies: an aid to the strategy of Graves' disease. Clin. Endocrinol. 21: 247-255.

Magnusson, R.P., Gestautas, J., Taurog, A., and Rapoport, B. (1987): Molecular cloning of the structural gene for porcine thyroid peroxidase. J. Biol.Chem. 262: 13885-13888.

Mariotti, S., Anelli, S., Ruf, J., Bechi, R., Czarnocka, B., Lombardi, A., Carayon, P., and Pinchera, A. (1987): Comparison of serum thyroid microsomal and thyroid peroxidase autoantibodies in thyroid diseases. J. Clin. Endocrinol. Metab. 65: 987-993.

Pacini, F., Mariotti, S., Formica, N., Elisei, R., Anelli, S., Capotorti, E., and Pinchera, A. (1988): Thyroid autoantibodies in thyroid cancer : incidence and relationship with tumour outcome. Acta Endocrinol. (Copenh.) 119: 373-380.

Résumé

Avec une nouvelle trousse commerciale, DYNO-test anti-TPO, les auto-anticorps antiperoxydase thyroïdienne (TPOAb) ont été déterminés et comparés aux anticorps microsomiaux (MAb) dans 4 groupes de sujets : des personnes âgées, de plus de 60 ans et euthyroïdiennes, des patients atteints de thyroïdite lymphocytaire, atrophique ou goitreuse, de maladie de Basedow, enfin de cancers différenciés de la thyroïde ayant des anticorps antithyroglobuline dans leur sérum. L'étroite corrélation entre les titres de TPOAb et MAb dans toutes les situations cliniques confirme le concept que la peroxydase représente l'antigène essentiel, sinon unique, des antigènes communément nommés microsomiaux. Dans la population âgée, la prévalence des TPOAb était en moyenne de 13,7 % avec un maximum à 22 % dans la tranche d'âge 70-80 ans. La TSH était significativement plus élevée dans les sérums positifs en TPOAb que dans le reste de la population. Les titres en TPOAb étaient le plus souvent très élevés dans les cas de thyroïdites lymphocytaires. Le plus souvent, les taux de TPOAb, plus bas dans les cas d'atrophies que dans les hypertrophies, infirment un effet cytotoxique de ces anticorps. Dans les cas de maladie de Basedow, les TPOAb étaient également présents chez les patients qui, ultérieurement, ont été guéris ou ont récidivé. Leurs taux ont baissé lors du traitement mais cette diminution n'était pas différente dans les deux évolutions. Chez les patients ayant un cancer différencié de la thyroïde et dont la surveillance après traitement a mis en évidence des anticorps anti-Tg dans le sérum, la corrélation entre ceux-ci et les TPOAb était très faible. La présence de TgAb semble plus reliée à celle de Tg elle-même qu'à une atteinte autoimmune plus générale. Enfin, l'évolution de la maladie ne peut être prévue par les anticorps antithyroïdiens car ils existaient aussi bien en cas de récidive que de rémission.

The value of ultrasonography in the detection of lymphocytic thyroiditis

R. Gutekunst, W. Hafermann, U. Löhrs and P.C. Scriba

Departments of Internal Medicine and Pathology, Medical University Lübeck, FRG

INTRODUCTION

Lymphocytic thyroiditis (LT) is believed to be a rare disease in Germany that is not well appreciated (13). The aim of this study was to évaluate different diagnostic procedures for the study of LT (10).

SUBJECTS and METHODS

The charts of 106 hospitalized and ambulatory patients with LT treated between January 1984 and December 1987 were reviewed. The diagnosis of LT was based on physical examination and confirmatory findings in at least two of the following four procedures: measurement of antimicrosomal antibodies [TPO(mic)]; TSH; ultrasonography (US) and fine needle aspiration cytology (FNA) of the thyroid. Only patients (n=92, 88 women, 4 men, age 11-81, mean age 47 yr) where all four diagnostic procedures were available, were included in the study.

Clinical manifestations were recorded; TPO(mic) was determined by immunofluorescence (20), TSH run in duplicate by a supersensitive luminescence immunoassay (24), T4 and T3 were measured using commercial kits (Henning Berlin, FRG). Thyroid size and morphology were investigated by ultrasound using SRT, linear Mhz 5, General Electric, Rancho Cordova, CA (9). Sonograms from population studies were used as controls (8). In addition both thyroid lobes were biopsied under sonographic control with a fine needle (od, 0.6-0.7mm). The smears were air dried and stained by the May-Grünwald-Giemsa technique for morphological evaluation.

RESULTS

Clinical manifestations

	PERCENT	n=92
NO SYMPTOMS	29.3	27
INCREASE IN WEIGHT	44.6	41
GOITRE	37.0	34
MENTAL COMPLAINTS	34.8	32
MYXEDEMA	23.9	22
PARAESTHESIA	19.6	18
FATIGUE	18.5	17
ARTHRALGIA	18.5	17
GLOBUS HYSTERICUS	17.4	16
EPIGASTRIC DISCOMFORT	15.2	14
ANAEMIA	11.9	11
DYSPHAGIA	8.7	8
HYPERCHOLESTEROLEMIA	6.5	6
THYROTOXICOSIS	6.5	6

TPO(mic)
In 12 (13%) patients TPO(mic) were undetectable. TPO(mic) titers of 1:32 were found in 5 (5.4%), 1:100 in 11 (12%), 1:320 in 19 (20.7%), 1:1000 in 31 (33.7%) and >1:1000 in 14 (15.2%) patients respectively. The frequency distribution is shifted towards higher titers.

TSH
In 4 patients (4.3%) TSH serum levels were <0.3 µU/ml (normal range 0.3-3.9). Three of those patients had elevated T3, but only one of those three had an elevated serum T4 level. Forty-one (44.6%) patients had TSH levels 0.3-3.9, 26 (28.3%) 4-20, 14 (15.2%) >20 - 50, and 7 (7.6%) >50 µU/ml.

Ultrasonography
Thyroid volume: 43 (48.9%) women had normal thyroid volume (<18ml, range 3-17.8, mean 12), and 45 (51.1.%) had enlarged glands (range 18.2- >140, mean 35.3). The four men had thyroid volume (normal >25ml) of 8, 23, 27 and 64 ml.
Echopatterns: all except 5 (5.4%) patients had scattered sonolucent echopatterns. In 13 (14%) patients solid nodules were detected. (Fig. 1 A and B).

Figure 1. Transverse sonograms of the thyroid (T):

A. normal echopattern compared to the sonolucent muscles (M) from a healthy person.

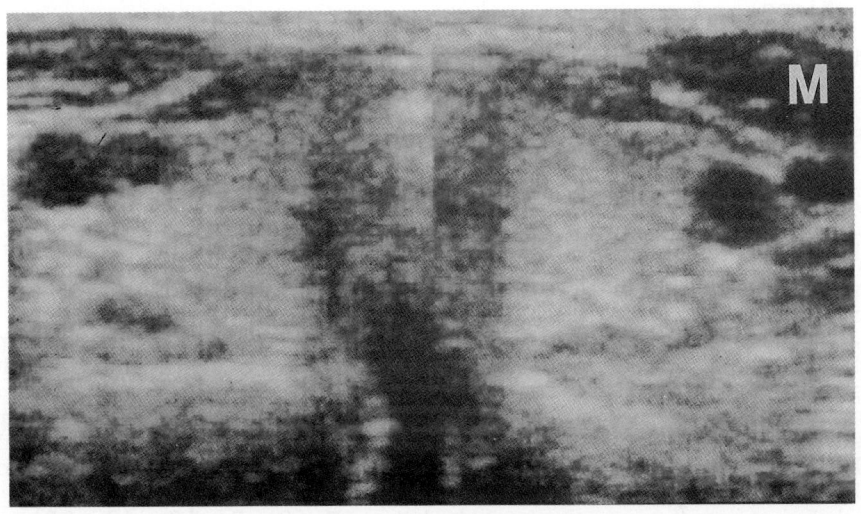

B. sonolucent echopattern from a patient with LT.

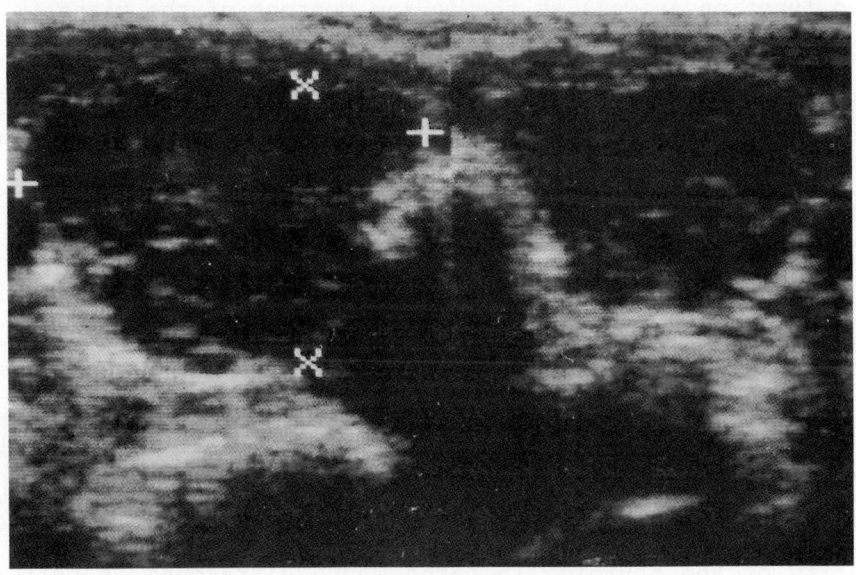

Cytology
Thirty (32.6%) patients had hypercellular smears; 54 (58.7%) smears presented a scanty to moderate overall cellularity; and 8 (8.7%) smears showed sparse lymphocytes and were not diagnostic for LT alone.

Correlations
There were no correlations between the cellularity of the smear, thyroid function and/or the TPO(mic) titer.

DISCUSSION

As in previous studies (2, 12, 17, 18) we also found great clinical variation. A quarter of the patients had no complaints or physical findings. Many symptoms were nonspecific and subject to the individual bias of the physician.
Determination of serum TPO(mic) is not always conclusive for the diagnosis of LT. In this study TPO(mic) were absent in 13% and low in 17.4% (<1:320), generally considered as negative (1). More than thirteen percent of all cases would have been missed without ultrasound and/or FNA. On the other hand, in 2 - 20% of the healthy population TPO(mic) can be found without apparent thyroid disease (1, 3 - 5, 7, 11, 21, 22); in our area 3% (20). Our data clearly support the assumption, that serum findings only incompletely reflect thyroid status.
Thyroid function is poorly related to LT (2, 3, 12, 17, 18). The prevalence of hypothyroidism underestimates the prevalence of LT. Since TSH and TPO(mic) titers are poorly correlated, the sensitivity of the combination of elevated TSH and detectable TPO(mic) for detection of LT in population studies must be even lower.
Scintiscanning is impractical and rather unreliable as a diagnostic tool for LT, since the uptake of radionuclides depends on thyroid function as well as the iodine content of the gland (13).
Although ultrasound does not differentiate between LT and Graves' disease (6, 15, 19, 23), it surely is a useful tool for screening in unselected groups. If a selected population of patients with thyroid diseases is considered, the specificity of ultrasound alone for detecting LT must be low, since this group will contain many patients with Graves' disease. However the combination of ultrasound and clinical evaluation will result in a high specificity even in a selected group.
FNA has a high diagnostic accuracy. Interpretation of the varying amounts of lymphocytes is however difficult (14). These findings could either indicate different LT diseases or merely reflect various inflammatory stages. If only one lobe is aspirated LT may be confused with focal lymphocytic reactions, which are common in endemic goitres (16). Only in rare instances can lymphocytes be found in focal sonolucent or solid alterations. To confirm the diagnosis of LT, FNA from one site probably suffices, if the scan is homogeneously sonolucent. Otherwise both lobes have to be aspirated.
In conclusion, this study confirms that sonography combined with clinical evaluation is rather specific for LT. Ultrasound additionally provides information about the size, topography and the nodularity of the thyroid. In cases where ultrasound is performed primarily, one can proceed to further examinations. Otherwise, it can support the laboratory and/or clinical findings that suggest

LT. When clinical features are inconclusive LT can only be confirmed by appropriate combination of serological and morphological tests. These conclusions have to be confirmed in a prospective study.

SUMMARY

The value of ultrasound (US) compared to established diagnostic procedures was investigated by retrospectively reviewing medical records of 92 patients (88 women and 4 men, age 11-81 yr, mean age 47 yr) with lymphocytic thyroiditis (LT). Clinical manifestations of the disease, serum antimicrosomal antibodies and TSH were determined in all patients. The thyroid was examined by US. Both lobes were aspirated by a fine needle under sonographic control and smears examined cytologically. A total of 27 (29.3%) patients had no clinical symptoms. TPO(mic) were undetectable in 12 (13%) patients, 16 (17.4%) had low titers 1:32-1:100, and 64 (69.6%) ≥1:320. TSH (normal range 0.3-3.9 µU/ml) was <0.3 in 4 (4,3%), 0.3-3.9 in 41 (44.6%), 4-20 in 26 (28.3%), and >20 in 21 (22.8%) cases. US revealed a scattered sonolucent echo in 87 (94.6%) patients, and in 45 (48.9%) a normal thyroid volume (women <18, men <25 ml). Cytology was diagnostic in 84 (91.3%) patients.

In conclusion, US can suggest LT. If TPO(mic) are undetectable or TPO(mic) titers are not significant and/or clinical symptoms are uncertain, fine needle aspiration (FNA) can confirm the sonographic finding. LT can only be confirmed by appropriate combination of serological and morphological tests. Finally, LT si obviously be more common in iodine deficient areas than generally assumed.

REFERENCES

1. Amino, N. (1986) Thyroid-directed antibodies In Werner's The Thyroid (eds S. H. Ingbar & L. E. Bravermann), pp. 546-559. J. B. Lippincott Company Philadelphia.
2. Bastenie, P. A., Bonnyns, M. & Vanhaelst, L. (1980) Grades of subclinical hypothyroidism in asymptomatic autoimmune thyroiditis revealed by the thyrotropin releasing hormone test. Journal of Clinical Endocrinology and Metabolism 51, 163-167.
3. Betterle, C., Callegari, G., Presotto, F., Zanette, F., Pedini, B., Rampazzo, T., Slack, R. S., Girelli, M. E. & Busnardo, B. (1987) Thyroid autoantibodies: A good marker for the study of symptomless autoimmune thyroiditis. Acta Endocrinologica 114, 321-327.
4. Bjoro, T., Gaardener, P. I., Smeland, E. B. & Kornstad, L. (1984) Thyroid antibodies in blood donors: Prevalence and clinical significance. Acta Endocrinologica 105, 324-329.
5. Boyages, S. C., Bloot, A. M., Maberly, G. F., Eastman, D. J., Mu, L., Qidong, Q., Derun, L., van der Graag, R. D. and Dreshage, H. A. (1989) Thyroid Autoimmunity in Endemic Goitre caused by exessive iodine intake. Clinical Endocrinology 31, 453-465.
6. Espinasse, P., Espinasse, D., Estour, B. & Navarro, D. (1980) Echography in thyroiditis. Ultrasound 1, 345-349.

7. Gordin, A., Maatela, J., Miettinen, A., Heleniust, T. & Lamberg, B. A. (1979) Serum thyrotropin and circulating thyroglobulin and thyroid microsomal antibodies in a Finnish population. Acta Endocrinologica 90, 33-42.
8. Gutekunst, R., Smolarek, H., Hasenpusch, U., Stubbe, P., Friedrich, H. J., Wood, W. G. & Scriba, P. C. (1986) Goitre epidemiology: thyroid volume, iodine excretion, thyroglobulin and thyrotropin in Germany and Sweden. Acta Endocrinologica 112, 494-501.
9. Gutekunst R, Becker W, Hehrmann R, Olbricht Th, Pfannenstiel P (1988) Ultraschalldiagnostik der Schilddrüse. Deutsche Medizinische Wochenschrift 113, 1109-1112.
10. Gutekunst, R., Hafermann, W., Mansky, T, Scriba, P. C. (1989) Ultrasonography related to clinical and laboratory findings in lymphocytic thyroiditis. Acta Endocrinologica (Copenh) 121, 129-135.
11. Hawkins, B.R., Dawkins, R.L., Burger, H.G., Mackay,I. R., Cheah, P.S., Whittingham, S., Patel, Y. & Welborn, T. A. (1980) Diagnostic significance of thyroid microsomal antibodies in randomly selected population. Lancet II, 1057-1059.
12. Hayashi, Y., Tamai, H., Fukata, S., Hirota, Y., Katayama, S., Kuma, K., Kumagai, L.F. & Nagataki, S. (1985) A long term clinical, immunological, and histological follow-up study of patients with goitrous chronic lymphocytic thyroidits. Journal of Clinical Endocrinology and Metabolism 61, 1172-1178.
13. Klein, E. (1980) Die Entzündungen der Schilddrüse In Die Krankheiten der Schilddrüse (eds K. Oberdisse, K. Klein & D. Reinwein), pp. 595-622. Georg Thieme Verlag Stuttgart, New York.
14. Löwhagen, T. & Linsk, J. A. (1983) Aspiration biopsy cytology of the thyroid gland. In Clinical aspiration cytology (eds J. A. Linsk & S. Franzen) pp 61-83. J. B. Lippincott Company, London.
15. Müller-Gärtner H. W. (1986) Grauwerthistogrammana-lyse in der Schilddrüsensonographie. Fortschritte Rönt-genstrahlen 145, 283-287.
16. Oechslin, E. & Hedinger, Chr. (1985) Thyroiditis lymphomatosa Hashimoto und endemische Struma. Schwei-zerische Medizinische Wochenschrift 115, 1182-1191.
17. Papendieck, L. G. de, Iorcansky, S., Rivarola, M.A. & Bergada, C. (1982) Variations in clinical, hormonal and serological expression of chronic lymphocytic thyroiditis (CLT) in children and adolescents. Clinical Endocrinology 16, 19-28.
18. Scherbaum, W. A., Stöckle, G., Wichmann, J. & Berg, P. A. (1982) Immunological and clinical characterization of patients with untreated euthyroid and hypothyroid autoimmune thyroiditis. Antibody spectrum, response to TRH and clinical study. Acta Endocrinologica 100, 373-381.
19. Simeone, J. F., Daniels, G. H., Mueller, P. R., Maloof, F., van Sonnenberg, E., Hall, D. A., O`Connell, R. S., Ferrucci, J. T. & Wittenberg, J. (1982) High-resolution real-time sonography of the thyroid. Radiology 145, 431-435.
20. Stöcker, W. (1985) Rationelle Histochemie mit einer neuen Mikroanalysemethode. Acta Histochemica Suppl 31, 269.

21. Tanner, A. R., Scott-Morgan, L., Mardell, R. & Lloyd, R. S. (1982) The incidence of occult thyroid disease associated with thyroid antibodies identified on routine autoantibidy screening. Acta Endocrinologica 100, 31-35.
22. Tunbridge, W. M. G., Evered, D. C., Hall, R., Appleton, D., Brewis, M., Clark, F., Grimley-Evans, J., Smith, P., Stephenson, J. & Young, E. (1981) Natural history of autoimmune thyroiditis. British Medical Journal 282, 258-262.
23. Wiedemann, W. (1984) Autoimmunerkrankungen In Sonographie und Szintigraphie der Schilddrüse, (ed W. Wiedemann) pp. 168-177. Thieme Verlag Stuttgart, New York.
24. Wood, W. G., Waller, D. & Hantke, U. (1985) An evaluation of six solid-phase thyrotropin (TSH) kits. Journal of Clinical Chemestry and Clinical Biochemistry 23, 461-471.

Résumé

Une étude rétrospective des dossiers médicaux de 92 patients (88 femmes et 4 hommes, âgés de 11 à 81 ans, moyenne d'âge: 47 ans), présentant une thyroïdite lymphocytaire (LT) a permis une comparaison entre le diagnostic établi par ultrasons (US) et un diagnostic établi par des méthodes habituelles. Les manifestations cliniques de la maladie, les anticorps anti-microsomiaux sériques et la TSH ont été évaluées chez tous les patients. Des prélèvements par aiguille fine sous contrôle échographique ont été effectués sur les lobes, et un examen cytologique a été effectué sur les prélèvements. Un total de 27 patients (29.3%) ne présentaient aucun aucun symptome clinique. La TPO n'était pas décelable chez 12 patients (13%), 16. (17.4%) présentaient une concentration basse de TPO 1:32 - 1:100, et 64 (69.6%) un taux > 1/320. La TSH (zone normale 0.3 - 3.9 uU/ml) était < 0.3 dans 4 cas (4,3%), 0.3 - 3.9 dans 41 cas (44.6%), 4 - 20 dans 26 cas (28.3%), et > 20 dans 21 cas (22.8%. Les US ont révélé une réponse positive diffuse chez 88 patients (94.6%) et un volume thyroïdien normal chez 45 sujets (48.9%) (femmes <18, hommes <25ml). Chez 84 patients (91.3%), le diagnostic a pu être confirmé par un examen cytologique. En conclusion, les US laissent supposer une thyroïdite lymphocytaire. Si les anticorps anti-TPO sont indétectables ou présentent des titres non significatifs et/ou si les symptômes cliniques sont incertains, une aspiration par aiguille fine peut confirmer les résultats échographiques. Les thyroïdites lymphocytaires peuvent seulement être confirmées par une combinaison appropriée de tests sérologiques et morphologiques. En conclusion, les thyroïdites lymphocytaires sont plus répandues dans les zones déficientes en iode qu'on ne l'a généralement supposé.

Autoantibodies to thyroid peroxidase and microsomal antigen in autoimmune thyroid diseases

K. Weber and H. Schatz

Department of Medicine, University Hospital Bergmannsheil, University Bochum, FRG

In the present study we were interested in the prevalence of anti-TPO-antibodies in patients with autoimmune thyroid disease.

We obtained 287 serum samples, including normal subjects (n=48), autoimmune thyroiditis (n=48), Graves' disease (n=191). Diagnosis of autoimmunity was confirmed by clinical, immunological and ultrasonographical findings. Anti-microsomal antibodies were determined by passive haemagglutination (MA-PH) and radio ligand assay (MA-RLA), anti-TPO-antibodies by means of a newly developed radio immuno assay (TPO-RIA) using the inhibition of binding of labeled thyroid peroxidase to a solid-phase-bound monoclonal antibody by autoantibodies.
Upper limits for normals: TPO-RIA 100 U/ml, MA-RLA 500 U/ml, MA-PH 1:100.

Diagram 1 shows the number of patients positive or negative in our assays classified for diseases:

	\multicolumn{3}{c}{normals}	\multicolumn{3}{c}{autoimmune thyroiditis}	\multicolumn{3}{c}{Graves' disease}
	TPO-RIA	MA-RLA	MA-PH	TPO-RIA	MA-RLA	MA-PH	TPO-RIA	MA-RLA	MA-PH
positive	0	0	3	43	41	39	130	122	122
negative	48	48	45	5	7	9	61	69	79

Patients negative in one and positive in another assay are shown in diagram 2:

		MA-RLA		MA-PH	
		positive	negative	positive	negative
TPO-RIA	positive	157	16	145	28
	negative	6	60	6	60

CONCLUSIONS:
Determination of antibodies to microsomal antigen has proved to be a valuable tool in diagnosis of autoimmune thyroid disease. Because of its unknown nature specific assays were not available. Current systems use preparations from thyrotoxic glands isolated by centrifugation. These crude fractions may contain undefined antigens. Recently, microsomal antigen was identified as thyroid peroxidase, a membrane-bound glycosylated protein. Replacing the preparation of undefined antigens by purified thyroid peroxidase, one would expect a decrease in antibodies detectable. In contrast, our study demonstrates an increased number of patients found antibody-positive by use of TPO-RIA. For explanation we consider a better access to antigenic epitopes by purification of the antigen. Preliminary results of longitudinal surveys (data not shown) point out that TPO-RIA is more sensitive to detect the onset of autoimmune thyroid disease, as some patients, first anti-TPO-antibody positive, but negative in MA-PH and, partly, MA-RLA, became anti-microsomal-antibody positive later on.

Auto-anticorps anti-thyroperoxidase (anti-TPO) en pathologie thyroïdienne

L. Baldet, J. Faure and C. Jaffiol

Service d'Endocrinologie, Hôpital Lapeyronie, 555, route de Ganges, 34059 Montpellier Cedex, France

Cette étude a pour objet d'évaluer la fréquence des anti-TPO en pathologie thyroidienne et leur intérêt pour la surveillance évolutive de la maladie de Basedow.

Les titres d'anti-TPO ont été déterminés au moyen de la trousse Dyno-test anti-TPO (Laboratoire Henning) et les résultats exprimés en unité par millilitre (U/ml). Les sérums testés proviennent de sujets témoins (16 cas), de patients ayant une hypothyroidie idiopathique (22 cas), de basedowiens (37 cas) chez lesquels les anti-TPO ont été mesurés avant et sous traitement par Carbimazole et malades présentant une maladie thyroidienne non autoimmune (28 cas).

Chez les témoins, les titres d'anticorps anti-TPO sont de 20.9 $\pm$ 14.9 U/ml (m $\pm$ SD) conduisant à considérer comme pathologique toute valeur supérieure à 75 U/ml (m + 3 SD). Au cours des affections thyroidiennes autoimmunes (hypothyroidie idiopathique et maladie de Basedow) des titres pathologiques sont observés avec une fréquence élevée : 16 sur 22 hypothyroidies, 12 sur 15 maladies de Basedow ; les titres d'anti-TPO présentent d'importantes variations (hypothyroidiens 16 à 18900 U/ml - basedowiens 16 à 17000 U/ml). Les titres d'anticorps anti-TPO ne varient pas lors des premiers mois de traitement par Carbimazole, se normalisent chez 8 sur 10 sujets en rémission et redeviennent pathologiques chez tous les sujets présentant une rechute (7 cas). Des titres très élevés sont observés chez 3 patients atteints d'une ophtalmopathie évolutive (13800 à 35000 U/ml) et 2 sujets développant une hypothyroidie spontanée aprés hyperthyroidie basedowienne (4900 et 13400 U/ml). Au cours des affections thyroidiennes non autoimmunes, la fréquence des anticorps anti-TPO est rare (3/12 dans les goitres euthyroidiens - 0/10 dans les hyperthyroidies nodulaires - 1/6 dans les hypothyroidies post chirurgicales).

Cette étude préliminaire confirme la fréquence des anticorps anti-TPO au cours des affections thyroidiennes auto-immunes. Une étude prospective de plus longue durée est nécessaire pour juger de la valeur pronostique de ces anticorps au cours de la maladie de Basedow.

Etude comparative des méthodes de dosage des auto-anticorps anti-thyroïdiens en pathologie thyroïdienne (à propos de 203 observations)

P. Caron[1], T. Babin[1] and M. Hoff[2]

[1] Service d'Endocrinologie, [2] Laboratoire des radioisotopes, CHU Rangueil, 1 Avenue Jean Poulhes 31054 Toulouse Cedex, France

La caractérisation de la thyropéroxydase humaine (hTPO) au sein des antigènes microsomiaux thyroïdiens a permis l'individualisation des auto-anticorps anti-thyropéroxydase (Ac anti-TPO) parmi les anticorps anti-microsomes thyroïdiens (ACAM). En pratique, la fréquence des Ac anti-TPO au cours des affections thyroïdiennes reste à préciser.

La recherche des auto-anticorps anti-thyroïdiens a été réalisée de façon prospective chez 203 patients (188 femmes et 15 hommes, âge moyen 42 ans), consultant pour un goître homogène ou hétérogène normofonctionnel (n = 81), une dystrophie nodulaire euthyroïdienne (n = 14), une hypothyroïdie périphérique (n = 50), une hyperthyroïdie (n = 42), ou un symptome pouvant être rattaché à une affection thyroïdienne (asthénie, gynécomastie, troubles des règles, surpoids, n = 16). Les auto-anticorps anti-thyroïdiens ont été recherchés grâce aux techniques suivantes : Ac anti TPO (Dynotest anti-TPO, Lab Henning Berlin GMBH, seuil de positivité ≥100), anticorps antithyroglobuline (ACAT RIA, ≥400), anticorps antimicrosomes (ACAM RIA Promak-assay, Lab. Henning Berlin GMBH,≥500 ; ACAM IF par immunofluorescence indirecte, ≥ ++).

Les résultats sont donnés dans le tableau suivant:

	N	AC-	ACAT RIA	ACAM IF	ACAM RIA	Ac anti-TPO
hyper	42	35,7 %	14,3 %	38 %	54.8 %	61,9 %
hypo	50	48 %	16 %	32 %	42 %	48 %
goître	81	75,3 %	2,4 %	8,6 %	21 %	22,2 %
nodule	14	100 %	0 %	0 %	0 %	0 %
autres	16	81,2 %	0 %	0 %	6,2 %	12,5 %
	203	61,5 %	7,9 %	19,2 %	30,5 %	34,4 %

Chez 78 patients (38,5 %) présentant au moins un auto-anticorps à un titre significatif les ACAT RIA sont présents dans 19,2 % des cas, les ACAM IF dans 50 %, les ACAM RIA dans 79,5 % et les Ac anti-TPO dans 90 %. Par ailleurs, les taux des Ac anti-TPO sont corrélés à ceux des ACAM RIA ($r = 0,87$, $p < 10^{-4}$).

Au total : I) parmi les patients étudiés 38,5 % présentent un stigmate d'auto-immunité thyroïdienne. 2) les techniques utilisées de détection des auto-anticorps anti-thyroïdiens révèlent une pathologie autoimmune fréquente lors des hypo et des hyperthyroïdies. 3) les ACAM et les Ac anti-TPO dosés par RIA sont les plus fréquemment rencontrés au cours des affections autoimmunes. 4) la place respective des ACAM et des Ac anti-TPO dans l'auto-immunité thyroïdienne reste encore à déterminer.

Anticorps anti-thyroperoxidase et maladie de Basedow : intérêt dans la surveillance du traitement par anti-thyroïdiens de synthèse

C. Massart*, I. Guilhem**, J. Gibassier, M. Nicol* and H. Allannic**

Service d'hormonologie-enzymologie et service d'endocrinologie**, CHU de Pontchaillou, rue H. Le Guilloux, 35043 Rennes, France*

Les anticorps anti-thyroperoxydase (Ac anti-TPO) ont été dosés chez des Basedowiens traités par antithyroïdiens de synthèse (ATS). Tous les sujets (n=62) ont reçu du Carbimazole pendant 6 mois, deux groupes étant à considérer. Dans le groupe I (GrI,n=23), le Carbimazole a été proposé à la posologie moyenne de 25,2 mg±3,9(SD) par jour. Ces 23 sujets ont fait l'objet d'un suivi 2ans après arrêt du traitement; 10 patients ont rechuté, 13 sont en rémission. Dans le groupe II (GrII,n=39), le Carbimazole a été donné à la posologie fixe de 60 mg/j pendant 6 mois; l'évolution de ces patients n'est pas connue au delà de ces 6 mois.

Les Ac anti-TPO et anti-récepteurs à la TSH (Ac anti-TSH-R(s)) ont été dosés en début et fin de traitement chez tous les patients. Les Ac anti-TPO ont été dosés par immunoradiométrie (trousse Berhing) (normale<300 U/ml) et les Ac anti-TSH-R(s) selon une technique basée sur la production d'AMPc par stimulation de thyrocytes humains en culture.

Dans les 2 groupes confondus, les Ac anti-TPO s'élèvent à 9925U/ml ±1939(SEM) avant traitement. Ils se situent à 3949 U/ml ± 1002(SEM) en fin de traitement (p< 0,05). Le traitement par fortes doses permet une chute plus rapide que celui à doses habituelles: 4579 U/ml ± 1263(SEM) dans le GrI versus 3578 U/ml ± 1418(SEM) dans le GrII (p< 0,05). Dans le GrI, les sujets en rémission (n=13) ont un taux d'Ac anti-TPO en fin de traitement inférieur à celui des sujets en rechute: 3494 U/ml ± 1802(SEM) versus 5989 U/ml ± 1717(SEM) (p<0,01) mais seuls 4 sujets sur 13 (31%) ont un taux d'Ac anti-TPO normal en fin de traitement. Chez ces 4 sujets, les titres d'Ac anti-TPO avant traitement étaient normaux chez 2 et voisins de la normale (307 et 367 U/ml) chez les 2 autres. Il n'est pas mis en évidence de corrélation significative entre les taux d'Ac anti-TPO et ceux d'Ac anti-TSH-R(s) avant traitement (r= 0,195) et en fin de traitement (r= 0,105).

Au total: le traitement par ATS permet d'obtenir une chute progressive du taux des Ac anti-TPO chez les Basedowiens; la chute est d'autant plus importante que la posologie d'ATS est élevée. Les taux en fin de traitement sont plus bas chez les sujets qui demeureront en rémission. Un taux normal ou voisin de la normale d'Ac anti-TPO en début ou fin de traitement pourrait être considéré comme un facteur pronostique de rémission.

Evaluation d'une technique de dosage des anticorps anti-thyroperoxydase par radiocompétition

C. Poustis-Delpont*, S. Altare*, S. Hieronimus**, A.M. Guedj**, M. Harter** and P. Sudaka

* Laboratoire de Biochimie, Hôpital St. Roch, 5, rue P. Devoluy, 06000 Nice. ** Service d'Endocrinologie Nutrition et Médecine Interne, Hôpital de l'Archet, Nice, France

But : Evaluation des performances de la trousse : précision, seuil de détection, IC_{50}^*, exactitude.

Méthodes : a) <u>Principe du dosage</u> : Le principe de la trousse repose sur la compétition des anticorps anti-thyropéroxydase (TPO) du patient ou de la gamme d'une part, et des anticorps monoclonaux anti-TPO immobilisés au fond du tube de dosage d'autre part, vis à vis de la TPO marquée (I^{125}). Les anticorps anti-TPO sont calibrés selon l'étalon MRC 66/387.

b) <u>Méthodes statistiques</u> : étude de la moyenne, de l'écart-type et du coefficient de variation d'une série. Comparaison des séries grâce au test t de STUDENT.

Résultats : La précision de la trousse a été évaluée à 5,2 et 6,5 % pour 2 lots différents. Le seuil de détection a été déterminé avec un intervalle de confiance de 95 %. Il est de 50 U/ml pour un traceur fraîchement iodé, et de 200 U/ml pour un traceur iodé depuis 6 semaines. l'IC_{50} n'est pas significativement différent entre les 2 trousses : il est de 1000 $\pm$ 50 et 1100 $\pm$ 100 U/ml respectivement. Le test de dilution révèle 93 % de récupération (Valeurs de 87 à 100 %).

Conclusion : La technique de radiocompétition appliquée au dosage des anticorps anti-TPO (Dyno-test, anti-TPO, Henning) apparait comme trés précise et reproductible. Le seuil de détection est inférieur à 100 U/ml avec un traceur fraîchement marqué. L'intérêt diagnostique est en cours d'évaluation chez des sujets témoins, porteurs de maladie de Basedow, de thyroïdite de Hashimoto ou d'hypothyroïdie périphérique.

---

*IC_{50} = concentration inhibant 50 % de la liaison.

Dosage des anticorps anti-TPO et anti-microsomes dans différentes pathologies thyroïdiennes

C. Schvartz*, H. Larbre**, B. Maes*, M.J. Delisle* and G. Deltour**

* Service UMNB2, Institut Jean Godinot BP 171 51056 Reims Cedex, France; ** Service UMNB3, Institut Jean Godinot BP 171 51056 Reims Cedex, France

BUT DE L'ETUDE
    Les antigènes microsomaux thyroïdiens ont été reconnus comme étant la thyroperoxydase thyroïdienne (TPO). Nous avons testé l'intérêt respectif des dosages d'anticorps anti-TPO et antimicrosomes thyroïdiens (anti-M) dans différentes populations définies après examen thyroïdien clinique, scintigraphique, hormonal et parfois échographique.
MATERIEL ET METHODES
    Les dosages ont été réalisés chez des patients normaux n = 37, des patients hypothyroïdiens n = 49 et des patients hyperthyroïdiens n = 44.
    Le dosage des anti-TPO est réalisé avec la trousse Dynotest anti-TPO Henning, dosage radio-immunologique par compétition. Le dosage des anti-M est pour sa part réalisé avec la trousse Promak Henning, dosage radio-immunologique par compétition. Toute valeur supérieure à 100 U/ml pour l'anti-TPO et 300 U/ml pour l'anti-M est considérée comme pathologique.
RESULTATS
    Pour la population normale, il existe une corrélation entre les deux dosages d'Ac (r = 0,80). Chez ces sujets, les anti-TPO et anti-M ont été retrouvés élevés dans 3 cas sur 37 dont une fois très fortement (anti-TPO = 1670 U/ml, anti-M = 7400 U/ml.)
    Chez les hypothyroïdiens, on retrouve deux populations : la première correspond à des thyroïdites de Hashimoto avec dosages d'anti-M élevés, de même que les anti-TPO, dans la deuxième où les anti-M sont bas, le dosage d'anti-TPO n'apporte pas plus d'élément d'orientation à un diagnostic de pathologie auto-immune que le dosage d'anti-M.

Les hyperthyroïdiens étudiés présentent des hyperthyroïdies apparemment diffuses et des dosages d'anticorps anti-récepteurs de la TSH (ARTSH) ont été couplés (dosage RIA par la trousse TRACK-HENNING). Il existe une différence du taux moyen d'anti-M entre les hyperthyroïdies ARTSH élevé (n = 15) avec anti-M : 1761 U/ml et ARTSH normal (n = 29) anti-M = 7420 U/ml. Cette différence n'est pas retrouvée pour le dosage de TPO (ARTSH élevé, TPO = 86 U/ml ; ARTSH normal, TPO = 1242 U/ml).

COMMENTAIRES

Ce résultat partiel pose les problèmes :
- de l'identité entre anticorps anti-M et anti-TPO
- de l'existence de mécanismes immunologiques différents dans ces deux groupes d'hyperthyroïdie.

Le dosage de TPO n'apporte pas d'éléments diagnostiques supplémentaires dans l'identification des pathologies auto-immunes thyroïdiennes, cependant nous avons noté les bonnes fiabilité et praticabilité de la trousse.

Intérêt clinique de la détermination des anticorps anti-thyroperoxydase : résultats préliminaires

M. Izembart and G. Vallée

Service Central de Radioisotopes, Hôpital Necker, 149, rue de Sèvres, 75747 Paris Cedex 15, France

Les anticorps antiperoxydase thyroidienne (ATPO) ont été mesurés par une technique radioimmunologique (dynotest anti-TPO Henning) chez 151 patients ayant eu dans le service un bilan thyroidien clinique, in vivo et in vitro. Tous ont eu une recherche des anticorps antimicrosomaux (ATM) par hemagglutination passive (HP).
Ces patients se répartissent en
- sujets normaux (19)
- patients porteurs d'une pathologie thyroidienne nodulaire (29) dont 15 adénomes toxiques et 10 nodules froids isolés
- patients atteints d'une maladie de Basedow (40) répartis en 28 patients choisis ATM négatifs (dont 15 sont aussi anticorps antithyroglobuline -ATT- négatifs par HP) et 12 patients positifs uniquement en ATM
- hypothyroidies ATM et ATT négatives (16)
- cancers thyroidiens différenciés (47), thyroidectomisés et traités par l'iode radioactif

<u>Résultats</u> La répartition des résultats des ATPO provenant du groupe des nodules est indiscernable de celle des sujets normaux (inférieur à 300 U/mL) sauf pour un nodule froid retrouvé positif. Dans le groupe des maladies de Basedow, les 12 patients positifs en HP sont supérieurs à 300 U/mL. Parmi les 28 patients négatifs en HP, 18 sont positifs en ATPO (dont 8 sur les 15 aussi négatifs en ATT). Dans les hypothyroidies, 5 sont trouvées positives en ATPO. Sur les 47 cancers testés, 33 sont retrouvés dans une zone inférieure à 300 U/mL : tous étaient ATM négatifs. Quatre sujets HP négatifs sont entre 300 et 600 U/mL et 10 supérieurs à 600 U/mL. Parmi ces 10 derniers patients, 5 sont positifs en HP et chez les 5 autres, actuellement négatifs, on retrouve une positivité des ATM lors de dosages antérieurs

<u>Conclusion</u> La valeur normale des ATPO par la technique utilisée se situe d'après cette expérience dans une zone inférieure à 300 U/mL. En prenant cette limite et sur cette petite série, la comparaison avec les résultats obtenus par la recherche des ATM par HP montre que 1/ les patients positifs en HP le sont aussi en

ATPO 2/ les patients classés dans le groupe nodulaire et négatifs en HP le sont aussi (sauf 1) en ATPO 3/ 18 des 28 maladies de Basedow négatives en ATM par HP sont retrouvées positives en ATPO 4/ 5 des 16 hypothyroïdies séronégatives en HP sont positives en ATPO 5/ en cancérologie, le dosage est suffisamment sensible pour suivre l'évolution des ATM après leur négativation en HP.

Ces essais préliminaires montrent donc que ce dosage très sensible permet de mettre en évidence des anticorps circulants chez des patients atteints d'une pathologie possiblement autoimmune mais qui étaient négatifs par la technique d'hemagglutination passive.

Comparaison entre le dosage des anticorps anti-TPO en radioimmunologie et le dosage des anticorps anti-microsomes en immunofluorescence

Y. Fulla*, L. Nonnenmacher* and B. Weill**

* Radioisotopes, ** Immunologie clinique, Hôpital Cochin 27, rue du Fg St-Jacques, 75674 Paris Cedex 14, France

Les anticorps anti-microsomes de la thyroïde fréquents en pathologie autoimmune thyroïdienne, sont habituellement détectés par immunofluorescence indirecte (IF) ou radioimmunologie (RIA). L'antigène microsomial ayant été caractérisé comme une péroxydase (thyropéroxydase: TPO), nous avons comparé les résultats du dosage radioimmunologique des anticorps anti TPO, à ceux de l'IF.

195 sérums ont été étudiés provenant de:
- 112 patients atteints cliniquement de thyroïdite de Hashimoto.
- 23 patients souffrant de maladie de Basedow, confirmée par la présence d'anticorps anti récepteur à la TSH.
- 30 sujets atteints de pathologie autoimmune non thyroïdienne.(anti-estomac, anti-muscle lisse, anti-membrane basale)
- 30 témoins sains.

Les résultats du RIA anti TPO (DYNOtest,Henning, Berlin) sont exprimés en unités/ml par rapport à un sérum de référence fourni avec la trousse.: le seuil de positivité est de 100 unités/ml. Les résultats de l'IF sont exprimés en dilution avec un seuil de positivité fixé à 1/10.

Dans les thyroïdites de Hashimoto, 92% de résultats positifs ont été observés en RIA-TPO et 91% en IF. Il y a donc une concordance de 96,5%. La sensibilité du RIA TPO est de: 96,5% et sa spécificité est de: 96,6%

Dans les maladies de Basedow, 95% des RIA TPO et 91% des tests IF étaient positifs (concordance de 95%)

Dans les 2 pathologies les discordances sont observées dans les deux sens et il n'y a pas de corrélation entre les taux d'anticorps détectés par les deux tests.

Le RIA TPO était négatif chez tous les patients atteints de maladie autoimmune non thyroïdienne et positif chez 3% (1 sujet) de la population témoin.

Il existe donc une excellente concordance entre la détection radioimmunologique des anticorps anti TPO et la détection des anticorps anti-microsomes par immunofluorescence.

L'absence de corrélation entre les taux d'anticorps dosés par ces deux méthodes s'explique par la nature différente des subtrats antigéniques utilisés.

Intérêt du dosage des anticorps anti-récepteurs de la TSH (TBII) dans la maladie de Basedow

S. Dimackie, P. Courrière, A. Boneu and G. Soula

Centre Claudius Regaud, 20, rue du Pont Saint-Pierre, 31052 Toulouse Cedex, France

Quand le système immunitaire d'un organisme fabrique des anticorps qui s'attaquent à ses propres cellules, on est en présence d'une maladie autoimmune ; la maladie de Basedow, qui se manifeste par une hyperthyroïdie, est due à la présence d'autoanticorps (TBII) qui, en bloquant les récepteurs de la TSH, stimulent la thyroïde.
La recherche de la présence de ces autoanticorps, pourrait donc permettre de mettre en évidence l'origine autoimmune d'une hyperthyroïdie.

Matériel et méthode

La trousse TRAK, commercialisée par les Laboratoires Berhing, utilise une méthode de dosage de type radiorécepteur : la mesure de la compétition entre les anticorps spécifiques présents dans un sérum et la TSH marquée à l'iode 125, vis à vis de son récepteur, permet de déterminer le pourcentage d'inhibition de la liaison dû à la présence des autoanticorps.

Les résultats sont exprimés en pourcentage d'inhibition ou facteur F ; la valeur 15 % a été prise comme valeur seuil.

Cette technique a été mise en oeuvre pour déterminer le taux de TBII chez 30 sujets atteints de la maladie de Basedow ; leur moyenne d'âge se situe autour de 40 ans. Le diagnostic a été confirmé par le dosage sérique de la TSH, de la T4 libre (LT4) et de la T3 totale (TT3), ainsi que par scintigraphie. Pour l'ensemble de ces malades, l'incidence des antécédents familiaux était de 43 %. Chacun d'eux a eu au moins 1 dosage de TBII.

Résultats

D'après l'état fonctionnel de leur thyroïde évalué par le dosage de la TSH ultra sensible), ces patients ont pu être divisés en 2 groupes.

1) Groupe A : 15 patients en rémission, en état d'euthyroïdie ou d'hyperthyroïdie.
2) Groupe B : 15 patients en état d'hyperthyroïdie (Basedow)

Les résultats obtenus montrent que, dans le groupe A, 1 seul malade présente un taux de TBII élevé ; pour les autre la moyenne se situe autour de 6 à 7 % d'inhibition.

Dans le groupe B, 11 valeurs sur 15 sont positives, la moyenne se situant autour de 28 % d'inhibition ; 2 valeurs sont très élevées ; les 4 valeurs négatives sont cependant très proches du seuil de 15 %.

Pour l'ensemble de ces patients, le taux de TBII est très bien corrélé avec les concentrations de TT3, LT4 et TSH.

Conclusion

En fonction de cette étude, nous pouvons conclure que le dosage de TBII par la trousse TRAK est un examen spécifique et sensible qui pourrait être utilisé à la fois pour confirmer le diagnostic de maladie de Basedow et pour le suivi du traitement. Mais il ne faut pas cependant négliger l'intérêt du dosage de la TSH ultra sensible, quand les valeurs sont à la limite.

Prevalence of postpartum thyroid dysfunction in the Netherlands

V.J.M. Popo[1], H.A.M. de Rooy[1], H.L. Vader[1] and D. Van der Heide[2]

[1] Department of Internal Medicine, Saint-Joseph Hospital, Aalsterweg 259, 5644 RC Eindhoven, The Netherlands. [2] University of Agriculture, Department of Human Physiology, Wageningen, The Netherlands

Thyroid dysfunction in the postpartum has been shown to occur frequently (3-16 %), postpartum thyroiditis being the main cause. Most of the prospective studies done so far only screened once or twice after birth, however two studies with frequent time of sampling used a selective group of women : mainly microsomal antibody-positive women were involved. Investigations into a relation between thyroid dysfunction and clinical symptoms were often biased by the fact that most of the women with thyroid dysfunction were referred to the hospital in order to get a correct diagnosis.

In an area in the south of Eindhoven 350 women were invited - during pregnancy - to participate in a screening program for thyroid function. They were randomized in an a-selective way. They were visited at home once during pregnancy at 32 weeks, then 4 weeks postpartum and further five times every six weeks (until 34 weeks postpartum). Every visit thyroid parameters were investigated : clinical symptoms, pulse-rate, weight, eye-signs, skin and thyroid palpation. Blood samples were taken in order to get £T3, £T4, TSH and microsomal antibody-titer evaluated.

There were 270 women who particiged the study. The women who did not participate were matched on age, parity, social class and obstetrical background features. There was no difference between the participating and non-participating group.

The study was completed by 255 women. Thyroid dysfunction proved to occur in 24 women (9.4 %). Most of the cases were found between 3 and 6 months after pregnancy. In the postpartum 40 women (15.6 %) had elevated microsomal-antibody titer. Except for pulse-rate, there was no clinical symptom related to thyroid dysfunction. Women with thyroid dysfunction did have a larger thyroid as found by palpation compared to women without thyroid dysfunction.

These results suggest that postpartum thyroid dysfunction in an a-selective population does occur quite often (9.4 %) - at least in this part of The Netherlands. There are no clinical signs and symptoms that are significantly related to thyroid dysfunction, except for pulse-rate and palpation.

Miscellaneous
Divers

Thyroid peroxidase autoantigen : localization of autoantigenic epitopes on recombinant protein and prediction of secondary structure

J.P. Banga, D.L. Ewins, P.S. Barnett, R.W.S. Tomlinson, D. Mahadevan, G.J. Barton, B.J. Sutton, J.W. Saldanha, E. Odell and A.M. McGregor

Department of Medicine, King's College School of Medicine, London; Imperial Cancer Research Fund Laboratories, Biomedical Computing Unit, London; Division of Biomolecular Sciences, King's College, London; United Medical and Dental Schools of Guy's and St Thomas', London Bridge, London, UK

SUMMARY

The cloning and expression of TPO as a recombinant protein has allowed progress on the characterisation of the autoantigenic epitopes recognised by autoantibodies. The main immunogenic region of the molecule recognised by autoantibodies has been localized to the carboxyl terminal. Multiple sequence alignment and secondary structure prediction methods used in conjunction with circular dichroic spectroscopy indicate that TPO structure is principally alpha-helical. Together with a knowledge of the exon-intron boundaries suggests a model for the domain organization of the TPO molecule. The ability in the future to map the autoantigenic epitopes on a three dimensional structural model of the TPO molecule will allow a greater understanding of the aetiological basis of autoimmune disease and allow the design of therapeutic strategies at an antigen specific level to be addressed.

INTRODUCTION

Thyroid peroxidase is the primary enzyme involved in thyroid hormone synthesis and a target autoantigen in destructive thyroid disease leading to thyroid failure in man (Banga et al, 1990a). The autoimmune response to TPO involves both the production of autoantibodies (aAbs) and T cell autoreactivity. A great deal of information is available on the autoantibody response to TPO in autoimmune thyroid disease (AITD). These autoantibodies are known to be polyclonal in nature where several antigenic sites, including the enzyme active site, are known to be recognized (Doble et al, 1988). Additionally, anti-TPO aAbs cross-react with other related peroxidases such as myeloperoxidase (MPO) which shares a high degree of sequence homology (Banga et al, 1989a). However, so far, there is a scarcity of information on the nature of the T cell autoreactivity or the epitopes on the TPO molecule recognized by T cells in AITD (Banga et al, 1990a).

The ability to dissect and study the autoimmune response in vitro requires a source of purified autoantigen. For TPO, a number of procedures have been developed for its purification but the purity and, in particular, the yield of the molecule has been relatively poor to be used for cellular investigations. To circumvent this, we have applied molecular biology techniques to clone and express TPO as a recombinant fusion protein in *E.coli*. In particular, we have taken advantage of polymerase chain reaction (PCR) to amplify various regions of the TPO molecule (averaging 120 amino acids) for expression as recombinant proteins. This has allowed us to identify the main immunogenic region on the TPO molecule recognized by autoantibodies from patients with AITD.

A detailed knowledge of the three dimensional structure and an accurate localization of the autoantigenic epitopes on the TPO molecule would greatly increase our understanding of the autoimmune response to this autoantigen. It would also allow the future design of therapeutic studies aimed for immune intervention at an antigen specific manner to be addressed (Banga et al, 1989b). Structural knowledge is usually obtained by X-Ray crystallography which requires access to milligram amounts of purified protein. Whilst this is currently not feasible for TPO, even with the availability of recombinant bacterial TPO protein, structure prediction methods developed over the past decade now allow protein structure to be predicted. Combining prediction methods can yield improvements in accuracy as can combining predictions on accurately aligned sequences. Accordingly, we have aligned the sequences of human TPO, porcine TPO and human MPO and applied different prediction methods on the aligned sequences to obtain a consensus structural prediction and the organization of domains of the TPO molecule. In view of the high sequence similarity between human TPO and MPO, we have also used purified MPO for circular dichroic (CD) spectroscopy; since purified preparations of intact TPO were not available, we have also used trypsinized, porcine TPO for CD spectroscopy. By combining the CD spectral information on MPO with the secondary structure prediction of TPO, we show that the structure of TPO is mainly alpha-helical with little beta sheet, and is organized into distinct domains.

METHODS

CD spectral analysis

Trypsinized pTPO was prepared as already described and was a gift from Professor A Taurog (Yokoyama and Taurog, 1988). hMPO was prepared from neutrophils (Banga et al, 1989a). The purity of these peroxidase preparations was assessed by SDS-polyacrylamide gel electrophoresis. For CD analysis, pTPO was resuspended at 0.1mg/ml in phosphate buffered saline whilst hMPO was at 0.1mg/ml in 0.1M Tris-Hcl pH 7.4. CD spectra were run at room temperature in 0.05cm "strain free" quartz 2 cells in a JASCO J600 CD spectrometer.

Multiple sequence alignment and prediction techniques

Sequence alignment was performed by the algorithm of Barton (1990) using the AMPS package. Alpha-helix and beta-strand regions were predicted using the algorithms of Lim (Lim, 1974), Chou and Fasman (Chou & Fasman, 1978) and Robson (Garnier et al, 1978), as programmed in the Leeds Prediction suite. Turns were predicted using the method of Wilmot and Thornton (Wilmot and Thornton, 1988) and that of Rose (Rose, 1987). B cell defined epitopes were predicted using the Hopp and Woods profile (Hopp and Woods, 1987). T cell defined epitopes were predicted using the motifs programme of Rothbard and Taylor (Rothbard and Taylor, 1988).

Expression of TPO as recombinant protein

Different segments of the TPO polypeptide were expressed as fusion proteins in *E.coli* using recombinant biology techniques and polymerase chain reaction as already described (Banga et al, 1989c, 1990b). The recombinant TPO proteins were assessed for their binding to autoantibodies to TPO from patients with thyroid autoimmune disease by immunoblotting techniques.

RESULTS AND DISCUSSION

SDS-polyacrylamide gel electrophoresis of pTPO and hMPO

Preparations of pTPO and hMPO were analysed by SDS-polyacrylamide gel electrophoresis to assess the purity of biochemically purified proteins. The trypsinized pTPO preparations under non-reducing or reducing conditions gave protein staining bands already described (Yokayama and Taurog, 1988) (Fig. 1, Lanes 1 NR and 1R respectively). hMPO preparation under reducing conditions gave a strong and a major protein staining band at 60Kd comprising the heavy polypeptide chain of the enzyme (Banga et al, 1989a). (Fig. 1, Lane 2R). Both the preparations of pTPO and hMPO were > 90% purity and used for CD analysis.

CD analysis of pTPO and hMPO

The far ultra-violet spectra of trypsinized pTPO and hMPO in aqueous solution exhibit a broad band of minimum in the 200-210nm range (Fig. 2). The values of alpha-helical content were calculated to be approximately 27-33% for trypsinized pTPO and 55-60% for hMPO, with the remainder of the protein in both preparations in random coil conformation. The lower alpha-helical content in the trypsinized pTPO preparations is probably due to the fact that it is a fragmented molecule which lacks approximately 90 residues at the NH_2 and COOH terminals and also contains a trypsin cleaved site after residue 561..

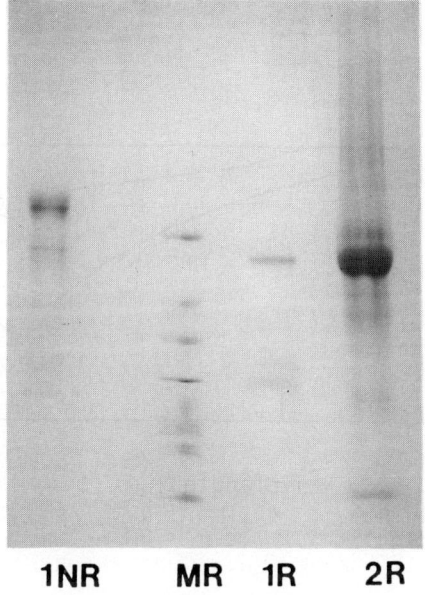

1NR   MR   1R   2R

Fig. 1   SDS-polyacrylamide gel electrophoresis of purified preparations of trypsinized, porcine TPO and human MPO which were used for CD spectroscopy. R refers to reducing conditions, NR refers to non-reducing conditions. Sample 1 is trypsinized, porcine TPO whilst sample 2 is MPO. M= molecule weight markers migrating at 66,45,36,29,24,20 and 14.2Kd.

Sequence alignment and secondary structure prediction techniques

Secondary structure prediction methods generally give around 55-65% accuracy for a three state prediction of helix, strand and non-helix/non-strand (i.e. coil) structure. Recently, it has become clear that the accuracy of the various secondary structure prediction methods can be greatly increased by (i) combining the prediction methods and (ii) combining predictions on accurately aligned sequences (Biou et al, 1988; Zvelebil et al, 1987). We have achieved this for TPO by aligning the sequences of hTPO, pTPO and hMPO by the algorithm of Barton and colleagues (Barton and Sternberg, 1987; Barton, 1990) (alignment not shown, but see Banga et al, 1990c). Five prediction methods were then performed independently on each aligned sequence and then the results combined into a consensus.

The overall result of predictions for TPO in the region of homology with MPO (residues 1-741) were alpha-helix 51%, beta sheet 8%, turn 41% and the remainder as random coil (Banga et al, 1990c). This compares favourably with the CD results of MPO which predict alpha-helical conformation of 55-60% and the remainder as random coil.

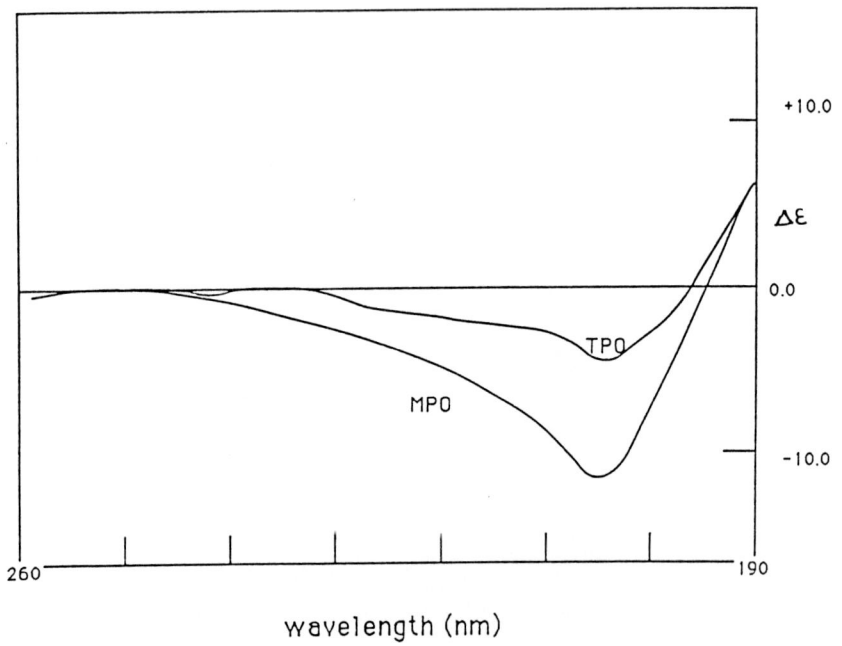

Fig. 2   Circular dichroic (CD) spectroscopy of trypsinized, porcine TPO and human MPO in the far ultraviolet region in aqueous solution. The difference in the two spectra are likely to reside in the fact that the trypsinized, porcine TPO is a fragmented molecule which is also truncated at the amino and carboxyl terminals.

The alignment of two or more sequences also allows further structural information to be obtained. The three proteins share a large number of identical amino acids (hTPO vs pTPO = 70% identity; hTPO vs hMPO as aligned by the algorithm of Barton (1990) = 50%) (for the alignment, see Banga et al, 1990c). Consideration of insertions or deletions in the aligned sequences shows areas in surface loop regions (Bashford et al, 1987). Four insertions between the hTPO and pTPO are apparent at positions E at 388 and L at 518 of hTPO and insertion of GK at 896 and LPG at 903 of pTPO and loops are predicted in these positions. When this analysis is extended to hMPO, a further 10 insertions are observed. The alignment of sequences also allows the conservation of cysteine residues to be ascertained. Sixteen cysteine residues are conserved between hTPO and pTPO. In the region of sequence homology with hMPO (residues 1-741), fourteen of these cysteine residues are conserved with hMPO (Banga et al, 1990c). The extensive conservation of cysteine residues strongly supports the contention that TPO and MPO are structurally homologous throughout the region of TPO that corresponds to MPO.

Recently the gene structures for hTPO and hMPO have been described where the hTPO gene comprises 17 exons and the hMPO gene consists of 12 exons (Kimura et al, 1989). When the exon-intron boundaries of these two genes are compared, exon 3-11 of TPO and exons 2-11 of MPO coincide exactly except that exon 8 of TPO corresponds to exons 7 and 8 of MPO (Kimura et al, 1989). The use of sequence alignment and exon-intron boundaries between related proteins has previously been used to successfully predict the domain organization of other proteins (Inna et al, 1983; Williams, 1984). Using this approach, the domain organization of TPO is predicted into nine distinct domains (Banga et al, 1990c).

The TPO region 799-847 has been shown to have a high sequence similarity to EGF (Libert et al, 1987). Additionally, there is absolute conservation of the six cysteine residues that are disulphide bonded in the EGF molecule - these cysteine residues in hTPO are at residue positions 799, 805, 819, 828 and 843 (Banga et al, 1990c). This allows the structure of TPO in this region to be predicted confidently by analogy with the NMR structure of EGF (Cooke et al, 1987). The structure of EGF consists of two B-strands and turns held together by a cluster of three disulphide bonds.

TABLE 1

Predicted B cell (antibody) and T cell epitopes of TPO

	ANTIBODY EPITOPE		T CELL EPITOPE	
	Residues	Sequence	Residues	Sequence
1.	684-697	DAQRRELEKHSLSR	562-568	EELTERL
2.	223-230	VTDDDRYS	47-53	KRLVDTA
3.	33-38	KPEESR	87-93	SGVIARA
4.	760-767	HCEESGRR	426-431	KALNAH
5.	60-65	RNLKKR	119-125	TDALSED
6.	359-365	RLRDSGR	94-99	AEIMET

Taken together, multiple sequence alignment and a combination of secondary structure prediction methods indicate that the TPO structure is principally alpha-helical. Together with a knowledge of the exon-intron boundaries suggests that the TPO molecule may fold into nine separate domains (Banga et al, 1990c).

Prediction of antibody and T cell defined epitopes

The TPO molecule is the target autoantigen in lymphocytic thyroiditis (Hashimoto's disease). We have used the Hopp and Woods hydrophilicity profiles to predict the amino acid residues in TPO which may be recognized by antibodies (Table 1). Since T cell help is required for antibody production, amino acid sequences that may serve as T cell epitopes are also described, using the motifs programme of Rothbard and Taylor (1988) (Table 1). The top six hydrophilic peaks for antibody epitopes and the top six T cell epitopes are predicted (Table 1).

Generation of recombinant preparations of TPO and mapping of autoantigenic sites

Different segments of the TPO molecule have been expressed as recombinant protein in *E.coli* as fusion proteins with glutathione-S-transferase (Banga et al, 1989c, 1990b). The recombinant overlapping TPO fusion proteins encompass the following amino acid residues 1-160, 145-250, 457-589, 577-677, 657-767 and 737-845. A larger fragment encompassing the latter three recombinants was also produced (residues 577-845). Using Western blotting and autoantibodies to TPO from patients with thyroid autoimmune disease, we recently showed that these sera recognize recombinant TPO proteins containing residues 657-767 and 145-250 of the fusion molecule. Interestingly, the latter recombinant TPO preparations harbour the two most hydrophilic peaks of position 684-697 and 223-230 respectively which have been predicted to contain the sequential antigenic determinants (Table 1) (Banga et al, 1989c, 1990b). Nine out of ten AITD sera contained autoantibodies to TPO which react with recombinant TPO fusion proteins derived from the COOH terminal of the molecule. These studies, together with another report (Ludgate et al, 1989), suggests that the main immunogenic region of the TPO polypeptide is localized towards the carboxyl region of the molecule.

ACKNOWLEDGEMENTS

Trypsinized, porcine TPO was kindly given by Professor A Taurog. We thank Drs J Fox and C Rawlings for advice and Dr A Drake and Mr J Hoardley for help with CD spectroscopy. Many thanks to Mrs J De Groote for organizing the manuscript preparation. Supported by grants from The Wellcome Trust and the Medical Research Council.

REFERENCES

Banga, J.P., Barnett, P.S., and McGregor, A.M. (1990a): Immunological and molecular characteristics of the thyroid peroxidase autoantigen. Autoimmunity (in press)

Banga, J.P., Barnett, P.S., Ewins, D.L., Page, M.J., and McGregor, A.M. (1990b): Mapping of autoantigenic epitopes on recombinant thyroid peroxidase fragments using the polymerase chain reaction. Autoimmunity (in press)

Banga, J.P., Mahadevan, D., Barton, G.J., Sutton, B.J., Saldanha, J.W., Odell, E., and McGregor, A.M. (1990c): Prediction of domain organization and secondary structure of thyroid peroxidase, a human autoantigen involved in destructive thyroiditis. FEBS Letts (in press)

Banga, J.P., Tomlinson, R.W.S., Doble, N., Odell, E., and McGregor, A.M. (1989a): Thyroid microsomal/thyroid peroxidase and autoantibodies show discrete patterns of cross-reactivity to myeloperoxidase, lactoperoxidase and horseradish peroxidase. Immunol. 67: 197-204

Banga, J.P., Barnett, P.S., Mahadevan, D., and McGregor, A.M. (1989b): Immune recognition of antigen and its relevance to autoimmune disease: recent advances at the molecular level. Eur. J. Clin. Invest. 19: 107-116

Banga, J.P., Barnett, P.S., Ewins, D.L., Page, M.J., and McGregor, A.M. (1989c): Autoantigenic epitopes on thyroid microsome/thyroid peroxidase antigen recognised by autoantibodies reside in the amino terminal, the carboxyl region and the central core of the molecule. Autoimmun. 5: 142-144

Barton, G.J. (1990): Protein multiple sequence alignment and flexible pattern matching. Meths. in Enzymol. 183: 403-428

Barton, G.J., and Sternberg, M.J.E. (1987): A strategy for the rapid alignment of protein sequences. J. Mol. Biol. 198: 327-337

Bashford, D., Chothia, C., and Lesk, A.M. (1987): Determinants of a protein fold: unique features of the globulin amino acid sequences. J. Mol. Biol. 196: 199-216

Biou, V., Gibrat, J.F., Lexin, J.M., Robson, B., and Garnier, J. (1988): Secondary structure prediction combination of three different methods. Prot. Eng. 2: 185-191

Chou, P.Y., and Fasman, G.D. (1978). Prediction of a secondary structure of proteins from their amino acid sequences. Adv. Enzymol. 47: 145-148

Cooke, R.M., Wilkinson, A.J., Baron, M., Pastore, A., Tappin, M.J., Campbell, I.D., Gregory, H., and Sheard, D. (1987): The solution structure of human epidermal growth factor. Nature 327: 339-341

Doble, N.D., Banga, J.P., Pope, R., Lalor, R., Kilduff, P., and McGregor, A.M. (1988): Autoantibodies to the thyroid microsomal/thyroid peroxidase antigen are polyclonal and directed to several distinct sites. Immunol. 64: 23-29

Garnier, J., Osguthorpe, D.L. and Robson, B. (1987): Analysis of the accuracy and implications of simple methods for predicting the secondary structure of globular proteins. J. Mol. Biol. 120: 97-120

Hopp, T.P., and Woods, K.R. (1981): Prediction of protein antigenic determinants from amino acid sequences. Proc. Natl. Acad. Sci. 78: 3824-3828

Inna, G., Piatigorsky, J., Norman, B., Slingsby, C., and Blundell, T. (1983): Gene and protein structure of a B-crystallin polypeptide in murine lens: relationship of exons and structural motifs. Nature 302: 310-315

Kimura, S., Hong, Y.S., Kotani, T., Ohtaki, S., and Kikkawa, F. (1989): Structure of the human thyroid peroxidase gene: comparison and relationship to the human thyroid peroxidase gene. Biochem. 28: 4481-4489

Libert, F., Ruel, J., Ludgate, M., Swillens, S., Alexander, N., Vassart, G., and Dinsart, C. (1987): Thyroperoxidase, an autoantigen with a mosaic structure made of nuclear and mitochondrial gene modules. EMBO J. 6: 4193-4196

Lim, V.I. (1974): Algorithms for prediction of -helical and B-structural regions in globular proteins. J. Mol. Biol. 88: 873-894

Ludgate, M., Mariotti, S., Libert, F., Dinsart, C., Piccolo, P., Santini, F., Ruf, J., Pinchera, A., and Vassart, G. (1989): Antibodies to human thyroid peroxidase in autoimmune thyroid disease: studies with a cloned recombinant complementary deoxyribonucleic acid epitope. J Clin. Endocrinol. Metab. 68: 1091-1096

Rose, G.D. (1978): Prediction of chain turns in globular proteins on a hydrophobic basis. Nature 272: 586-591

Rothbard, J.B., and Taylor, W.R. (1988): A sequence pattern common to T cell epitopes. <u>EMBO J 7:</u> 93-100

Williams, A.F. (1984): The immunoglobulin super family takes shape. <u>Nature 308:</u> 12

Wilmot, C.M., and Thornton, J.M. (1988): Analysis and prediction of the different types of B-turns in protein. <u>J. Mol. Biol. 203:</u> 221-232

Yokoyama, N., and Taurog, A. (1988): Porcine thyroid peroxidase: relationship between the native enzyme and an active, highly purified tryptic fragment. <u>Mol. Endocrinol. 2:</u> 838-849

Zvelebil, M.J.J., Barton, G.J., Taylor, W.J., and Sternberg, M.J.E. (1987): Prediction of protein secondary structure and active sites using the alignment of homologous sequences. <u>J. Mol. Biol. 195:</u> 957-961

Résumé

Le clonage de la TPO et son expression par recombinaison génétique a permis de progresser dans la caractérisation des épitopes auto-antigéniques reconnus par les auto-anticorps. La principale région immunogénique reconnue par les auto-anticorps a été localisée sur la partie C terminale de la molécule. Des méthodes d'alignements de séquences et de prédiction de structures secondaires combinées à la spectroscopie par dichroïsme circulaire indiquent que la structure de la TPO est principalement en hélice alpha. La connaissance supplémentaire des enchaînements des exons et des introns suggère un modèle d'organisation en domaines de la molécules de TPO. La possibilité future de positionner les épitopes auto-antigéniques sur un modèle structural tri-dimensionnel de la TPO permettra une meilleure compréhension de l'étiologie des maladies auto-immunes et permettra d'envisager des stratégies thérapeutiques spécifiques d'un antigène donné.

Colloques **INSERM**
ISSN 0768-3154

Other *Colloques* published as co-editions by John Libbey Eurotext and INSERM

153 Hormones and Cell Regulation (11th European Symposium). *Hormones et Régulation Cellulaire (11ᵉ Symposium Européen).*
Edited by J. Nunez and J.E. Dumont.
ISBN : John Libbey Eurotext 0 86196 104 8
INSERM 2 85598 324 X

158 Biochemistry and Physiopathology of Platelet Membrane. *Biochimie et Physiopathologie de la Membrane Plaquettaire.*
Edited by G. Marguerie and R.F.A. Zwaal.
ISBN : John Libbey Eurotext 0 86196 114 5
INSERM 2 85598 345 2

162 The Inhibitors of Hematopoiesis. *Les Inhibiteurs de l'Hématopoïèse.*
Edited by A. Najman, M. Guignon, N.C. Gorin and J.Y. Mary.
ISBN : John Libbey Eurotext 0 86196 125 0
INSERM 2 85598 340 1

164 Liver Cells and Drugs. *Cellules Hépatiques et Médicaments.*
Edited by A. Guillouzo.
ISBN : John Libbey Eurotext 0 86196 128 5
INSERM 2 85598 341 X

165 Hormones and Cell Regulation (12th European Symposium). *Hormones et Régulation Cellulaire (12ᵉ Symposium Européen).*
Edited by J. Nunez, J.E. Dumont and E. Carafoli.
ISBN : John Libbey Eurotext 0 86196 133 1
INSERM 2 85598 347 9

167 Sleep Disorders and Respiration. *Les Evénements Respiratoires du Sommeil.*
Edited by P. Lévi-Valensi and D. Duron.
ISBN : John Libbey Eurotext 0 86196 127 7
INSERM 2 85598 344 4

169 Neo-Adjuvant Chemotherapy. *Chimiothérapie Néo-Adjuvante.*
Edited by C. Jacquillat, M. Weil, D. Khayat.
ISBN : John Libbey Eurotext 0 86196 150 1
INSERM 2 85598 349 5

171 Structure and Functions of the Cytoskeleton. *La Structure et les Fonctions du Cytosquelette.*
Edited by B.A.F. Rousset.
ISBN : John Libbey Eurotext 0 86196 149 8
INSERM 2 85598 351 7

Colloques INSERM
ISSN 0768-3154

172 The Langerhans Cell. *La Cellule de Langerhans.*
Edited by J. Thivolet, D. Schmitt.
ISBN : John Libbey Eurotext 0 86196 181 1
INSERM 2 85598 352 5

173 Cellular and Molecular Aspects of Glucuronidation. *Aspects Cellulaires et Moléculaires de la Glucuronoconjugaison.*
Edited by G. Siest, J. Magdalou, B. Burchell
ISBN : John Libbey Eurotext 0 86196 182 X
INSERM 2 85598 353 3

174 Second Forum on Peptides. *Deuxième Forum Peptides.*
Edited by A. Aubry, M. Marraud, B. Vitoux
ISBN : John Libbey Eurotext 0 86196 151 X
INSERM 2 85598 354 1

176 Hormones and Cell Regulation (13th European Symposium). *Hormones et Régulation Cellulaire (13ᵉ Symposium Européen).*
Edited by J. Nunez, J.E. Dumont, R. Denton
ISBN : John Libbey Eurotext 0 86196 183 8
INSERM 2 85598 356 8

179 Lymphokine Receptors Interactions. *Interactions Lymphokines-récepteurs.*
Edited by D. Fradelizi, J. Bertoglio
ISBN : John Libbey Eurotext 0 86196 148 X
INSERM 2 85598 359 2

190 Growth Factors and Oncogenes. *Facteurs de Croissance et Oncogènes.*
Edited by M. Bolla, E.M. Chambaz, C. Vrousos
ISBN : John Libbey Eurotext 0 86196 222 2
INSERM 2 85898 392 4

191 Anticancer Drugs (1st International Interface of Clinical and Laboratory responses to anticancer drugs). *Médicaments anticancéreux (1ʳᵉ Confrontation internationale des réponses cliniques et expérimentales aux médicaments anticancéreux).*
Edited by H. Tapiero, J. Robert, T.J. Lampidis
ISBN : John Libbey Eurotext 0 86196 223 0
INSERM 2 85598 393 2

193 Living in the Cold (2nd International Symposium). *La Vie au Froid (2ᵉ Symposium International).*
Edited by A. Malan, B. Canguilhem
ISBN : John Libbey Eurotext 0 86196 234 9
INSERM 2 85598 395 9

Colloques INSERM
ISSN 0768-3154

194 Progress in Hepatitis B Immunization. *La Vaccination contre l'épatite B.*
Edited by P. Coursaget, M.J. Tong
ISBN : John Libbey Eurotext 0 86196 2494
INSERM 2 85598 396 7

198 Hormones and Cell Regulation (14th European Symposium). *Hormones et Régulation Cellulaire (14e Symposium Européen).*
Edited by J. Nunez, J.E. Dumont
ISBN : John Libbey Eurotext 0 86196 229 X
INSERM 2 85598 400 9

199 Placental Communications : Biochemical, Morphological and Cellular aspects. *Communications placentaires : aspects biochimique, morphologique et cellulaire.*
ISBN : John Libbey Eurotext 0 86196 227 3
INSERM 2 85598 401 7

Reproduction photomécanique
IMPRIMERIE LOUIS-JEAN
BP 87 — 05003 GAP Cedex
Tél. : 92.51.35.23
Dépôt légal : 401 — Juin 1990
Imprimé en France